ANIMAL AGENTS
AND
VECTORS OF
HUMAN DISEASE

CONTRIBUTOR MEMBERS

Department of Tropical Medicine, School of Public Health
and Tropical Medicine, and Department of Parasitology,
The Graduate School, Tulane University,
New Orleans, Louisiana

Antonio D'Alessandro-Bacigalupo, M.D., Ph.D., MPHTM, Professor of Tropical Medicine

Jack H. Esslinger, Ph.D., Associate Professor of Parasitology

Stephen P. Katz, Ph.D., Associate Professor of Parasitology

Maurice Dale Little, Ph.D., Professor of Parasitology

Emile A. Malek, Ph.D., Professor of Parasitology

Thomas C. Orihel, Ph.D., William Vincent Professor of Tropical Diseases and Hygiene

Robert G. Yaeger, Ph.D., Professor of Parasitology

ANIMAL AGENTS AND VECTORS OF HUMAN DISEASE

5TH EDITION

PAUL CHESTER BEAVER, Ph.D., Sc.D. (HON.)

Emeritus Professor of Parasitology, School of Public Health and Tropical Medicine, Tulane University, New Orleans, Louisiana

RODNEY CLIFTON JUNG, M.D., Ph.D., F.A.C.P.

Clinical Professor of Medicine, School of Medicine, and Clinical Professor of Tropical Medicine, School of Public Health and Tropical Medicine, Tulane University, New Orleans; Physician in Internal Medicine, Touro Infirmary, New Orleans; Senior Visiting Physician, The Charity Hospital of Louisiana at New Orleans; Consultant to United States Quarantine Division of Centers for Disease Control, Atlanta, Georgia; Former Director of Health, City of New Orleans, Louisiana

200th Anniversary
1785 - 1985

Lea & Febiger   *Philadelphia   1985*

Lea & Febiger
600 Washington Square
Philadelphia, PA   19106-4198
U.S.A.
(215) 922-1330

First Edition, 1955
Second Edition, 1962
  Reprinted, 1962
Third Edition, 1968
  Reprinted, 1968, 1969, 1973
Fourth Edition, 1975
  Reprinted, 1976, 1979, 1980, 1982
Fifth Edition, 1985

Library of Congress Cataloging in Publication Data
Main entry under title:

Animal agents and vectors of human disease.

  Rev. ed. of; Animal agents and vectors of human
disease/Ernest Carroll Faust, Paul Chester Beaver,
Rodney Clifton Jung. 4th ed. 1975.
  Includes bibliographies and index.
  1. Medical parasitology. 2. Animals as carriers of
disease. I. Beaver, Paul Chester, 1905–
II. Jung, Rodney Clifton, 1920–   . III. Faust,
Ernest Carroll, 1890–1978. Animal agents and vectors
of human disease. [DNLM: 1. Disease Vectors.
2. Parasites. QZ 85 A598]
RC119.A54   1985   616.9′6   85–183
ISBN 0-8121-0987-2

PRINTED IN THE UNITED STATES OF AMERICA

Print No.   4   3   2   1

Preface

The scope of this volume is the area of knowledge covering the animals that cause human disease or serve as vectors of organisms that cause disease in man. It is designed for medical students, upper division students in biology, including premedical students, and students in international health and other branches of public health. The first edition was based largely on a syllabus prepared for public health students in an interdepartmental course on infectious diseases entitled *Animal and Microbial Agents of Disease,* a prerequisite for courses in epidemiology. A companion volume on *Microbial Agents of Disease* was planned but did not reach publication.

In the preparation of the previous edition (4th), we were assisted by associates who read and offered suggestions on the content of chapters covering their respective fields of special interest. In the present edition seven of them are contributors, having largely revised the chapters that cover the subjects representing their research interests or their teaching responsibilities or both. With this arrangement, followed by detailed editing of all chapters, we were able to make the present edition smaller than previous ones without restricting its coverage or omitting important details. Basic information is given on all important endemic and zoonotic parasites, as well as on amphizoic forms such as *Naegleria, Acanthamoeba, Micronema, Pelodera,* and others. However, for further condensation, nonpathogenic and rare or minor parasites have been relegated to smaller type, and the cited references have been limited for the most part to recent and readily available sources where more detailed information and references to the older literature can be found.

For assistance in scanning journals and other sources for current information on animal agents and vectors, we are indebted to Miss Helen Day. For assistance in manuscript preparation and editing, we are grateful to Mrs. Ena Castillo. We acknowledge with special thanks the cooperation of the publisher, Lea & Febiger.

New Orleans, Louisiana   Paul C. Beaver
                                            Rodney C. Jung

Contents

Section IV.
ARTHROPODS AS AGENTS AND VECTORS

Section V.
AIDS TO DIAGNOSIS AND TREATMENT

Section 1

Introduction

Chapter 1

General Principles:

Parasite, Host, Community

Phenomena of Parasitism

Among the evolutionary processes that have been under way for countless millennia, perhaps the most interesting are the adaptations to a parasitic mode of life. Many examples are found among the groups of lower organisms, such as the viruses, rickettsiae, bacteria, fungi, and spirochetes. Even more interesting from the standpoint of evolutionary changes are the parasites belonging to the animal kingdom, because they have originated from so many phylogenetic stems. Parasitism varies widely with respect to the degree of adaptation, including morphologic simplification and physiologic readjustments that have resulted from dependent relationships.

The relationship between two dissimilar organisms that are adapted to living together is called *symbiosis* and the associates are *symbionts*. The association may be beneficial or harmful to either of the associates. A symbiotic association that is beneficial to both parties is termed *mutualism*. Some authorities define symbiosis as an association that is of mutual benefit to partners who have each lost the ability to live without the other, illustrated by the protozoan fauna in the digestive tract of termites and wood roaches (Baer, 1951). When one of the associated organisms is benefited and the other is neither benefited nor harmed, the relationship is termed *commensalism*; and when one, the *parasite*, lives in or on the other at the expense of the latter, the *host*, the relationship is termed *parasitism*.

The designation *parasitism* possibly suggests that the parasite is harmful to its host, but the successful parasite has reached a delicate equilibrium with its host so that each tolerates the other. If the

balance is upset, the host may spontaneously expel or destroy the parasite, or, at the other extreme, the association may be so detrimental to the host that the latter succumbs to the infection and the parasite perishes as a consequence.

Organisms that live on or in the skin of their hosts are *ectoparasites*. This relationship is an *infestation*. Most parasitic arthropods belong to this category. Parasites of the digestive tract, extraintestinal organs and tissues, and those that are intracellular within the host are referred to as *endoparasites* and produce *infection*, irrespective of their size.

Because the parasite has achieved a relatively secure ecologic niche within the host, it has gradually lost those morphologic features no longer useful for its survival through adaptive evolution, but it has developed physiologic and biochemical adaptations needed for its new associations.

The continued existence of a parasite as a species is dependent on adaptations for reaching and entering its host as well as maintenance of its position within the host once it has arrived. In order for some of its progeny to survive and reach the next host, it has elaborated its reproductive potential enormously. Considering the complexity of the life cycles of many parasites, and the chances of miscarriage in transfer of a particular stage of the parasite from one susceptible host to another, it is a matter of wonder that so many thousands of species have succeeded in their evolutionary transformation from a free-living to a parasitic mode of life. Parasites that are entirely dependent on their hosts are *obligate parasites;* those that are capable of living either free or in or on a host are *facultative parasites;* those that have become dependent on a single species of host are said to be *host-specific*.

An organism in which the adult or final stage of a parasite develops is the *definitive host,* and one in which an intermediate or larval stage develops is an *intermediate host.* A *paratenic host* is one in which the parasite is transported and neither gains nor loses infectivity for its definitive host. Transmitters of parasites from host to host are *vectors.* If the transmitter is not essential to the life cycle, it is a *mechanical vector;* if it is essential, it is a *biologic vector.* A *reservoir host* is an animal species on which the parasite depends for its survival in nature and thus serves as a source of infection for other susceptible hosts, including man. *Zoonosis* is the term applied to a disease of animals when it is transmitted to man; this may be a common or an incidental occurrence.

The Parasite and Its Environment

The host is the parasite's immediate ecologic niche, but the parasite must also maintain itself in a larger environment, the host community. This macrocosm consists not only of a variable number of susceptible hosts but also of other animals and plants, all responsive to climatic conditions such as temperature, rainfall, abundance or scarcity of food, and to overcrowding. Favorable or unfavorable factors that affect the host likewise affect the parasite and its ability to survive, multiply, and gain transfer from one host to the next. Infections maintained at a more or less stable rate of prevalence within the human population of an area are said to be *endemic;* those similarly maintained in animals are *enzootic.* When acquired by man, enzootic infection is said to be *zoonotic* or a *zoonosis.* In tropical Africa tsetse flies serve not only as biologic vectors for trypanosomes that produce disease in man but also for other species of pathogenic trypanosomes that infect cattle and thus endanger a major food supply of the people. Here the economic picture greatly complicates the problem of human trypanosomiasis, resulting in human malnutrition.

Nomenclature of Animal Parasites and Vectors

Four groups of animals are of major importance in medical parasitology, *viz.,* the protozoa, helminths, arthropods, and molluscs. These organisms are classified according to the Rules of Zoological Nomenclature (International Commission on Zoological Nomenclature, 1926, 1961). Within the animal kingdom there are first the larger divisions, phylum and subphylum, then successive lesser divisions consisting of classes, orders, and families, down to genus and species. All of these names must be of Greek or Latin origin or have a classical termination.

A *species* designates a population, the members of which have essentially the same genetic characters and are capable of continued reproduction of their kind but usually cannot interbreed with individuals of other species. A *genus* is a group of closely related species.

The scientific designation of a species is a combination of the generic and specific names, *viz.,* for the domestic dog, *Canis* (genus) *familiaris* (species). This is referred to as *binomial nomenclature,* which originated in the tenth edition of Linnaeus' *Systema Naturae* (1758). The generic name is always a noun, while the specific name may be an adjective agreeing in gender and number with the noun, a noun in apposition to the generic name, or a noun in the genitive case. Examples of these three categories are *Entamoeba histolytica, Giardia lamblia,* and *Plasmodium malariae.* Proper usage requires that the scientific binomial be printed in *italics.* The generic name begins with a capital letter, while the specific name, including the first letter, is in lower case, even if the name originates from a proper noun, such as a person or country. For additional information on the Rules of Zoological Nomenclature and their application, see Beaver, Jung, and Cupp's *Clinical Parasitology,* 9th ed. (1984), pages 15–17.

Pathogenesis and Symptomatology

Parasites that injure their hosts are *pathogens;* the development of this damage is *pathogenesis.* The degree of injury to the host depends on a variety of factors, including the potential virulence of the agent (*i.e.,* its intrinsic pathogenicity), the amount of inoculum and the rapidity with which it may multiply in host tissues, the site of inoculation, whether the exposure is single or repeated, the tolerance or resistance of the host to the particular strain of the agent, and the general threshold of resistance of the host. The type of damage produced may be primarily mechanical, lytic (enzymatic), toxic, or allergic in nature, or the lesion produced by the parasite may open a way for bacteria and other secondary pathogens to enter the tissues (Binford and Connor, 1976). In general, intestinal parasites compete with the host for nutritional substances.

The reaction of the host has a distinct bearing

on the immediate and subsequent effects of the pathogen. In some parasitoses the host may be essentially unresponsive. In other instances the host may elaborate specific antibodies that counteract the antigens introduced by the foreign agent, or may wall off the invader or its products by cellular infiltration, proliferation, and differentiation. The host response may be essentially local at the site of injury or it may include systemic humoral or cellular changes.

Symptoms are the manifestations of pathologic processes resulting from the effects of the agent. A person may carry a parasitic infection that is transmissible to others yet himself show no related signs or symptoms; such a person is referred to as a *carrier.*

Diagnosis

With few exceptions laboratory diagnosis is essential for a definitive diagnosis of parasitic diseases. This involves three distinct problems: the first is to detect the presence of eggs, larvae, cysts, or some other form of the parasite in feces, blood, sputum, urine, or tissues; the second, always more difficult, is to distinguish these stages from each other and from artifacts; and finally, when the parasitic infection has been detected and specifically identified, there remains the problem of establishing its role, if any, in the causation of disease in a given case. The coincidental presence of a parasitic infection may divert attention from the primary cause of illness. There is a wide diversity of forms to be found and recognized in diagnosing parasitic diseases (Fig. 1–1).

Treatment

In the treatment of parasitic diseases, as of other diseases, the objectives are not only to destroy the etiologic agent but also to relieve symptoms. At times supportive and alleviative therapy preceding or associated with specific chemotherapy is desirable, as in acute amebic dysentery and severe hookworm disease. In some types of parasitosis no chemotherapy is available, but surgical removal of the parasite may be curative or at least remedial.

Chemoprophylaxis is the use of drugs to prevent infection. For example, diamidine drugs are considered capable of preventing African trypanosomiasis in persons residing in endemic areas. When taken by persons exposed to the bites of malaria-bearing mosquitoes, chloroquine temporarily prevents attacks of vivax malaria but does not prevent

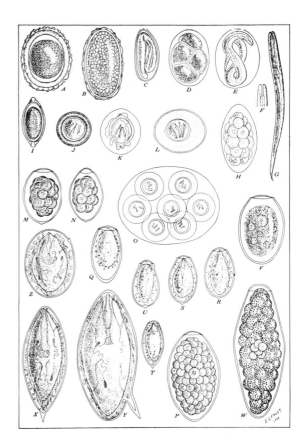

Fig. 1–1. Diagnostic stages (eggs and larvae) of some helminth parasites of man, seen in fecal (or other) specimens. *A, Ascaris lumbricoides,* fertile; *B, A. lumbricoides,* infertile; *C, Enterobius vermicularis; D, Ancylostoma duodenale* or *Necator americanus; E, A. duodenale* or *N. americanus* (from specimen after standing); *F, A. duodenale* or *N. americanus* (larva, showing long buccal cavity); *G, Strongyloides stercoralis; H, Trichostrongylus; I, Trichuris trichiura; J, Taenia saginata* or *T. solium; K, Hymenolepis nana; L, Hymenolepis diminuta; M, Diphyllobothrium latum; N, Spirometra* sp.; *O, Dipylidium caninum; P, Fasciolopsis buski* or *Fasciola hepatica; Q, Dicrocoelium dendriticum; R, Heterophyes heterophyes; S, Metagonimus yokogawai; T, Opisthorchis felineus; U, Clonorchis sinensis; V, Paragonimus westermani* (from sputum or feces); *W, Gastrodiscoides hominis; X, Schistosoma haematobium* (from urine or feces); *Y, Schistosoma mansoni; Z, Schistosoma japonicum. R, S, T,* and *U,* × *400; all other figures,* × *200.* (From Faust, E.C. 1949. *Human Helminthology,* 3rd ed. Philadelphia, Lea & Febiger, p. 585.)

the infection, and delayed attacks may occur after discontinuance of the dosing. This is *suppression.* On the other hand, primaquine, which destroys the hepatic stages of the malarial parasite, is a chemoprophylactic because it prevents infection.

Epidemiology

Epidemiology is the science concerned with the factors that determine the prevalence of infection and the incidence of disease. It is the natural history of the disease, including not only infection in man but also in animals and agents that serve as reservoirs and vectors. *Prevalence* is defined as the number of infected individuals at a given time in a designated area. *Incidence* is the rate or frequency with which a disease or event (new infection) occurs. If the infection maintains itself in a human community, it is *endemic;* if there is high prevalence, it is *hyperendemic;* if it appears irregularly in scattered individuals, it is *sporadic;* and if it develops a high prevalence through unusually rapid transmission, it is *epidemic.* Comparable terms for diseases in animals are *enzootic, hyperenzootic, sporadic,* and *epizootic,* respectively. An unusual number of infections acquired simultaneously from the same source and not transmitted from person to person, for example, trichinosis from eating pork sausage, is referred to as an *outbreak.*

Parasitic diseases may be grouped epidemiologically as follows:

1. *Filth-borne* or *contaminative,* as in the case of the intestinal protozoa, some of the intestinal helminths, sarcoptic mange, and louse infestation.

2. *Contracted from soil* or *water,* with exposure through ingestion of the infective stage, as the eggs of *Ascaris* and *Trichuris,* or through the skin, as with the infective larvae of hookworms or blood flukes.

3. *Food-borne infections* contracted (a) from raw or inadequately processed flesh containing the larval stage of the parasite, *viz., Trichinella* in pork, fish tapeworm in freshwater fish, or (b) from ingestion of encysted larvae on aquatic plants, *viz.,* sheep liver fluke.

4. *Arthropod-borne infections,* in which the arthropod is an essential intermediate host and vector, *viz., Anopheles* and malaria, tsetse flies and African trypanosomiasis.

5. *Infestation by arthropods,* which may be specific, semispecific or accidental, depending on the degree of adaptation of the arthropod to the host.

6. *Arthropod envenomation,* including a wide range, from mild allergy to fatal envenomation or hypersensitization (not a parasitosis but conveniently included in this outline).

Control and Prevention

Since parasitic diseases involve the individual, the community in which he lives, and large geo-political areas, programs of control and prevention involve all of these entities.

The Individual. In the parasitized individual, chemotherapy can be employed to eradicate the infection, not only to relieve suffering but also to prevent transmission to others in the community. Education in methods of personal hygiene and provision of means for taking precautions against exposure can have a marked effect on individual transmission of infection.

The Community. Public health services assist the community in obtaining safe water supplies, sanitary disposal of human excreta, and in instituting measures directed against arthropod vectors and molluscan intermediate hosts, in order to break the life cycles of disease-producing organisms and thus reduce the hazards of individual and group exposure. At times mass chemotherapy may be effective in preventing insects from acquiring and transmitting the disease, as in areas of endemic malaria and filariasis.

National and International Aspects. Parasitic and other infectious diseases know no national boundaries. For this reason, in 1920 the Health Section of the League of Nations was established to promote exchanges of information on communicable diseases. The Panamerican Sanitary Bureau provided an even earlier demonstration of the value of international cooperation in the field of public health, while more recently The World Health Organization has attacked these problems on a global scale. Whatever the size of the community or larger population group may be, an unavoidable aspect of public health is the economic one. The methods of control or attempted eradication of a parasitic disease must be practical and within the financial ability of the group or its sponsors. Hence it is necessary to employ the most practical methods in order to obtain the greatest possible degree of control.

REFERENCES

Baer, J.G. 1951. *Ecology of Animal Parasites.* Urbana, University of Illinois Press.

Beaver, P.C., Jung, R.C., and Cupp, E.W. 1984. *Clinical Parasitology,* 9th ed. Philadelphia, Lea & Febiger.

Binford, C.H., and Connor, D.H. 1976. *Pathology of Tropical and Extraordinary Diseases: An Atlas,* vols. 1 and 2. Washington, D.C., Armed Forces Institute of Pathology.

International Commission on Zoological Nomenclature, 1926. Rules and Regulations. Proc. Biol. Soc. Washington, *39:*75–104.

———, 1961. *International Code of Zoological Nomenclature.* London, International Trust for Zoological Nomenclature.

Section II

Protozoa and Protozoan Infections

Chapter 2

Introduction to Protozoa

The protozoa are single-celled eukaryotic organisms that constitute a subkingdom of the Animalia in which each cell unit performs all of the necessary functions of life. Thousands of species of protozoa have been described, the majority of which are free-living; yet many representatives of the subgroups Sarcomastigophora and Ciliophora are parasitic, and all species of the subgroups Apicomplexa and Microsporidia are parasitic.

Morphology and Biology

Species of protozoa range in size from forms visible to the naked eye to others so small that high-power magnification with the light microscope is required for identification. The morphology of the protozoa is as variable as their size. Some are practically spherical or regularly ovoid in contour, some have a bilateral symmetry, and others have a torsion along the longitudinal axis. Ameboid forms have no consistent contour in their trophozoite stage because of the constant movement of their protoplasm.

All protozoa have certain morphologic features that can be readily observed (Kudo, 1966; Levine, 1973). Most essential is the *nucleus*, which contains the chromosomes that regulate growth and reproduction and determine the genetic characteristics of the species. Among the parasitic protozoa, the number of chromosomes may vary in different families of the same class, but it is relatively constant in species of the same genus. In the alveolar type of nucleus, which is characteristic of the intestinal amebae, there is a *karyosome*, which is situated in a relatively viscous nucleoplasm. The nucleoplasm is bounded by a distinct membrane that may have minute pores connecting it with the *endoplasm*, the inner portion of the cytoplasm. This latter consists of moderately dense, finely granular protoplasm that functions in the digestion

of ingested food and other processes. Here also food reserves in the form of *glycogen* may be accumulated in the trophic stage. Surrounding the endoplasm is a portion of the cytoplasm, the *ectoplasm*, which serves for locomotion, for obtaining and ingesting food, and for respiration and excretion; it may also have a protective function. The limiting cell membrane, the *plasma membrane*, controls the intake of food and discharge of waste products and maintains normal concentration of the plasma. In the amebae and other intestinal forms, the endoplasm contains food vacuoles. Certain parasitic protozoa such as species of *Balantidium* also have contractile vacuoles that preserve normal osmotic pressure. Specialized structures that are characteristic of the different groups of parasitic protozoa will be considered in subsequent chapters of this section.

Considerable adaptation has been developed among the parasitic protozoa with respect to their immediate environment and their microclimate, including temperature at different stages in the parasite's life cycle, anaerobic metabolism, hydrogen ion concentration, available food, and in some species a variety of hosts or multiple habitats within the same host. Intracellular parasites have acquired special ways of entering host cells and are able not only to use nutrients already available there but also may induce the cell to assist actively in their nutrition (Trager, 1974).

Life Cycles and Reproduction

The life cycle of the parasitic protozoa may be very simple, consisting only of a trophic stage in a single host, in which propagation is by asexual mitotic binary fission. This type of propagation is illustrated by *Entamoeba gingivalis* as well as by the flagellate species *Trichomonas tenax, T. hominis, T. vaginalis* and *Dientamoeba fragilis.*

Somewhat more advanced in their cycles are *Entamoeba histolytica*, *E. hartmanni*, *E. coli*, *Endolimax nana*, and *Iodamoeba buetschlii*, which have an encysted resting stage that provides for survival during transfer from one host to the next. Moreover, in the case of *E. histolytica*, *E. hartmanni*, *E. coli*, and *Endolimax nana*, there is multiplication of the nuclei during the encysted stage. Asexual binary fission in the examples cited and in many other protozoa is continued indefinitely without the intervention of a sexual stage. The ciliate *Balantidium coli* only occasionally undergoes conjugation, whereas an essential part of the life cycle of the coccidia and malarial parasites is the sexual phase.

In the amebae there is no characteristic plane of binary division. In the flagellates division is along a longitudinal axis, and in the ciliates it is transverse. In the flagellates the trophic nucleus functions in the ordinary processes of metabolism and growth; a second organelle-apparatus, the *kinetoplast*, initiates binary fission. In *Balantidium coli* the macronucleus performs the first-named function, and the micronucleus is responsible for the second. Asexual multiplication of the malaria parasites and their relatives results in the simultaneous production of several to many daughter cells.

A type of life cycle in which two successive hosts are required is a delicately adjusted sequence in which one of the hosts is a secondary adaptation. Where blood-sucking insects are hosts and vectors, as in the life cycle of the *Leishmania*, *Trypanosoma*, and *Plasmodium* species, not only does this adaptation provide a mechanism for transfer from one vertebrate host to the next but it also furnishes an opportunity for multiplication of progeny and hence a better chance for some of the offspring to reach the vertebrate host. Some coccidia, such as *Toxoplasma* and *Sarcocystis*, have a cyst stage that persists in the tissues of the vertebrate host for months or years, thus assuring survival of the species.

Classification of Protozoa

The classification presented here is based on that of the Society of Protozoologists (Levine *et al.*, 1980) for the protozoa that are parasites of man. The pathogenic species are indicated by an asterisk (*).

Subkingdom PROTOZOA Goldfuss, 1817. Consisting of a single cell that performs all necessary functions of metabolism and reproduction.

Phylum SARCOMASTIGOPHORA Honigberg and Balamuth, 1963. Species with single-type nucleus; sexual reproduction, when present, is essentially syngamous; flagella, pseudopodia, or both types of locomotor organelles present.

Subphylum MASTIGOPHORA Diesing, 1866. Trophozoites with one or more flagella; asexual reproduction basically by longitudinal binary fission; sexual reproduction in some groups.

Class ZOOMASTIGOPHOREA Calkins, 1909. Chloroplasts absent; one to many flagella; ameboid forms with or without flagella in some groups.

(A) Species living in the digestive and genital tracts; transmission from person to person without biologic vector:

Giardia lamblia Stiles, 1915

Trichomonas hominis (Davaine, 1860) Leuckart, 1879

Trichomonas tenax (O.F. Müller, 1773) Dobell, 1939

**Trichomonas vaginalis* Donné, 1837

**Dientamoeba fragilis* Jepps and Dobell, 1918

Chilomastix mesnili (Wenyon, 1910) Alexeieff, 1912

Enteromonas hominis da Fonseca, 1915

(B) Parasites of the blood stream and tissues requiring a blood-sucking invertebrate as biologic vector:

**Leishmania tropica* (Wright, 1903) Luhe, 1906

**Leishmania braziliensis* Vianna, 1911

**Leishmania mexicana* (Biagi, 1953)

**Leishmania aethiopica* Bray, Ashford and Bray, 1973

**Leishmania donovani* (Laveran and Mesnil, 1903) Ross, 1903

**Trypanosoma gambiense* Dutton, 1902

**Trypanosoma rhodesiense* Stephens and Fantham, 1910

**Trypanosoma cruzi* Chagas, 1909

Trypanosoma rangeli Téjera, 1920

Subphylum SARCODINA Schmarda, 1871. Pseudopodia or locomotive protoplasmic flow without discrete pseudopodia; flagella, when present, usually restricted to developmental or other temporary stages; body naked or with test or skeleton; asexual reproduction by fission; sexual reproduction, if present, associated with flagellate or, more rarely, ameboid gametes.

Superclass RHIZOPODA von Siebold, 1845. Locomotion by lobopodia, filopodia, or reticulopodia or by protoplasmic flow without production of discrete pseudopodia.

Class LOBOSEA Carpenter, 1861. Pseudopodia lobose or more or less filiform but extended from a broader hyaline lobe; usually uninucleate; multinucleate forms not flattened or with much-branched plasmodia.

Subclass GYMNAMOEBIA Haeckel, 1862. Without test.

Order AMOEBIDA Ehrenberg, 1830. Typically uninucleate; mitochondria typically present; no flagellate stage.

Suborder TUBULINA Bovee and Jahn, 1966. Body a branched or unbranched cylinder; no bidirectional flow of cytoplasm; nuclear division mesomitotic.

Entamoeba histolytica Schaudinn, 1903

Entamoeba coli (Grassi, 1879) Smith and Barrett, 1914

Entamoeba hartmanni von Prowazek, 1912

Entamoeba gingivalis (Gros, 1849) Smith and Barrett, 1914

Endolimax nana (Wenyon and O'Connor, 1917) Brug, 1918

Iodamoeba buetschlii (von Prowazek, 1912) Dobell, 1918

Suborder ACANTHOPODINA Page, 1976. Subpseudopodia more or less finely tipped, sometimes filiform, often furcate hyaline, produced from a broad hyaline lobe; not regularly discoid; cysts usually formed; nuclear division mesomitotic or metamitotic.

Acanthamoeba culbertsoni (Singh and Das, 1970) Sawyer and Griffin, 1970, and other pathogenic *Acanthamoeba* species.

Order SCHIZOPYRENIDA Singh, 1952. Body a monopodial cylinder, usually moving with more or less eruptive, hyaline, hemispheric bulges; typically uninucleate; nuclear division promitotic; temporary flagellate stage in most.

Naegleria fowleri Carter, 1970.

Phylum APICOMPLEXA Levine, 1970. Apical complex (visible with electron microscope) generally consisting of polar ring(s), rhoptries, micronemes, conoid and subpellicular microtubules present at some stage; micropore(s) generally present at some stage; sexual reproduction by syngamy.

Class SPOROZOEA Leuckart, 1879. Conoid, if present, a complete cone; reproduction generally both sexual and asexual; oocysts generally contain infective sporozoites produced by sporogony; locomotion by body flexion, gliding, or undulation of longitudinal ridges; flagella present only in microgametes of some groups; pseudopods, if present, used for feeding, not locomotion; homoxenous or heteroxenous.

Subclass COCCIDIA Leuckart, 1879. Gamonts ordinarily present, small when mature, typically intracellular; syzygy, if present, involves gametes; anisogamy marked; life cycle characteristically consists of merogony, gametogony, and sporogony; most species in vertebrates.

Order EUCOCCIDIIDA Leger and Duboscq, 1910. Merogony present; in vertebrates or invertebrates, or both.

Suborder EIMERIINA Leger, 1911. Macrogamete and microgamont develop independently; microgamont typically produces many microgametes; zygote not motile; sporozoites typically enclosed in sporocyst within oocysts; homoxenous or heteroxenous.

Cryptosporidium sp.

Isospora belli Wenyon, 1923

Sarcocystis hominis (Railliet and Lucet, 1891) Levine, 1977

Sarcocystis suihominis Heydorn, 1971.

Sarcocystis "lindemanni"

Toxoplasma gondii Nicolle and Manceaux, 1909

Suborder HAEMOSPORINA Danilewsky, 1885. Macrogamete and microgamont develop independently; conoid ordinarily absent; microgamont produces eight flagellated microgametes; zygote motile (ookinete); sporozoites naked, with three-membraned wall; merogony in vertebrate, sporogony in invertebrate host; transmitted by blood-sucking insects.

Plasmodium vivax (Grassi and Feletti, 1890) Labbé, 1899

Plasmodium falciparum (Welch, 1897)

Plasmodium malariae (Laveran, 1881) Grassi and Feletti, 1890

Plasmodium ovale Stephens, 1922

Subclass PIROPLASMIA Levine, 1961. Merozoite pyriform, round, rod-shaped or ameboid; conoid absent; oocysts, spores, and pseudocysts absent; usually without subpellicular microtubules, with polar ring and rhoptries; locomotion by body flexion, gliding, or in sexual stages (in Babesiidae and Theileriidae, at least) by large axopodium-like "Strahlen"; asexual and probably sexual reproduction present; parasitic in erythrocytes and sometimes in other circulating and fixed cells; heteroxenous, with merogony in vertebrate and sporogony in invertebrate; sporozoites with one-membraned wall; transmitted by ticks.

Babesia sp.

Phylum CILIOPHORA Doflein, 1901. Simple cilia or compound ciliary organelles typical in at least one stage of life cycle; subpellicular infraciliature present even when cilia absent; usually with two types of nuclei; binary fission, transverse; contractile vacuole typically present.

Class KINETOFRAGMINOPHOREA de Puytorac *et al.*, 1974. Oral cilia only slightly distinct from somatic cilia; cytostome often apical (or subapical) or mid-ventral, on surface of body or at bottom of atrium or vestibulum; cytopharyngeal apparatus commonly prominent..

Subclass VESTIBULIFERIA de Puytorac *et al.*, 1974. Vestibulum, if present, apical or near-apical, with cilia derived from anterior parts of somatic kineties (rows of cilia) leading to cytostome.

Order TRICHOSTOMATIDA Bütschli, 1889. Somatic kineties not reorganized at level of vestibulum other than more packed alignment or addition of supernumerary segments of kineties; many species commensal in vertebrate hosts.

Suborder TRICHOSTOMATINA Bütschli, 1889. Ciliature not reduced.

Balantidium coli (Malmsten, 1857) Stein, 1862.

Classification uncertain.

Pneumocystis carinii Delanoë and Delanoë, 1912.

REFERENCES

Kudo, R.R. 1966. *Protozoology*, 5th ed. Springfield, Ill., Charles C Thomas.

Levine, N.D. 1973. *Protozoan Parasites of Domestic Animals and of Man*, 2nd ed. Minneapolis, Burgess Publishing Co.

———, et al. 1980. A newly revised classification of the protozoa. J. Protozool., *27*:37–58.

Trager, W. 1974. Some aspects of intracellular parasitism. Science, *183*:269–273.

Chapter 3

Flagellate Protozoa (Mastigophora)

A. D'Alessandro-Bacigalupo

The flagellate protozoa are distinguished by having in their trophozoite stage one to several thread-like extensions of the ectoplasm, the *flagella* (singular, *flagellum*), each of which contains an axial structure *(axoneme)* arising from a basal body, associated with a *kinetoplast* or similar structure. The flagellum, basal body, and kinetoplast constitute the *neuromotor apparatus,* of which the former two are the motor component and the latter the energizing portion.

The flagellate protozoa that are parasites of man are conveniently discussed as (1) flagellates of the digestive tract and genital organs, and (2) flagellates of the blood and tissues.

FLAGELLATES OF THE DIGESTIVE TRACT AND GENITAL ORGANS

Flagellates inhabiting the mouth, intestine, and genital tract are typically lumen parasites. Although no member of the group is a tissue invader, *Giardia lamblia* in the duodenum and *Trichomonas vaginalis* in the vagina may evoke symptoms. There is some evidence that *Dientamoeba fragilis* also may cause symptoms.

Giardia lamblia
(Giardiasis)

Giardia lamblia Stiles, 1915 has a cosmopolitan distribution and is common in both warm and temperate climates.

Morphology and Life Cycle. *G. lamblia* has trophozoite and cystic stages. The *trophozoite* (Fig. 3–1*A,B*) is delicate but very active; it measures 9 to 21 μm in length by 5 to 15 μm in width and is only about 2 to 4 μm thick. When seen from the ventral aspect, the trophozoite appears broadly rounded anteriorly and tapering to a point posteriorly; when viewed in profile, it is relatively thin and in its anterior half is concave ventrally, forming an adhesive disc. It bears four pairs of *flagella,* all arising from a complex system of *axonemes* extending along the midline. Approximately in the center of the trophozoite there is a deeply staining, short, rod-shaped organelle that is believed to be the *parabasal body.* In the anterior portion of the body there are *two ovoid nuclei,* each with a central *karyosome,* one nucleus lying on each side of the midline. By means of the eight flagella *Giardia* is able to move very actively, and by applying its cup-shaped anterior ventral disc it becomes firmly attached to epithelial surfaces. Multiplication is by longitudinal binary fission.

The *cyst* measures 8 to 12 μm in length by 7 to 10 μm in breadth. In preparation for encystment, the flagella are retracted into their respective axonemal components, which now appear as stiffly curved fibrils situated in parallel pairs. Meanwhile the protoplasm is condensed and a thin hyaline membrane is secreted around it. The ripe cyst contains four nuclei (Fig. 3–1*C*).

The primary habitat of the trophozoites is the epithelial brush border of the upper two thirds of the small intestine, where myriad active organisms may be present (Fig. 3–1*D*). The stage commonly recovered in the feces is the cyst; trophozoites are seen in the stool only when it is diarrheal.

Pathogenesis and Symptomatology. *G. lamblia* infections usually are asymptomatic but oc-

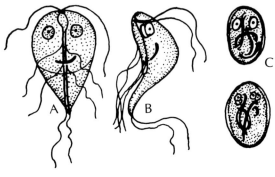

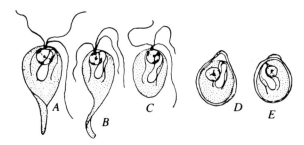

Fig. 3–2. *Chilomastix mesnili. A, B, C,* Trophozoites. *D, E,* Cysts. (× 1200.) (By E.C. Faust.)

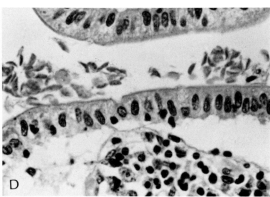

Fig. 3–1. *Giardia lamblia. A,* Trophozoite, ventral view. *B,* Trophozoite, lateral view. *C,* Cysts, immature *(above)* and mature, with 4 nuclei *(below).* (× 1360.) *D,* Trophozoites in section of mucosal biopsy, present in numbers sufficient to cover brush border of villi. (× 400.) (*A* through *C* from Beaver, P.C., Jung, R.C., and Cupp, E.W. 1984. *Clinical Parasitology,* 9th ed. Philadelphia, Lea & Febiger, p. 44. *D,* By P.C. Beaver.)

casionally cause diarrhea, epigastric pain, abdominal cramps, weight loss, and steatorrhea (Meyer and Jarroll, 1980). Scanning electron micrographs have shown that although the trophozoites do not invade tissues, they form a pavement-like sheet covering and damaging the mucosa, causing functional derangement and reducing brush border enzymes. Diarrhea and malabsorption may be caused by this mechanism, together with factors such as synergism with other agents like *Salmonella* and rotavirus (Craft, 1982).

Diagnosis and Treatment. Diagnosis is based on recovery of typical cysts and less frequently of trophozoites in the stools. Concentration methods are effective. Trophozoites may also be obtained by duodenal aspiration or biopsy. The infection may disappear spontaneously but usually is eradicated following therapy with quinacrine (Atabrine) or with metronidazole, which is effective and better tolerated. Furazolidone is also effective. As a suspension it is the drug of choice for small children.

Epidemiology. Infection with *Giardia lamblia* results from ingestion of viable cysts from human sources, *i.e.,* human feces. Giardiasis is most common in warm, moist climates throughout the world and particularly in children in institutions and large families. In heavily infected groups infection begins in early infancy and reaches peak prevalence in juveniles. Thereafter it rapidly declines to about one third or one fourth of the maximum, a level that tends to be maintained in later years. It occurs sporadically or in epidemic form among travelers and resort populations of all ages. Oral-anal sex is an important risk factor for *Giardia* and other enteric infections (Phillips *et al.,* 1981). Cats, dogs, and other animals can carry the infection but their role in the epidemiology of giardiasis has not been demonstrated.

Control. Ordinary chlorination of water does not kill *Giardia* cysts. Commercial iodine preparations or boiling can be used to disinfect unsafe water for drinking. Group, family, and personal hygiene, as with other fecal-borne infections, assist in control.

Chilomastix mesnili

Chilomastix mesnili (Wenyon, 1910) Alexeieff, 1912 is a common cosmopolitan protozoon of the human intestinal tract. It has both a trophozoite and a cystic stage. Infection usually is acquired from cysts in contaminated food or drink.

The actively moving trophozoite (Fig. 3–2*A,B*) is rounded anteriorly and is spirally twisted posteriorly to a tapering end. It measures up to 20 μm in length when in progressive forward movement but only 3 to 10 μm when relatively quiescent, with the posterior end contracted and rounded (Fig. 3–2*C*). In the anterior rounded portion there is a distinct longitudinal cleft, the *cytostome.* Arising from the anterior pole are *one long and two short flagella,* a delicate *flagellum* that lies within the cytostome, and two stiffer *curved fibrils,* one on each side of the cytostome. The *nucleus* is situated at the extreme anterior end. *Chilomastix mesnili* moves forward with a jerky movement in a spiral path. Multiplication is by longitudinal binary fission.

The *cyst* (Fig. 3–2*D,E*) is lemon-shaped and measures 7 to 10 μm in length by 4 to 6 μm in breadth. It has a relatively thick hyaline wall and the characteristic internal features of the trophozoite, *viz.,* cytostome, curved fibrils, and nucleus.

The natural habitat of *C. mesnili* is the colon. In unformed

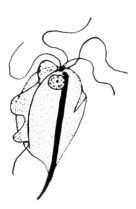

Fig. 3–3. *Trichomonas hominis*, trophozoite. (× 1600.) (By E.C. Faust.)

stools a majority of the organisms are motile trophozoites. In formed stools only cysts are seen.

C. mesnili is not pathogenic; hence the only significance attached to its presence in the intestine is the evidence that material contaminated by human feces has been ingested.

Trichomonas Species

Trichomonas species in the trophozoite stage (Fig. 3–3) are rounded anteriorly and have a somewhat pointed posterior end; a semirigid translucent rodlike *axostyle* that arises near the median anterior pole extends through the entire body and protrudes from the posterior end. Also present are a small *cytostome* on one side of the anterior end; a spherical *nucleus* in the midline near the anterior pole; a *kinetoplast* between the nucleus and the anterior margin of the organism from which arise three to five *free flagella;* and an additional *marginal flagellum* on an *undulating membrane,* which spirals down the side of the body. Multiplication is by longitudinal binary fission. For those species that parasitize man a cyst stage has not been described. The species that occur in man are *T. hominis, T. tenax,* and *T. vaginalis.*

Trichomonas hominis

Trichomonas hominis (Davaine, 1860) Leuckart, 1879 has a cosmopolitan distribution. It inhabits the lumen of the cecum. It measures 5 to 14 μm by 7 to 10 μm. There are 3 to 5 *free flagella* (usually 4). Its *undulating membrane* has a characteristic wavelike movement. The flagellum on the margin of the undulating membrane extends a short distance behind the membrane. The *nucleus* is near the anterior pole. At times the organism exhibits pseudopodial prolongations of its cytoplasm and might be mistaken for a very active minute ameba were it not for the undulations of its membrane and the *axostyle* that protrudes a short distance through the posterior extremity (Fig. 3–3).

There is no proof that *T. hominis* is pathogenic. Since it has only a trophozoite stage, it is presumably transmitted in a rounded-up unencysted stage. It is most commonly diagnosed

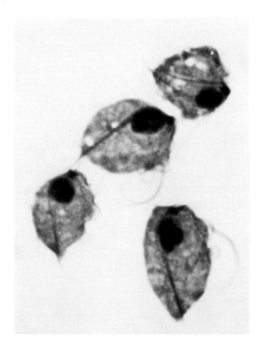

Fig. 3–4. *Trichomonas vaginalis.* Trophozoites from a culture that was inoculated with vaginal discharge. The nucleus, axostyle, and free flagella (4) are evident in each. The short undulating membrane is most clearly evident in the one at the lower left. (By P.C. Beaver.)

in unformed stools that contain considerable mucus. It is not clinically important.

Trichomonas tenax

Trichomonas tenax (O. F. Müller, 1773) Dobell, 1939 apparently is a cosmopolitan parasite of man, although relatively few surveys have been conducted to determine its geographic distribution. The active organism has four anterior *free flagella* of equal length, a relatively short *undulating membrane,* a slender *axostyle* that protrudes a considerable distance beyond the posterior end of the body, and a subspherical *nucleus. T. tenax* is slightly smaller than *T. hominis.* Its normal habitat is the mouth, particularly in diseased gums, in tartar around the teeth, and in carious teeth. It is not pathogenic but its presence indicates poor oral hygiene.

Trichomonas vaginalis
(Trichomonas vaginitis, trichomoniasis)

Trichomonas vaginalis Donné, 1837 is cosmopolitan in distribution. The motile organism (Fig. 3–4) generally is considerably larger than *T. hominis* and *T. tenax,* reaching maximum measurements of 27 μm in length and 18 μm in breadth. There are four anterior flagella of equal length, a fifth flagellum on the margin of a relatively short *undulating membrane* but not extending beyond the posterior limit of the membrane, a long delicate *axostyle* protruding a considerable distance beyond the posterior tip of the organism, and a large *nu-*

cleus and a small kinetoplast. This species is found only in the trophozoite stage and multiplies by longitudinal binary fission.

T. vaginalis is a frequent inhabitant of the human vagina and of the male genital tract (probably localized in the prostate gland and the urethra). Transmission of the infection is principally through sexual intercourse. The organism can survive for a few hours on dry fomites and for longer periods if moist.

T. vaginalis infection in the male is often asymptomatic, although at times it is associated with urethritis (Fullilove, 1983). In the female the infection also may be asymptomatic or may produce a vaginitis complicated by bacterial, yeast, or spirochetal infection. The chief complaints are leukorrhea and dysuria. Excessive discharge together with genital sprays may produce urticaria and acute vulvitis (Fouts and Kraus, 1980). The symptoms vary from mild to severe, but the disease is more annoying than disabling. Phagocytosis and killing of gonococci by *T. vaginalis* have been reported (Francioli *et al.*, 1983).

Diagnosis of *T. vaginalis* infection is based on recovery of the organism in urethral and prostatic discharges and urine in the male, and in vaginal discharge in the female. Direct examination of fresh microscopic films of the exudates usually is done routinely. Sometimes the organism is identified in Papanicolaou preparations made for other purposes. Isolation in cultures is an efficient method of demonstrating the organism (Fouts and Kraus, 1980).

Metronidazole orally, 250 mg 3 times daily for 7 days, is the treatment of choice. Vaginal inserts of 500 mg metronidazole used daily concurrently with the oral regimen provide increased efficacy in resistant infections. Alcohol should not be ingested during the course of treatment.

Dientamoeba fragilis
(Dientamoebiasis)

Dientamoeba fragilis Jepps and Dobell, 1918 was first described by Wenyon in 1907. Until 1974, when Honigberg placed it together with *Trichomonas* species in the order Trichomonadida, it was generally regarded as an ameba.

Only the trophozoite stage is known. It is amebalike, usually 5 to 12 μm in diameter. In fresh preparations it may be actively motile, with hyaline pseudopodia and distinct ectoplasm and endoplasm. In stained preparations two nuclei usually

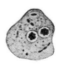

Fig. 3–5. *Dientamoeba fragilis.* Uninucleate and binucleate trophozoites. (× ca. 1200.) (From Dobell, C.C., and O'Connor, F.W. 1921. *The Intestinal Protozoa of Man.* New York, Wm. Wood & Co., Figs. 40–42.)

are evident, with no chromatin at the nuclear membrane and a relatively large, central karyosome that often appears to be four distinct granules (Fig. 3–5). *D. fragilis* colonizes the cecum and upper colon and does not invade the mucosa. In diarrheal or semiformed stools, it may be present in large numbers.

Occasionally pathogenicity of *D. fragilis* has been suspected when it has been the only organism identified in cases of anorexia, abdominal discomfort, and diarrhea. In such cases it may sometimes be desirable to prescribe treatment with tetracyclines or luminal amebicides, as recommended for *Entamoeba histolytica*.

Occasional Intestinal Flagellates

From time to time other species of harmless flagellate parasites of the large intestine of man are found in fecal specimens. These include *Retortamonas* and *Enteromonas* species, all of which are small forms with changing shapes and no axostyle.

FLAGELLATES OF BLOOD AND TISSUES

Species of flagellate protozoa that inhabit the blood and tissues of man are *Leishmania tropica*, *L. major*, *L. aethiopica*, *L. braziliensis*, *L. mexicana*, *L. donovani*, *Trypanosoma rhodesiense*, *T. gambiense*, *T. cruzi*, and *T. rangeli*. Some authorities assign species status to taxa that are considered subspecies by others. These will be alluded to under the respective species. All these organisms require two hosts in their life cycle, man or another susceptible mammal on the one hand and a bloodsucking insect on the other. For the species of *Leishmania* the insect is a sand fly (usually *Phlebotomus* or *Lutzomyia*); for *T. rhodesiense* and *T. gambiense*, a tsetse fly *(Glossina);* and for *T. cruzi* and *T. rangeli*, a triatomine bug.

In infections with species of *Leishmania* as well as *T. gambiense* and *T. rhodesiense*, the organisms multiply as flagellates in the midgut of the insect, then migrate forward to the insect's proboscis, referred to as the *anterior station*. In *T. cruzi* the parasites pass through the posterior part of the digestive tract *(posterior station)* and are evacuated in liquid feces soon after the bug feeds. They then enter the mucous membrane or skin at the site where the bug punctured the host's tissues. Mature promastigotes of *Leishmania* in the sand fly are infective for the vertebrate host, being injected at the time of feeding. In *T. rangeli,* after multiplying in the digestive tract the parasites migrate to the hemolymph and then to the salivary glands and are inoculated via the mouthparts into the vertebrate host. The essential features in the life cycle of the *Leishmania* and *Trypanosoma* species that infect man are compared in Table 3–1.

Leishmania Parasites as a Group

The genus *Leishmania* is named in honor of William Leishman, who discoverd the species *(L. donovani)* that causes kala-azar. In man and reservoir hosts (dogs, rodents), the organism in the amastigote form is a parasite of macrophage cells, in which it multiplies by binary fission, causing the death of the host cells.

Morphology and Life Cycle. The *Leishmania* of man, although morphologically very similar, have long been grouped into three species: *L. tropica,* which causes Old World cutaneous leishmaniasis; *L. braziliensis,* which causes New World cutaneous and mucocutaneous leishmaniasis; and *L. donovani,* which causes visceral leishmaniasis. However, there are at least four clinical types of cutaneous leishmaniasis in the New World, each probably caused by a distinct species or subspecies of *Leishmania,* and three distinct types of cutaneous leishmaniasis in the Old World. All these differ clinically, epidemiologically, immunologically, and biochemically. Visceral leishmaniasis, too, varies in its clinical picture in different geographic areas, and the respective agents can be distinguished by a number of laboratory procedures. For these reasons it is convenient to consider the *Leishmania* of man as grouped into complexes of species and subspecies. The approximate areas of geographic distribution of the two principal clinical types of *Leishmania* infections are shown in Figure 3–6.

When a sand fly ''bites'' an infected person or reservoir host, it sucks up parasitized macrophages or temporarily free parasites (amastigotes) in the blood or tissue juices (Table 3–1*A*). Soon after the amastigotes reach the midgut of the fly, they transform into the flagellated promastigote forms (Table 3–1*B*), which after rapid multiplication transform into infective promastigotes and migrate forward

(Sacks and Perkins, 1984). From the foregut they are regurgitated or otherwise introduced into the skin of the next individual when the sand fly takes another blood meal (Fig. 3–7).

Two stages in the life cycle are known: the *amastigote* in man and reservoir mammals and the *promastigote* in the sand fly and in cultures (Figs. 3–7, 3–8, 3–9). The amastigote is spherical or sub-spherical and measures 2 to 5 μm in its greatest dimension. It lives and reproduces by longitudinal binary fission in macrophages of skin, mucosa, lymph nodes, and reticuloendothelial system. In preparations stained with Giemsa's or Wright's stain, the cytoplasm is pale blue and the relatively large nucleus is red. In the cytoplasm, usually lying in the median line of the cell, is a deep red rodlike structure called the *kinetoplast*; a delicate filament called the *axoneme* extends from near the kinetoplast to the cell membrane. Ultrastructures include a Golgi apparatus, mitochondrium, endoplastic reticulum, lipid droplets, and subpellicular microtubules.

The promastigote is pyriform or spindle-shaped, measuring roughly 15 to 25 μm by 1.5 to 3.5 μm, with a single flagellum as long as or longer than the cell (Fig. 3–9). The nucleus is near the middle of the cell, and the kinetoplast is at the base of the flagellum (Table 3–1*B*).

Pathogenesis. Depending on the parasite strain and the host response, the primary lesions may be either obvious (usually in cutaneous leishmaniasis) or inapparent (usually in visceral leishmaniasis). This is attributable to the degree of delayed hypersensitivity developed and the destruction of the granulomas formed by macrophages containing amastigotes, which may be killed by sensitized lymphocytes. Although antibodies are usually produced, they are nonprotective and they are useful only for diagnostic tests. In addition, the lesions may become chronic, producing *diffuse leishmaniasis* (leproid or keloid with many macrophages filled with amastigotes lacking cellular reaction) in anergic individuals, and *espundia* and *recidiva* or *lupoid* leishmaniasis (relapsing cutaneous lesions with few or no amastigotes) in hypersensitized individuals. Apparently, immunity to homologous strains whose lesions were allowed to run their natural course is long-lasting, but reinfection with other strains may occur.

Diagnosis. Leishmaniasis diagnosis is based on the demonstration of the parasite obtained from lesions or organs in smears and in culture, or in

Table 3–1.   Stages of Leishmania and Trypanosoma in Man and Insect Host

Stage of the Parasite	Amastigote (*Leishmania*)	Promastigote (*Leptomonas*)	Epimastigote (*Crithidia*)	Trypomastigote (*Trypanosoma*)
Name of Parasite				
Leishmania tropica	*Intracellular* in macrophages of skin and subcutaneous tissue	In midgut, later in proboscis of sand fly *(Phlebotomus): transfer stage* to man	Lacking	Lacking
Leishmania braziliensis	*Intracellular* in macrophages of skin; may invade mucosa	In midgut, later in proboscis of sand fly *(Lutzomyia): transfer stage* to man	Lacking	Lacking
Leishmania donovani	*Intracellular* in macrophages; mainly in spleen, liver, marrow, and lymph nodes	In midgut, later in proboscis of sand fly *(Phlebotomus): transfer stage* to man	Lacking	Lacking
Trypanosoma rhodesiense	Lacking	Lacking	In proventriculus, gut, and salivary glands of tsetse fly *(Glossina)*	In salivary glands of tsetse fly; *transfer stage* to man; first in blood, then in lymph nodes
Trypanosoma gambiense	Lacking	Lacking	In proventriculus, gut, and salivary glands of tsetse fly *(Glossina)*	In salivary glands of tsetse fly; *transfer stage* to man; first in blood, then in lymph nodes, later in central nervous system
Trypanosoma cruzi	*Intracellular* in cells of many organs	Transitional stage only	In midgut of triatomine bug	In feces of bug; *transfer stage* to man; in blood during early stages
Trypanosoma rangeli	No intracellular stage demonstrated	Transitional stage only	In midgut, hemolymph and salivary glands of triatomine bug	In feces, hemolymph and salivary glands of bug; *transfer stage* to man; in blood of definitive host

hamsters inoculated with patients' specimens. In most regions more than one type of *Leishmania* strain may be present, and therefore isolations should be identified by means of isoenzyme characterization, monoclonal antibodies, and DNA analysis (Peters *et al.*, 1983). The leishmanin intradermal test may be positive in patients with active (except in *L. tropica*), healed, or cured lesions and negative in early infections and in anergic persons such as those with diffuse or visceral leishmaniasis. False positive tests may be seen in pa-

tients with tuberculosis, leprosy, and mycoses. Several serologic tests are available, but the immunofluorescent antibody test is the most used for diagnosis and for assessment of cure after treatment.

Old World Cutaneous Leishmaniasis

Three varieties of cutaneous leishmaniasis have been distinguished in the Eastern Hemisphere: an urban or "dry" type caused by *Leishmania trop-*

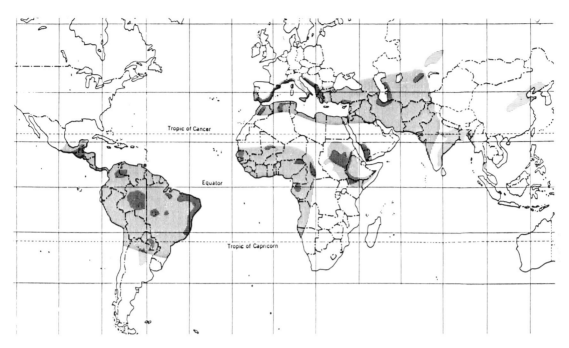

Fig. 3–6. Leishmaniasis. Approximate world distribution of cutaneous and mucocutaneous infections *(vertical shading)* and visceral infections *(horizontal shading)*. (Adapted by R.C. Jung from original by E.C. Faust.)

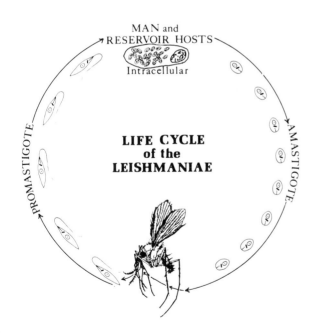

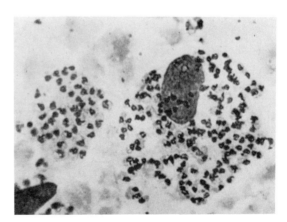

Fig. 3–7. *Leishmania.* Diagram of life cycle of species that cause disease in man. *Above,* intracellular amastigotes in macrophage of mammalian host. *Below,* sand fly *(Phlebotomus or Lutzomyia),* intermediate host and vector. *Right,* amastigotes taken up with blood meal from infected mammal. *Left,* promastigotes in vector, to be introduced into skin of mammal at time of subsequent blood meal. (Adapted by R.C. Jung from original by E.C. Faust.)

Fig. 3–8. *Leishmania tropica.* Amastigotes in macrophages from skin lesion. (× 1200.) (Courtesy of Armed Forces Institute of Pathology.)

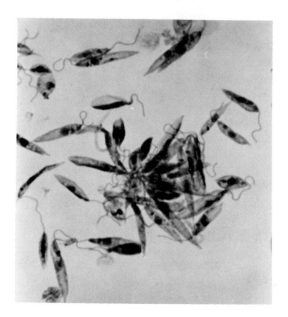

Fig. 3–9. *Leishmania tropica.* Promastigotes in Giemsa-stained smear from culture of forms inoculated directly in scrapings from skin lesion. (× 1000.) (From Beaver, P.C., Jung, R.C., and Cupp, E.W. 1984. *Clinical Parasitology,* 9th ed. Philadelphia, Lea & Febiger, p. 60.)

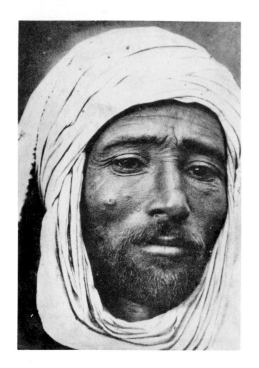

Fig. 3–10. *Leishmania tropica.* Early lesion on face, North Africa. (From Sergent, E., et al., 1925. Le clou de Míla. Arch. Inst. Pasteur Alger., *3*:1–8, Fig. 5.)

ica, a rural or ''wet'' type caused by *L. major,* and a diffuse cutaneous type caused by *L. aethiopica.* Clinical, epidemiologic, immunologic, and biochemical differences among these varieties indicate that each is a distinct entity.

Leishmania tropica

(Syn. *L. tropica minor)*
(Dry or urban cutaneous leishmaniasis,
Oriental sore, Aleppo button, Jericho boil,
Delhi boil)
and

Leishmania major

(Syn. *L. tropica major*)
(Rural or wet cutaneous leishmaniasis)

Leishmania amastigotes causing cutaneous leishmaniasis probably were first seen by Cunningham in 1885. French workers in North Africa and Adler and Theodor in Palestine in 1926 found that *Phlebotomus papatasi* is the vector of *L. tropica* in the Mediterranean area.

Pathogenesis and Symptomatology. Tissue reaction is initiated with the introduction of promastigotes into the dermis. Macrophages in the vicinity pick up the parasites, which rapidly transform into amastigotes and multiply, destroying the host cells. Soon there is a dense concentration of macrophages

in the invaded area, all of which are liable to infection and destruction. The lesion then becomes necrotic at the center, and the margins containing parasitized macrophages may become infiltrated with giant and plasma cells.

The lesion appears first as a macule, then as a papule with a slightly raised center covered by a thin blisterlike layer of epidermis. The lesion then breaks down, with discharge of a small amount of clear or purulent exudate. At its craterlike base in the dermis a granulating layer is formed, and the margin becomes indurated by infiltration of fibroblasts (Fig. 3–10). In the *urban disease* ulceration is slow and may not occur. There is comparatively little surrounding tissue reaction. The course of the healing process may take more than a year. In the *rural disease* ulceration, often multiple, is prone to occur early, there is a greater degree of surrounding reaction, and if secondary bacterial infection does not interfere healing may take place within 6 months.

The *incubation period* may be as short as 2 weeks or as long as 3 years, but it usually is between 2 and 6 months. In uncomplicated cases, there are no systemic manifestations, and since the infection is typically self-limiting, patients seldom seek medical assistance. However, the common occurrence of pyogenic complications causes painful, disfiguring, local ulcers, neutrophilic leukocytosis and fever, and at times septicemia.

Diagnosis. Clinically the uncomplicated lesion may be mistaken for a variety of infections of the skin; hence demonstration of the parasite is essential. As soon as the ulcer opens, material aspirated or scraped from a slit incised at the margin of the ulcer may be smeared onto a clean glass slide and stained by Giemsa's or Wright's technique. The amastigote stage of the parasite will be found within macrophages or spread out from ruptured cells (Fig. 3–8). The specimens also may be cultured or inoculated into hamsters.

Treatment. Pentavalent antimonials are the drugs of choice. Sodium antimony gluconate (Pentostam, Solustibosan) and meglumine antimonate given intramuscularly are usually effective in cases with multiple lesions. For treatment of a single lesion without significant secondary infection, cryotherapy may be the method of choice, or sodium antimony gluconate or quinacrine may be injected into the margin of the ulcer. Leishmaniasis recidiva responds poorly to treatment and frequently relapses.

Secondary bacterial infection of the ulcer, when present, should be eliminated by treatment with appropriate antibacterial agents.

Epidemiology. Old World cutaneous leishmaniasis (Fig. 3–6) has an extensive distribution from western and northwestern India and West Pakistan into countries bordering on the Mediterranean. It also occurs in several foci in tropical Africa and the southern U.S.S.R. Cutaneous leishmaniais is found in relatively barren, sandy, arid regions where there is moisture at the time the sand fly vectors are breeding. Reservoir hosts are dogs (urban) or wild rodents (zoonotic or rural).

The vectors most widely distributed in the endemic-enzootic zones are *Phlebotomus papatasi* and *P. sergenti.* The stable fly *(Stomoxys calcitrans)* may transmit the organism from an open ulcer to clean skin by mechanical transfer. Infection usually confers life-long immunity.

Control. Mass chemotherapy is not practical for control. Producing an ulcer by injection of a pure culture of *L. tropica* into a covered area of the skin will provide lasting immunity; however, it may cause leishmaniasis recidiva. Dog reservoirs should be destroyed. Residual insecticide sprayed on the doors, windows, and on the inside walls of human habitations and adjacent buildings is effective in killing the adult sand flies.

Leishmania aethiopica
(Cutaneous and diffuse or disseminated cutaneous leishmaniasis of Ethiopia, anergic cutaneous leishmaniasis)

Leishmania aethiopica was described as a distinct species only recently, in 1973, by R.S. Bray and associates. It occurs in the highlands of Ethiopia, in Kenya, and possibly in Yemen. Morphologically it is indistinguishable from *L. tropica,* and in its life cycle and epidemiology it causes a zoonosis resembling that caused by *L. major.* Animal reservoirs are species of hyrax and the vectors are species of *Phlebotomus.*

Clinically, three types have been described—lepromatoid, intermediate, and tuberculoid. The first is indistinguishable from disseminated cutaneous leishmaniasis of the New World. The three types resemble the respective varieties of leprosy. In the tuberculoid type, lymphangitis and elephantiasis may occur. Primary mucocutaneous leishmaniasis has also been reported.

To establish a diagnosis, amastigotes must be demonstrated in scrapings of skin slits, in aspirates, or in biopsy specimens. The lepromatoid type of infection is usually resistant to antimonials, although intravenous sodium stibogluconate has given good results (Chulay *et al.,* 1983). Amphotericin B has been used as the drug of choice, but it is relatively toxic, and tolerance of individuals is widely variable. Pentamidine isethionate is useful given weekly for 3 months longer than it takes to eliminate the parasite. However, relapses are frequent.

New World Cutaneous and Mucocutaneous Leishmaniasis

The history of attempts to clarify the taxonomic status of parasites causing various clinical types of American cutaneous leishmaniasis is long and complicated. In one or more of its various clinical forms, leishmaniasis is found in all of the countries from the southern United States (Texas and Florida) to Paraguay and northern Argentina. Canine cutaneous leishmaniasis extends as far north as Oklahoma. In the northern part of its range, in Central America and southern Mexico, infections seldom produce secondary mucocutaneous disease and clinically they resemble Oriental sore.

Classification. The classification proposed by

Lainson (1983) for the American species and sub-species that cause cutaneous and mucocutaneous leishmaniasis is as follows:

LEISHMANIA BRAZILIENSIS COMPLEX

1. *L. braziliensis braziliensis,* causing espundia in Brazil and adjacent tropical forest areas.
2. *L. braziliensis guyanensis,* causing pian bois in the Guianas and adjacent areas of Brazil and Venezuela.
3. *L. braziliensis panamensis,* causing cutaneous infection without metastasis in Panama and adjacent Colombia and Central America.
4. *L. braziliensis peruviana,* causing uta without nasopharyngeal involvement in Peru and Argentina on the western slope of the Andes.

LEISHMANIA MEXICANA COMPLEX

1. *L. mexicana mexicana,* causing chiclero ulcer in Mexico, Guatemala, and Belize.
2. *L. mexicana amazonensis,* causing cutaneous and, rarely, diffuse leishmaniasis with no nasopharyngeal involvement in the Amazon Basin.
3. *L. mexicana pifanoi,* causing disseminated (anergic) cutaneous disease in Venezuela.

In addition, cases of diffuse leishmaniasis have been described in Brazil, Peru, Bolivia, and the Dominican Republic, but specific characterization of the agents involved is not yet available (Schnur et al., 1983).

There are other subspecies of *Leishmania. L. mexicana enriettii* is known only from laboratory guinea pigs; *L. m. aristidesi* was isolated from rodents and opossums in Panama; and *L. hertigi* was isolated from porcupines in Panama, Costa Rica, and Brazil. Differentiation between the *L. mexicana* and *L. braziliensis* complexes is based on the size of amastigotes and promastigotes and on the behavior of the parasites in blood-agar culture, hamsters, and sand flies. Growth of the larger *L. mexicana* is rapid and luxurious and the infection develops faster, is more marked, and causes numerous metastases containing abundant amastigotes. The reverse is true in *L. braziliensis.* In the vector, *L. mexicana* grows in the midgut and *L. braziliensis* in both the mid- and hindgut. In addition, serologic and biochemical tests differentiate the two groups, generally in agreement with clinical and epidemiologic differences. The life cycle both in the vector and in the mammalian host is similar to that of the other *Leishmania* species.

Pathogenesis and Symptomatology. American strains of *Leishmania* causing cutaneous infections

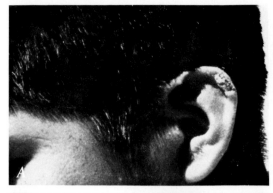

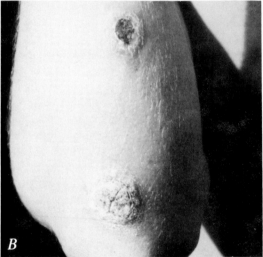

Fig. 3–11. *A.* Chiclero ulcer on the pinna. *B.* Pian bois on the forearm. (From Beaver, P.C., Jung, R.C., and Cupp, E.W. 1984. *Clinical Parasitology.* 9th ed. Philadelphia, Lea & Febiger, p. 68.)

differ in their tendency to involve the mucous membranes of the mouth and nasopharynx by extension or metastasis. The character of the lesions also varies, ranging from transient and trivial to extensive and mutilating. Secondary infections add to the severity of lesions both in the skin and mucous membranes. Racial differences in pathogenesis have been noted, mutilation of the face being most common and extensive in Negroes. In general the papular lesions, nodules, and ulcers of the skin are the same as those of Oriental sore, but in American cutaneous leishmaniasis the types of lesions and course of the disease vary widely and markedly so that distinct diseases with established names and boundaries of distribution are recognized.

Chiclero ulcer, caused by *L. mexicana mexicana,* typically affects the face and ears and does not spread to the nasopharynx (Fig. 3–11). Usually the disease is mild and self-limiting, consisting of a single papule, nodule, or ulcer, though in some cases much of the pinna is destroyed. The name derives from the high frequency of occurrence of the infection among chicle collectors in the forest areas of southern Mexico, Guatemala, and Belize.

Pian bois, caused by *L. braziliensis guyanensis,* is characterized by a high frequency of multiple ulcers of the body and extremities resulting from extensive metastasis that tends to extend along lymph channels (Fig. 3–11*B*). Transmitted primarily by *Lutzomyia umbratilis,* it occurs in the Guianas and northern Amazon Basin.

"Panamanian" cutaneous leishmaniasis, caused by *L. braziliensis panamensis,* is present in Panama, Colombia and neighboring countries. Transmitted by *Lu. trapidoi* and other species of sand flies, it typically consists of shallow ulcers on exposed parts, occasionally forming secondary nodules along lymph channels, but is reported as not spreading to the nasopharynx. It is closely related biologically and biochemically to *L. b. guyanensis.* However, *L.b. panamensis* and possibly *L.b. guyanensis* have been observed to invade the nasopharyngeal mucosa (Saravia et al., 1985).

Uta, caused by *L. braziliensis peruviana,* is a relatively mild disease with few lesions that usually are self-limiting. The vectors are *Lutzomyia verrucarum* and *Lu. peruensis,* common in dry areas of the western slope of the Andes.

Espundia, caused by *L. braziliensis braziliensis* and transmitted by several species of sand flies, has been considered somewhat synonymous with mucocutaneous leishmaniasis. It is well known for its tendency to mutilate the face; it is often resistant to treatment and follows a chronic course. Involvement of the larynx as well as the nasopharynx is common. Cartilage and mucous membranes but not bone are destroyed (Fig. 3–12). It has been reported widely in tropical forest areas of South America. *L. b. braziliensis* has been identified from British military personnel returning from Belize (Evans *et al.,* 1984). However, isolation and characterization of the involved parasites can be difficult.

Disseminated (anergic) cutaneous leishmaniasis, presumed to be caused by *L. mexicana pifanoi* and *L. mexicana amazonensis,* found in Venezuela and Brazil, resembles the lepromatoid type of leishmaniasis that occurs in Ethiopia. The disease is linked with a deficient cell-mediated immunity associated only with *L. mexicana* complex. These uncommon forms are usually incurable.

An utalike disease in the Andes of Western Venezuela, caused by *L. garnhami,* is relatively benign, with cutaneous ulcers that are self-terminating but in most cases remain active for more than a year without metastasis or mucosal involvement. The vector is still unidentified and biochemical taxonomic studies are still lacking. *L. garnhami* was described in 1979 and further studied by Scorza *et al.* (1983). Because of its biological characteristics, Lainson (1983) preferred to use the name *L. m. garnhami.*

L. mexicana venezuelensis has recently been isolated from people with single or disseminated lesions in Lara State in Venezuela. The isoenzyme and monoclonal antibodies are different from all other *L. mexicana* (Lainson, 1983). The vector may be *Lu. olmeca.*

Diagnosis. Accurate diagnosis is a prerequisite for treatment. The organism can be demonstrated in smears from skin slit scrapings, aspiration or biopsy specimens from the lesions' borders, in cultures, or in hamster inoculation; intradermal and immunologic tests are useful (see Technical Aids, pp. 258 and 260). Efforts should be made to ensure that healing of lesions is accompanied by negative results of an indirect fluorescent antibody test (IFAT) and absence of organisms in biopsies from the "cured" lesion site.

Differential diagnosis includes tuberculosis, blastomycosis, leprosy, scleroma, treponemal infections, carcinoma, tropical ulcer, and sickle cell and varicose ulcers.

Treatment. The drug of choice is meglumine antimonate, since sodium stibogluconate is not generally available in endemic areas. Long-term uninterrupted doses may be more efficient than the traditional repeated short courses if renal function of the patient is good. Pentavalent antimonial compounds are eliminated in the urine. Daily intramuscular injections of 20 mg Sb^v/kg to a maximum of 850 mg for a minimum of 20 days are indicated. In cases refractory to antimonial drugs, the second choice is amphotericin B, given as for visceral leishmaniasis. Other drugs such a pyrimethamine, metronidazole, and nifurtimox have been used with variable degrees of success.

Epidemiology. Most of the American leishmaniases are zoonoses infecting several species of rodents and other mammals, usually showing no skin lesions. The vectors are forest species of sand flies. Man typically becomes infected when his occupation takes him into the forest. The main vectors

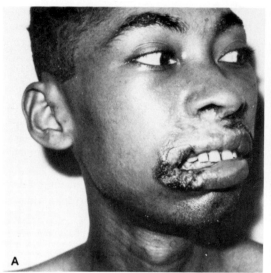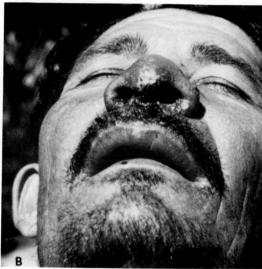

Fig. 3–12. *Leishmania braziliensis*. Characteristic lesion of espundia: ulceration of the nose, palate, pharynx, and lips. (By A. D'Alessandro.) (From Beaver, P.C., Jung, R.C., and Cupp, E.W. 1984. *Clinical Parasitology*, 9th ed. Philadelphia, Lea & Febiger, p. 69.)

of *L. braziliensis* are more anthropophilic than are those of *L. mexicana,* and therefore the number of people infected with the former is higher. Both cutaneous and mucocutaneous leishmaniasis are widely distributed in the lowland forests of Central and South America. On the other hand, uta is found in high Andean valleys, where the vectors are species of *Lutzomyia,* breeding in close proximity to man's habitation, and dogs are reservoir hosts. Diffuse cutaneous leishmaniasis occurs mostly in Venezuela and Brazil.

Control. Since most forms of the disease are not contracted in the villages, residual insecticide spraying of homes is not a major weapon. However, area power dusting with insecticides, along with residual spraying of dwellings, has been shown to be successful in destroying the adult flies that transmit uta.

Visceral Leishmaniasis

Leishmania donovani
(Kala-azar, Dum-Dum fever, visceral leishmaniasis)

Leishmania donovani (Laveran and Mesnil, 1903) Ross, 1903, the causative agent of kala-azar, was first demonstrated by William Leishman in 1900 in smears from the spleen of an English soldier who died of a fever near Calcutta, India. In 1903, Charles Donovan found the same organism

in smears from splenic puncture of a person with the disease in Madras, India. Ross created the genus *Leishmania* in honor of the original discoverer. Leonard Rogers (1903) first cultured the organism and demonstrated that it had a flagellate stage. It was not until 1942 that a sand fly *(Phlebotomus argentipes)* was shown to be the natural vector in India. In the New World, visceral leishmaniasis is caused by *L. donovani chagasi* and in the Mediterranean basin by *L. donovani infantum.*

Morphology and Life Cycle. With the light microscope, the amastigote and promastigote forms of *L. donovani* are indistinguishable in size or other morphologic characteristics from those of *L. tropica* (Figs. 3–8, 3–9) and *L. braziliensis.* In its tissue relations in man and most susceptible laboratory animals, however, *L. donovani* has a predilection for the reticuloendothelial cells of the spleen, liver, bone marrow, and visceral lymph nodes, and its primary colonization in the skin usually is inapparent. In the dog, conspicuous lesions are on the skin, so that in this reservoir host cutaneous leishmaniasis due to infection with *L. tropica* and kala-azar caused by *L. donovani* are difficult to distinguish.

Pathogenesis and Symptomatology. The promastigote stage of the parasite is introduced into the outer dermis by an infected sand fly. In China, India, and the Mediterranean endemic areas, the primary lesion is inapparent. In the U.S.S.R., 1-

to 2-mm papules appear on the exposed skin in infants some time before *Leishmania donovani* infection can be otherwise demonstrated. After colonizing in the dermis, some of the organisms gain access to the bloodstream or lymphatics and are transported to the viscera, where they lodge in fixed tissue macrophages and rapidly multiply. As the number of amastigotes becomes greatly augmented, there is intense phagocytic activity and a remarkable increase in the number of macrophages, increasing neutropenia and anemia, and resistance to intercurrent infection is markedly reduced. Although the parasites are found in all soft tissues of the body, they are particularly abundant in those rich in reticuloendothelial cells. Hence the fundamental histopathologic condition results from this parasite-host cell relationship.

The *spleen* is greatly enlarged. The *liver* is likewise enlarged and firm but somewhat friable, with an increase in size and number of parastized Kupffer cells. The *bone marrow* exhibits markedly increased production of macrophages and decreased erythropoietic function. Thromobocytopenia results in multiple hemorrhages, particularly from mucous membranes. Lymph nodes and tonsils are also involved. In fatal cases the dermis contains large masses of amastigotes.

The *incubation period* varies from 10 days to many months. The *onset* may be sudden, with acute manifestations, but in the usual case it is insidious, on the average about 90 days following exposure.

In the typical acute case, temperature of an undulant type fluctuates daily from 36.7 to 40°C (90 to 104°F), often with two peaks daily. The appetite is usually good. Wasting may be partly masked by edema of the face, trunk, and feet. The abdomen is protuberant, and both the liver and spleen can be palpated far below the costal margin. In spite of the enlarged liver there is no periportal cirrhosis and hence no ascites (Fig. 3–13). Bleeding typically occurs from the gums, lips, nares, and the intestinal mucosa. The blood picture is one of anemia, leukopenia with monocytosis and lymphocytosis, thrombocytopenia, and occasionally agranulocytosis. Complications usually observed in kala-azar are principally diarrhea or dysentery and bronchopneumonia; less frequently there is cancrum oris.

Diagnosis. For assurance that the patient is suffering from kala-azar, the organism itself must be demonstrated microscopically in a biopsy specimen of bone marrow or spleen (Fig. 3–8), by cultivation

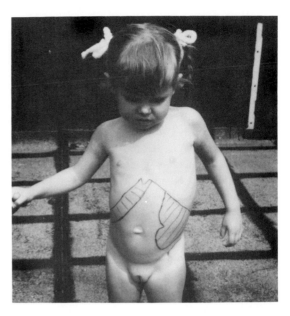

Fig. 3–13. *Leishmania donovani.* Enlargement of spleen and liver characteristic of kala-azar in a child. The disconsolate expression is typical. (Courtesy of P.E.C. Manson-Bahr.) (From Beaver, P.C., Jung, R.C., and Cupp, E.W. 1984. *Clinical Parasitology,* 9th ed. Philadelphia, Lea & Febiger, p. 73.)

in vitro (Fig. 3–9), or by inoculation in hamsters. Immunologic diagnosis consists of (1) aldehyde, formol-gel, antimonyl tests; and (2) indirect fluorescent antibody and other serologic tests. The leishmanin skin test is negative in patients with active disease.

Treatment. Supportive treatment and good nursing care are needed in most cases, particularly those with complications of bronchopneumonia, severe diarrhea, dysentery, or cancrum oris. Three types of drugs are employed in the treatment of kala-azar: antimonials, the drugs of first choice, the diamidines, and amphotericin B, the latter two being used in relapses and unresponsive patients. In general, treatment should be given until the aspirate is free of parasites for at least 2 weeks. If relapses occur, the drug should be given for twice as long as the first treatment.

ANTIMONIALS. Of the pentavalent antimonials, meglumine antimonate *(Glucantime)* and sodium antimony gluconate *(Pentostam, Solustibosan)* have been the most useful, given as for cutaneous leishmaniasis (p. 23).

DIAMIDINES. The diamidines, including stilbamidine, hydroxystilbamidine and pentamidine, are employed routinely in the Sudan in the treatment of kala-azar, since this particular strain of *L. donovani* does not respond satisfactorily to antimony therapy. Likewise, in India, China, and the Mediterranean endemic areas cases refractory to antimony are usually benefited by diamidine therapy.

Amphotericin B will sometimes effect a cure after failure of antimonial and diamidine treatments. However, the drug is toxic and should not be used except after repeated unsuccessful treatments with the other drugs.

In India, East Africa, and China, a sequela to antimony treatment is known as post-treatment kala-azar dermal leishmaniasis, in which a verrucous condition develops in the skin. Histologically these excrescences contain amastigotes in focal concentrations of macrophages. This phenomenon is interpreted as an indication of inadequate treatment, with a residuum of parasites that continue to propagate. Such cases may be an important source of infection. Repeated treatment with antimonials is required.

Epidemiology. Kala-azar is endemic in northern China, eastern India, Afghanistan and Turkestan, the Sudan, many foci around the Mediterranean Sea, Ethiopia, the east and west coasts of Africa, Paraguay, Bolivia, northern Argentina, eastern Brazil, and minor foci elsewhere in South and Central America (Fig. 3–7).

In most of these areas, the infection is endemic or hyperendemic but on occasion it may become epidemic. In Mediterranean countries and China, it is primarily a disease of infants and young children. In India and South America, young adults are most frequently infected. In the Sudan, a particularly fulminating type is observed, commonly in young adults. Previous infection confers immunity.

In endemic areas of North China, Baghdad, and the Mediterranean, dogs are common reservoir hosts; naturally infected dogs and foxes have been found in Brazil. The only known vector in South America is *Lu. longipalpis*. Lesions caused by *L. donovani* in dogs are notably cutaneous, so that the sand fly has direct access to infected macrophages.

Control. Since it has been demonstrated that residual spraying of insecticides in and around human habitations is both highly efficacious and economical in sand fly control, this measure has replaced all others as the main weapon of attack against kala-azar. In areas where dogs constitute a source of infection for the sand flies, campaigns to destroy street dogs and others with obvious skin lesions can be effective.

Trypanosomes

Some species of trypanosomes apparently live in their natural vertebrate hosts without causing evident disease. Others cause variable degrees of tissue pathology. Three species of trypanosomes that commonly parasitize man are all pathogenic and not infrequently cause death: *Trypanosoma (Trypanozoon) brucei rhodesiense* (= *Trypanosoma rhodesiense*), *Trypanosoma (Trypanozoon) brucei gambiense* (= *Trypanosoma gambiense*), and *Trypanosoma (Schizotrypanum) cruzi* (= *Trypanosoma cruzi*).

Trypanosoma, Salivarian and Stercorian Groups

Trypanosoma brucei brucei (= *T. brucei*) (found commonly in game animals but not infective to man), *T. rhodesiense*, *T. gambiense*, and *T. (Herpetosoma) rangeli* constitute a group in which the forms of the parasite that are infective for the mammalian host develop in the salivary glands (the anterior station) of the vector and are referred to as the *salivarian trypanosomes*. *T. cruzi* is of a distinctly different type in two respects: (1) it is leishmania-like in having dividing amastigote tissue forms, and (2) the infective stage of the parasite develops in the hindgut of the vector and emerges from the intestine (posterior station) in the feces and thus is referred to a a *stercorian* trypanosome.

Trypanosoma rhodesiense, T. gambiense, and *T. brucei* are confined to Africa and use *Glossina* (tsetse flies) as their vector. When these trypanosomes are sucked into the labial cavity from the mammalian host, they pass directly through the proventriculus into the midgut, where multiplication occurs in an elongated trypanosome stage. Thereafter the organisms migrate through the gut posteriorly and then through the proventriculus and buccal cavity up the hypopharynx into the salivary glands, where a second multiplication occurs. These forms are epimastigotes, with a posterior nucleus (Table 3–1C), but they later transform into small infective-stage *metacyclic* trypanosomes (metatrypomastigotes), which accumulate in the salivary gland ducts (Table 3–1D). In these species the hypopharynx serves only for transit and not for multiplication or metamorphosis of the parasites (Fig. 3–14). Recent observations suggest that the flagellates may reach the wall of the salivary glands, going through the intestinal wall and the body cavity of the fly. Mechanical transmission by *Glossina* has also been reported.

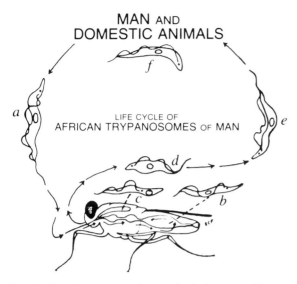

MAN AND
DOMESTIC ANIMALS

LIFE CYCLE OF
AFRICAN TRYPANOSOMES OF MAN

Fig. 3–14. *Trypanosoma brucei-rhodesiense-gambiense* complex. Diagram of life cycle in tsetse fly, mammals, and man. *a,* Trypanosome stage taken from mammalian host by tsetse fly. *b,* Multiplication of trypanosome stage in midgut of fly. *c,* Mutiplication of crithidial stage in salivary glands, followed by transformation into metacyclic trypanosome stage. *d,* Metacyclic trypanosomes transferred from fly to mammal. *e* and *f,* Trypanosome stage in bloodstream of mammal.

In the mammalian host *T. brucei, T. rhodesiense,* and *T. gambiense* are trypomastigote forms (Fig. 3–15) circulating primarily in the bloodstream, where they multiply by longitudinal binary fission. They measure 14 to 33 μm in length and 1.5 to 3.5 μm in breadth. They are polymorphic and morphologically indistinguishable but different biologically and biochemically. If the host-parasite adaptation is good, they produce little humoral or tissue damage. This is illustrated by *T. brucei* in African game animals. *T. rhodesiense* is a mutant of *T. brucei,* which has become more or less adapted to man. Here the adjustment is poor, and the parasite typically produces an overwhelming

infection with fatal consequences to the victim. It is also likely that *T. gambiense* was originally derived from a parent stock of *T. brucei* but at a much earlier period, so that the adjustment to the human host has been somewhat more satisfactory.

Trypanosoma rhodesiense
(Rhodesian trypanosomiasis,
East African sleeping sickness)

Trypanosoma rhodesiense Stephens and Fantham, 1910 was discovered in 1909 in the blood of a patient in Rhodesia who had symptoms suggestive of a fulminating early stage of African "sleeping sickness." Three years later, Kinghorn and Yorke demonstrated that it is transmitted to man by the tsetse fly, *Glossina morsitans.*

Morphology and Life Cycle. Morphologically the infective trypanosome stage of *T. rhodesiense* cannot be distinguished from that of *T. gambiense* (Fig. 3–16). When a tsetse fly takes a blood meal containing *T. rhodesiense* from animal reservoirs or man, the trypanosomes reach the midgut, multiply, and then migrate to the salivary glands and reach the infective stage. The development within the fly requires approximately 3 weeks. When the infective stage trypanosomes are introduced into the human host, they multiply in the blood, lymph nodes, and spleen.

Pathogenesis and Symptomatology. On introduction into the human skin from the proboscis of an infected tsetse fly, *T. rhodesiense* first lodges in the local tissues where the trypanosomes may set up a painless, boil-like interstitial inflammatory reaction. When present it subsides within a week or two as the trypanosomes gain entry to the circulating blood. Then they enter the lymph nodes, where a second focus of inflammation occurs, with hyperplasia of the endothelial lining of the blood

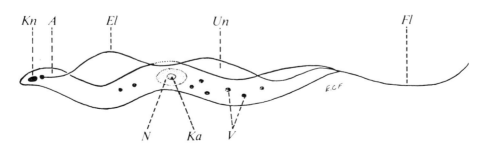

Fig. 3–15. Trypanosome, typical morphology. *A,* Axoneme, arising from the basal body. *Fl,* Flagellum. *Ka,* Karyosome. *Kn,* Kinetoplast. *N,* Nucleus. *Un,* Undulating membrane. *V,* Volutin granules. (Adapted from Beaver, P.C., Jung, R.C., and Cupp, E.W. 1984. *Clinical Parasitology,* 9th ed. Philadelphia, Lea & Febiger, p. 78.)

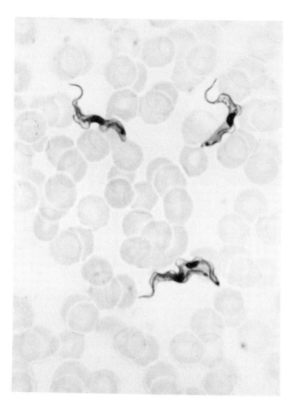

Fig. 3–16. *Trypanosoma rhodesiense.* Trypanosomes (trypomastigotes) in Giemsa-stained blood smear. Dividing form at bottom has 2 kinetoplasts, 2 nuclei, and 2 flagella. (× 1200.) (By R.G. Yaeger.)

sinuses and perivascular infiltration of leukocytes. This process is rapid, fulminating, and often causes death in a few months. Only rarely does the victim survive long enough for the trypanosomes to invade the central nervous system and produce the signs characteristic of the third stage of *T. gambiense* infection (so-called "sleeping sickness").

Following an incubation period of 1 to 2 weeks, the patient suffers from headache, febrile paroxysms that recur frequently, extreme weakness, and rapid loss of weight. Lymph node enlargement is not pronounced; skin rashes, edema, and myocarditis may be present. Central nervous system signs are not common but when they are present the diagnosis is clearer. Death supervenes within a year in untreated cases due to intercurrent infections and encephalomyelitis with mental deterioration and coma (Foulkes, 1981).

Diagnosis. During febrile episodes the trypanosomes appear in thick smears of circulating blood; at other times specific diagnosis must be based on recovery of the organisms in lymph node or spinal fluid aspirates. Elevated serum and cerebrospinal fluid IgM levels are indicative of African trypanosomiasis; increase in protein content in the cerebrospinal fluid after treatment may indicate a relapse. Serologic tests (IFAT, ELISA) can be useful, especially for screening populations and for assessing cure (IFAT).

Treatment. Early treatment is imperative. Suramin, although more toxic, is preferable to pentamidine because of its greater efficacy. Patients with late infections, recognized principally by increased cells and protein in the cerebrospinal fluid, should be treated with melarsoprol. Follow-up examination to detect relapses should be continued for 2 to 3 years.

Epidemiology. *T. rhodesiense* has a geographic distribution limited to the upland savannas of East Africa (Fig. 3–17). It is an infection of antelopes, at present not frequently in close contact with man. The vector of Rhodesian trypanosomiasis is usually the savanna *Glossina morsitans,* both sexes of which transmit the infection. Less commonly *G. pallidipes* and *G. swynnertoni,* usually referred to as game tsetses, and rarely *G. palpalis* and *G. brevipalpis,* serve as vectors. The main vectors breed in relatively dry habitats, preferring warm to cold environmental temperatures.

Small numbers of people are infected with *T. rhodesiense* compared with *T. gambiense,* but the usually fatal course of the Rhodesian disease serves to emphasize its importance. It occurs typically in sporadic form, but at times epidemics develop. It is a disease of hunters, fisherman, and tourists visiting game areas (Cochran and Rosen, 1983). Healthy human carriers are uncommon.

Control. Recommended procedures for control include the following: (1) remove people from forested or heavy bush regions (especially around lakes) to open country; (2) clear out brush around settlements, (3) settle individual families in uninfected territory concentrated in large villages, and (4) use of traps, impregnated or not with insecticides, to reduce the tsetse population (Ryan *et al.,* 1981). Attempts to eradicate the disease by destruction of infected game animals have not succeeded. Successful efforts often require international cooperation. Prophylactic treatment is unreliable.

Trypanosoma gambiense
(Gambian trypanosomiasis,
African sleeping sickness)

Trypanosoma gambiense Dutton, 1902 was first seen by Forde in 1901 in the blood of a European

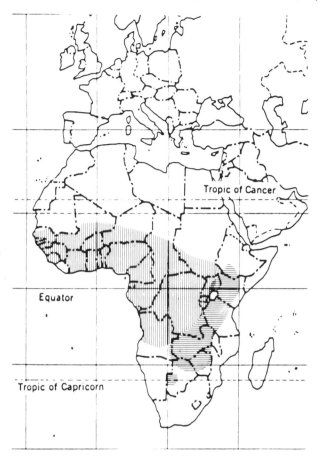

Fig. 3–17. *Trypanosoma gambiense (vertical shading)* and *Trypanosoma rhodesiense (horizontal shading),* distribution in Africa. The regions overlap in a small area northwest of Lake Victoria in Uganda. (From Beaver, P.C., Jung, R.C., and Cupp, E.W. 1984. *Clinical Parasitology,* 9th ed. Philadelphia, Lea & Febiger, p. 80.)

in Gambia, West Africa. In 1903, Castellani found trypanosomes in the cerebrospinal fluid of patients in Uganda suffering from "sleeping sickness." In the same year, Bruce and Nabarro discovered that the organism was transmitted from man to man by a tsetse fly, *Glossina palpalis.*

Morphology and Life Cycle. *T. gambiense* is indistinguishable in morphology and life cycle from *T. rhodesiense.*

Pathogenesis and Symptomatology. At the site of inoculation in the skin, the trypanosomes provoke an interstitial inflammation that gradually subsides in 1 to 2 weeks. Meanwhile the parasites gain access to the bloodstream and initiate a parasitemia. Although they never invade the cytoplasm of cells, their metabolites are toxic to cells, particularly those of the endothelial lining of the smaller blood vessels. The parasites come more and more to lodge in lymph nodes, later in the arachnoid spaces of the central nervous system, and then in the brain substance. Thus, following the initial lesion in the skin, three progressive stages of tissue relationship occur, *viz.,* parasitemia, lymphadenitis, and central nervous system

involvement. A remarkable variation exists in the virulence of this species, from a low-grade to an exalted pathogenicity resembling that of *T. rhodesiense.*

A primary dermal lesion is seen in European patients but rarely in native Africans. Within 6 to 14 days (the *incubation period*) the trypanosomes appear in circulating blood. In natives, this is characteristically a symptomless stage. But as soon as the parasites invade lymph nodes, causing painful enlargement, there is a febrile attack of about a week's duration and then an afebrile period, typically followed by one or more bouts of fever. The trypanosomes are found in the blood only during the febrile episodes. The most pronounced lymphadenitis occurs in the posterior cervical triangle (Winterbottom's sign), but the axillary lymph nodes and those of the groin are also frequently enlarged, as are the spleen and liver. At this stage, common complaints are headache, arthritic pain, weakness of the legs, and cramps. Later dyspnea, precordial pain, disturbed vision, mental confusion, delayed sensation response to pain, anemia, and extreme weakness are apt to appear. At times

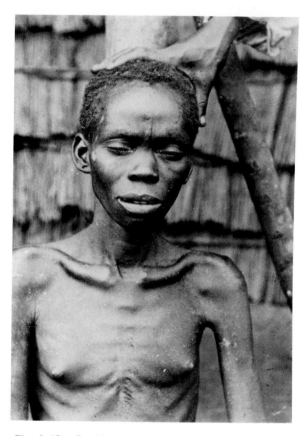

Fig. 3–18. Gambian trypanosomiasis. Typical somnolence and emaciation. (Courtesy of Cuthbert Christie.) (From Beaver, R.C., Jung, R.C., and Cupp, E.W. 1984. *Clinical Parasitology*, 9th ed. Philadelphia, Lea & Febiger, p. 83.)

there is spontaneous improvement in the symptoms, followed by another acute febrile attack. Again, during this stage of the disease the patient may die from fulminating toxemia, as in Rhodesian trypanosomiasis.

The syndrome resulting from invasion of the central nervous system is commonly referred to as "sleeping sickness," but this designation only suggests one of the more advanced neurologic symptoms. Sleepiness occurs and becomes so pronounced that the patient falls asleep while eating or even while standing (Fig. 3–18). In the more advanced stage the patient sleeps continuously, emaciation becomes extreme, convulsions occur, and then profound coma and finally death, which frequently results from intercurrent infection.

Diagnosis. A presumptive diagnosis should always be supplemented by demonstration of the trypanosome in blood, tissue fluid aspirated from enlarged lymph nodes, bone marrow biopsy, or spinal fluid. Since the trypanosomes rapidly disintegrate following their removal from the tissues, the microscopic preparations should be examined fresh for motile forms or fixed and stained immediately. Cultivation on suitable media and animal inoculation may be useful.

Treatment. Treatment should be undertaken at the earliest possible moment following proof that the disease is Gambian trypanosomiasis, since delay reduces the chances of recovery. The drugs most valuable in treatment are tryparsamide and certain other arsenicals, suramin sodium, and diamidine compounds. These drugs are all more or less toxic. Since those that are effective against trypanosomiasis that has reached the central nervous system are the most toxic, selection is based on whether or not there is increased protein or cells in the cerebrospinal fluid.

Suramin and pentamidine are effective during the earlier stages of the infection. In the later stages melarsoprol offers the greatest hope of improvement. Alternatively, treatment with tryparsamide concurrently with suramin may be used. Tryparsamide is not available in the United States.

Epidemiology. Gambian trypanosomiasis is widely distributed throughout the central half of Africa (Fig. 3–17). In recent years this infection on the north shore of Lake Victoria has been replaced by the Rhodesian type.

The amount of infection is determined by the number of *Glossina palpalis* (or at times *G. fuscipes* or *G. tachinoides*) that have an opportunity to feed on humans infected with *T. gambiense*. All of the endemic territory is in rain forests, where there is luxuriant vegetation as well as moist ground in which the flies breed, in particular in riverine and lakeside areas.

Age, sex, race, and occupation have no relation to susceptibility to Gambian trypanosomiasis, although they may favor exposure. The principal mammalian host of *T. gambiense* is man himself. However, domestic animals are highly susceptible to infection. There is no proof that wild game animals serve as reservoirs.

Control. The following measures have been found practical in reducing the incidence of Gambian trypanosomiasis in endemic areas: (1) discovery, isolation, and specific treatment of all human cases, including mildly symptomatic and asymptomatic carriers in the area, (2) protection of the people from *Glossina,* including the use of fly traps (Ryan *et al.,* 1981), (3) quarantine of people coming from infected into uninfected territory, (4) campaigns to destroy the breeding and resting places of the tsetse flies, and (5) administration of prophylactic doses of pentamidine once every 5 or 6 months to individuals liable to exposure. Domestic mammals that acquire the disease not only serve as reservoirs but infected cattle become emaciated or die, and hence a principal food supply is greatly depleted. No satisfactory prophylactic has yet been developed against Gambian trypanosomiasis in these animals, although spraying of dieldrin on tsetse fly habitats in Kenya promises some success.

Trypanosoma (Herpetosoma) rangeli

Trypanosoma rangeli, a flagellate harmless to man and wild and domestic animals, overlaps in many geographic areas of the New World with the pathogenic *T. cruzi.* The two parasites therefore must be differentiated. The most susceptible vectors in nature are species of the triatomine genus *Rhodnius,* the most widespread species being *R. prolixus.* Very probably *T. rangeli* occurs within the known geographic boundaries of this genus, from southern Mexico to Bolivia. Thousands of cases are known, particularly in Guatemala, Panama, Colombia, and Venezuela, where *Rhodnius* colonize in human dwellings. Animals naturally or experimentally infected include marsupials, edentates, rodents, carnivores, and primates (D'Alessandro, 1976).

In human blood films the trypanosome averages 31 μm in length, with a relatively broad undulating membrane and a free flagellum rarely more than half the length of the body. In *Rhodnius,* the flagellates multiply in the midgut but then migrate into the hemolymph and enter the salivary glands, where the epimastigotes transform to become infective metatrypomastigotes that are injected with saliva during probing or feeding. Differential diagnosis with *T. cruzi* is based on morphologic characteristics and biological behavior in the insect vector. No intracellular amastigotes have been demonstrated. Biochemically *T. rangeli* can be differentiated from *T. cruzi* by means of isoenzyme profiles (Miles *et al.,* 1983). Although there is no specific serologic test for this parasite, apparently those used for Chagas' disease do not cross-react with *T. rangeli* infection if pure *T. cruzi* antigen is employed.

Trypanosoma (Schizotrypanum) cruzi
(Chagas' disease,
American trypanosomiasis)

In 1909 Carlos Chagas discovered a flagellate in the hindgut of a large blood-sucking triatomine, *Panstrongylus megistus.* After obtaining experimental infection in a monkey, he found in bug-infected human dwellings a cat and a sick child with an illness known today as Chagas' disease in extensive areas of the hemisphere (Fig. 3–19).

Morphology and Life Cycle. Two main stages of *T. cruzi,* trypomastigote and amastigote, are found in the mammalian hosts, and epimastigotes and trypomastigotes are found in the triatomine bug (Table 3–1). During or following a blood meal, the infected bug discharges feces containing infective metacyclic trypomastigotes which enter the

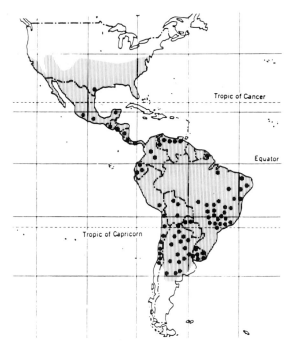

Fig. 3–19. *Trypanosoma cruzi,* distribution of infection (Chagas' disease). Shading indicates estimated extent of infection in reservoir hosts. Dots indicate distribution of human infections. (By R.C. Jung.) (From Beaver, P.C., Jung, R.C., and Cupp, E.W. 1984. *Clinical Parasitology,* 9th ed. Philadelphia, Lea & Febiger, p. 88.)

host through the bite wound or intact mucous membranes (conjunctiva, mouth). The parasites are engulfed by macrophages and become amastigotes *via* an epimastigote stage (Pan, 1978). After 4 or 5 days of multiplication by binary fission, amastigotes again become trypomastigotes, disrupt the cell, and enter the bloodstream and other tissues where the cycle continues, apparently for as long as the host lives. In the blood of man and reservoir or laboratory animals, the trypomastigote is spindle-shaped and measures about 20 μm in length. Dividing forms are absent. Early in the infection the trypanosomes are slender and then become broader. Both forms have the nucleus at the center of the cell and a characteristic large and round subterminal kinetoplast. The undulating membrane is narrow, with few convolutions and a free flagellum. The general appearance of the usual broad form is S- or C-shaped. In its intracellular phase, *T. cruzi* is a typical amastigote, about 1.5 μm to 5 μm in diameter, with a large nucleus and a deeply staining rodlike or spherical kinetoplast (Fig. 3–20A,C,D). In tissues the accumulation of multiplying parasites produces pseudocysts; the amastigotes are indistinguishable from those of *L. don-*

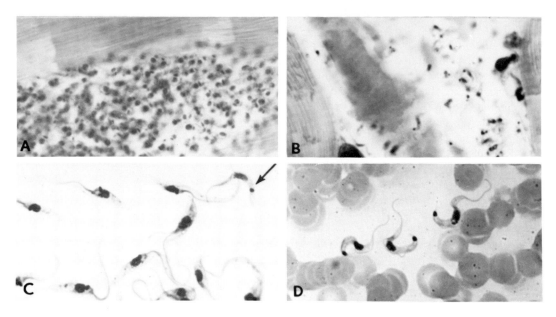

Fig. 3–20. *Trypanosoma cruzi. A,* Intracellular amastigotes in skeletal muscle. H & E stain. *B,* Slender trypomastigotes breaking out of muscle fiber. H & E stain. *C,* Culture forms, including metacyclic trypomastigote *(arrow)* with kinetoplast posterior to nucleus and epimastigotes with kinetoplast immediately anterior to the nucleus. (These and transitional forms are found in the intestine of the triatomid bug as well as in cultures.) Giemsa stain. *D,* Trypomastigotes in blood. Giemsa stain. ($\times$ 1200.) (By R.G. Yaeger.)

ovani, but *L. donovani* invades only macrophages whereas *T. cruzi* invades the cells of any tissue, most frequently macrophages and smooth, cardiac and skeletal muscle and central and peripheral neuroglia.

T. cruzi is taken up by triatomine bugs as a free blood trypomastigote. In the midgut as well as in cultures it becomes an epimastigote, multiplying by binary fission. Then it proceeds to the hindgut, where it transforms into metacyclic trypomastigotes, infective to the vertebrate host by contamination (Fig. 3–20*C*). Usually the infection in the triatomine bug is lifelong in both sexes and all stages of development. Other less frequent modes of human infection are by blood transfusion and by congenital or transmammary transmission. More rarely infections may be acquired by eating food contaminated with infective bug feces or by ingesting infected meat. Accidental laboratory infections have beeen reported.

Pathogenesis and Symptomatology. When first-generation trypanosomes emerge from macrophages, they cause a localized tissue reaction and through lymphatic multiplication an acute regional lymphadenitis. The incubation period ranges from 5 to 12 days. In 95% of infections there is no history of clinically recognizable primary infection or acute period, but when this does occur it usually

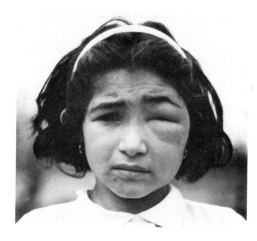

Fig. 3–21. *Trypanosoma cruzi.* Romaña's sign in a Paraguayan girl with acute Chagas' disease. Edema of left eyelid and cheek was accompanied by preauricular lymph node enlargement and conjunctivitis. (By A. D'Alessandro.) (From Beaver, P.C., Jung, R.C., and Cupp, E.W. 1984. *Clinical Parasitology,* 9th ed. Philadelphia, Lea & Febiger, p. 93.)

is in children. The most frequently observed form is the Romaña sign, characterized by unilateral, painless, erythematous palpebral edema, at times extending to the entire side of the face (Fig. 3–21) and accompanied by enlarged preauricular or submaxillary lymph nodes, conjunctivitis, and dacryoadenitis. Less frequent is the chagoma, an erythematous, itching but painless infiltration of the dermis with central desquamation and, rarely, ulceration of the skin. The chagoma is localized on exposed parts of the sleeping individual. It may last several weeks. Through the blood the infection may reach any organ, causing signs and symptoms such as fever, hepatosplenomegaly, generalized lymphadenitis and edema, muscular pain, vomiting and diarrhea, bronchitis and myocarditis of variable intensity; although sometimes fatal, myocarditis usually is completely reversible. Meningoencephalitis, although seldom present, is usually fatal. Anemia, leukocytosis with lymphocytosis and monocytosis, and increased IgM levels are usually present.

In infected individuals, the early stage usually is followed by a lifelong asymptomatic period, the infection being mainly demonstrated serologically. In areas of high endemicity, however, 10% to 30% of the infected people, usually between 20 and 50 years of age, may develop late or chronic Chagas' disease. The organ most typically involved is the heart, with diffuse multifocal myocarditis, mononuclear cell infiltration, destruction of the heart cells, edema, and fibrosis. Amastigotes rarely are demonstrable. Thrombosis in the heart wall is frequent, as is thinning of the heart apex with formation of an aneurysm. EKG changes are the first to appear with abnormalities in conduction, usually right bundle branch block and premature ventricular contractions. These changes may be accompanied by an enlarged heart and symptoms of palpitation, dyspnea, precordial pain, and heart failure. Sudden death is frequent, due to ventricular fibrillation, pulmonary embolism, or rupture of an aneurysm of the apex. A noninflammatory Chagas-like idiopathic cardiomyopathy is clinically hard to differentiate from this myocarditis but can be distinguished at autopsy (D'Alessandro et al., 1974). In some areas dilatation of hollow viscera (megaesophagus, megacolon, megaureter) is part of the clinical picture of chronic Chagas' disease. All these lesions are caused by different degrees of destruction of the parasympathetic neurons of these organs, but the pathogenesis of the process is undetermined.

Diagnosis. During the early stage of *T. cruzi* infections, diagnosis may be made by demonstrating typical trypomastigotes in blood films or amastigotes in muscle biopsies. During the late stage the parasitemia is low. The best method available to demonstrate *T. cruzi* is *xenodiagnosis*. Clean triatomines are allowed to engorge on the patient, and if the infection is present, flagellates are found in the bug's feces, usually 30 days later. Late *T. cruzi* infections are detected by serologic tests (CF, IHA, IFAT, ELISA) (Brener, 1982).

Treatment. Symptomatic relief is all that is available during the chronic stage of Chagas' disease. However, nifurtimox (Lampit, Bayer 2502), 10 mg/kg daily for 60 to 90 days, may terminate the early stage of the disease.

Epidemiology. *Trypanosoma cruzi* is restricted to the Western Hemisphere. Its distribution extends from central Chile and Argentina to the southwestern United States (Fig. 3–19). It has been reported as a natural human infection as far north as Corpus Christi, Texas, and northern California (Schiffler et al., 1984). More than 80 species of vectors are known; they are of sylvatic origin and their degree of adaptation to human dwellings varies. The best adapted are *Triatoma infestans, Rhodnius prolixus, Panstrongylus megistus,* and *Triatoma dimidiata*. Over 100 species of 8 orders of domestic and wild animals are reservoir hosts. They include dogs, cats, opossums, raccoons, armadillos, anteaters, carnivores, rodents, monkeys, and bats. Endemic transmission occurs only when colonies of triatomine bugs are established in human dwellings. Flying adults may rarely be responsible for infections. The unavailability of refuge and animal blood sources in the wild environment resulting from irrational colonization and exploitation of land and the poor quality of human dwellings built at such sites are the two most important factors influencing domiciliary colonization by triatomine bugs (D'Alessandro et al., 1984). *T. cruzi* affects 10 to 12 million people, and the population at risk has been estimated to be about 32 million.

In recent years, isoenzyme profiles have demonstrated at least three *T. cruzi* strains or zymodemes: Z1 and Z3 associated with arboreal and terrestrial mammalian transmission, and Z2 associated with domiciliary parasites. Although all three zymodemes can produce human infections, so far no proven association between zymodemes and human clinical features has been established (Miles, 1983).

Control. Housing improvement is the determining factor in avoiding bug colonization. Residual spraying with a kerosene detergent emulsion of Gamexane (gamma isomer of hexachlorocyclohexane, HCH), sprayed at 0.8 g/m² once or twice a year, will keep the human habitation free of or with fewer bugs. Fenitrothion and other insecticides are also used. Dieldrin-resistant *R. prolixus* has been found in Venezuela. The use of gentian violet or amphotericin B in endemic areas to kill *T. cruzi* in blood before transfusion is effective as a preventive measure.

SUMMARY

1. *Giardia lamblia* in the small intestine and *Trichomonas vaginalis* in the urogenital organs are worldwide in distribution. Giardiasis, transmitted by cysts in feces, usually is asymptomatic but it may produce diarrhea. *T. vaginalis* infection, transmitted by sexual intercourse and usually asymptomatic in males, is a frequent cause of vaginitis. Treatment of giardiasis with quinacrine or metronidazole and treatment of vaginal trichomoniasis with metronidazole usually is satisfactory.

2. The *Leishmania* that cause disease in man are *L. tropica, L. major, L. aethiopica, L. braziliensis, L. mexicana,* and *L. donovani,* all of which are transmitted by sand flies, usually *Lutzomyia* or *Phlebotomus.* When introduced into the skin by the sand fly, the flagellates are engulfed by macrophages, transform into amastigotes, multiply by binary fission, destroy the host cell, and are engulfed by other macrophages and continue to multiply. In the Eastern Hemisphere, *L. tropica* and *L. major* cause an ulcer at the site of inoculation (cutaneous leishmaniasis), and *L. donovani* is a parasite of the reticuloendothelium, especially of the spleen, liver, bone marrow, and visceral lymph nodes (visceral leishmaniasis or kala-azar). Reservoir hosts for *L. major* are rodents, and for *L. tropica* and *L. donovani,* dogs. In the Western Hemisphere, *L. donovani* causes visceral leishmaniasis in scattered foci east of the Andes from northern Argentina to Central America; reservoir hosts are dogs and foxes. New World cutaneous and mucocutaneous leishmaniasis is caused by subspecies complexes of *L. mexicana* and *L. braziliensis,* respectively. Distinct forms of cutaneous leishmaniasis are *chiclero ulcer* and *uta,* with ulcers developing at the site of inoculation; *pian bois* with multiple ulcers formed by metastasis; and *espundia,* well known for its mutilating metastatic lesions of the mouth, nose, and pharynx. A disseminated lepromatoid type of leishmaniasis is produced by *L. aethiopica* in Africa and two subspecies of *L. mexicana,* mainly in Brazil and Venezuela. Diagnosis of all types of leishmaniasis is made by demonstration of the parasite in macrophages. All types of leishmaniasis generally are responsive to antimony therapy.

3. *Trypanosoma rhodesiense* in the upland savannas of east Africa and *T. gambiense* in the rain forest areas of west and central Africa cause sleeping sickness. Tsetse flies (*Glossina*) are intermediate hosts and infection is transmitted through the mouthparts. Untreated patients with *T. rhodesiense* infection characteristically die early, while in *T. gambiense* infection the disease usually is chronic and the parasites tend to invade the central nervous system. African trypanosomiasis is diagnosed by early recovery of the trypanosomes in the blood and later in tissue fluids aspirated from lymph nodes; in *T. gambiense* infection, trypanosomes are recovered from the spinal fluid. African trypanosomiasis, especially the Rhodesian type, must be treated early.

4. American trypanosomiasis, caused by *Trypanosoma cruzi,* is transmitted by triatomine bugs, the parasites being discharged in the bug's feces when a blood meal is taken. Organisms from the primary lesion, a chagoma, reach the liver, spleen, lymph nodes, myocardium, and central nervous tissue or other organs, where they invade fixed cells and multiply as amastigotes, causing cardiomyopathy, mega disease (megaesophagus, megacolon), and other conditions. During the early stages Chagas' disease is diagnosed by recovery of trypanosomes in blood or amastigotes in invaded cells, and in the late stages by xenodiagnosis or serologic tests. No satisfactory specific treatment is available for the late stages, although nifurtimox may terminate the acute infections.

REFERENCES

Brener, Z. 1982. Recent developments in the field of Chagas' disease. Bull. W.H.O., *60*:463–473.

Chulay, J.D., Anzeze, E.M., Koech, D.K., and Bryceson, A.D.M. 1983. High-dose sodium stibogluconate treatment of cutaneous leishmaniasis in Kenya. Trans. R. Soc. Trop. Med. Hyg., *77*:717–721.

Cochran, R., and Rosen, T. 1983. African trypanosomiasis in the United States. Arch. Dermatol., *119*:670–674.

Craft, J.C. 1982. *Giardia* and giardiasis in childhood. Pediatr. Infect. Dis., *1*:196–211.

D'Alessandro, A. 1976. Biology of *Trypanosoma (Herpetosoma) rangeli* Tejera, 1920. In Biology of the Kinetoplastida, Vol. 1. Edited by W.H.R. Lumsden and D.A. Evans. London, Academic Press, pp. 328–402.

———, Barreto, P., Saravia, N., and Barreto, M. 1984. Epidemiology of *Tryypanosoma cruzi* in the Oriental Plains of Colombia. Am. J. Trop. Med. Hyg., *33*:1084–1095.

———, Sanchez, G., and Duque, E. 1974. *Trypanosoma cruzi* and virological studies in idiopathic cardiomyopathies in Cali. Am. J. Trop. Med. Hyg., *23*:856–860.

Evans, D.A., Lanham, S.M., Baldwin, C.I., and Peters, W. 1984. The isolation and isoenzyme characterization of *Leishmania braziliensis* subsp. from patients with cutaneous leishmaniasis acquired in Belize. Trans. R. Soc. Trop. Med. Hyg., *78*:35–42.

Foulkes, J.R. 1981. Human trypanosomiasis in Africa. Br. Med. J., *283*:1172–1174.

Fouts, A.C., and Kraus, S.J. 1980. *Trichomonas vaginalis:* Reevaluation of its clinical presentation and laboratory diagnosis. J. Infec. Dis., *141*:137–143.

Francioli, P., Shio, H., Roberts, R.B., and Muller, M. 1983. Phagocytosis and killing of *Neisseria gonorrhoeae* by *Trichomonas vaginalis.* J. Infec. Dis., *147*:87–94.

Fullilove, R.E., Jr. 1983. *Trichomonas vaginalis* in men. J. Med. Soc. New Jersey, *80*:94–96.

Lainson, R. 1983. The American leishmaniases: Some observations on their ecology and epidemiology. Trans. R. Soc. Trop. Med. Hyg., *77*:569–596.

Meyer, E.A., and Jarroll, E.L. 1980. Giardiasis. J. Epidemiol., *111*:1–12.

Miles, M.A. 1983. The epidemiology of South American trypanosomiasis—biochemical and immunological approaches and their relevance to control. Trans. R. Soc. Trop. Med. Hyg., *77*:5–23.

———, Arias, J.R., Valente, S.A.S., Naiff, R.D., de Souza, A.A., Povoa, M.M., Lima, J.A.N., and Cedillos, R.A. 1983. Vertebrate hosts and vectors of *Trypanosoma rangeli* in the Amazon basin of Brazil. Am. J. Trop. Med. Hyg., *32*:1251–1259.

Pan, S. Chia-Tung. 1978. *Trypanosoma cruzi:* Ultrastructure of morphogenesis *in vitro* and *in vivo.* Exp. Parasitol., *46*:92–107.

Peters, W., Evans, D.A., and Lanham, S.M. 1983. Importance of parasite identification in cases of leishmaniasis. J. Roy. Soc. Med., *76*:540–542.

Phillips, S.C., Mildvan, D., William, D.C., Gelb, A.M., and White, M.C. 1981. Sexual transmission of enteric protozoa and helminths in a venereal-disease-clinic population. N. Engl. J. Med., *305*:603–606.

Ryan, L., Molyneux, D.H., Kuzoe, F., and Baldry, D. 1981. Traps to control and estimate populations of *Glossina* species. Tropenmed Parasitol., *32*:145–148.

Sacks, D.L., and Perkins, P.V. 1984. Identification of an infective stage of *Leishmania* promastigotes. Science, *223*:1417–1419.

Saravia, N.G., Holguin, A.F., McMahon-Pratt, D., and D'Alessandro, A. 1985. Mucocutaneous leishmaniasis in Colombia: *L. braziliensis* subspecies diversity. Am. J. Trop. Med. Hyg., *33*:1084–1095.

Schiffler, R.J., Mansur, G.P., Navin, T.R., and Limpakarn-janarat, K. 1984. Indigenous Chagas' disease (American trypanosomiasis) in California. JAMA, *251*:2983–2984.

Schnur, L.F., Walton, B.C., and Bogaert-Diaz, H. 1983. On the identity of the parasite causing diffuse cutaneous leishmaniasis in the Dominican Republic. Trans. R. Soc. Trop. Med. Hyg., *77*:756–762.

Scorza, J.V., Valera, M., Moreno, E., and Jaimes, R. 1983. Epidemiologic survey of cutaneous leishmaniasis: An experience in Merida, Venezuela. Bull. Pan. Am. Health Org., *17*:361–374.

Chapter 4

Amebae

R. G. Yaeger

The name "ameba" refers to protozoa belonging to several genera of the subphylum Sarcodina, superclass Rhizopoda, the members of which move by means of cytoplasmic extensions that are projected and retracted in response to external stimuli. Many species are free-living while others are parasitic, typically in the digestive tract of invertebrates and vertebrates.

All amebae have a *trophozoite* stage in which there is multiplication by binary fission as long as environmental conditions are favorable. Many species also have an encysted stage that is more resistant to unfavorable conditions and that provides an opportunity for transfer from one host to the next in the case of the parasitic amebae. In preparation for encystation, the ameba discharges undigested food, rounds up to form the *precyst,* and then secretes a covering membrane to become the *cyst.* A few species exhibit a maturing process of the cyst, whereby the nucleus divides one or more times. Among the parasitic forms the cyst is voided in the host's feces, and excystation occurs only after the mature cyst has been taken into a suitable host and has reached a suitable level of the intestine. Thereupon the ameba becomes active, ruptures the cyst membrane, and escapes. It then divides into trophozoites which take in nourishment, as do all trophozoites, and which then divide repeatedly to establish a colony in the host's digestive tract (Fig. 4–1).

The species of amebae that parasitize man are *Entamoeba histolytica, Entamoeba hartmanni, Entamoeba coli, Entamoeba gingivalis, Endolimax nana,* and *Iodamoeba buetschlii. (Dientamoeba fragilis,* an amebalike flagellate, was formerly classified as an ameba [see p. 16]. *Entamoeba polecki,* a natural parasite of the hog, occasionally is di-

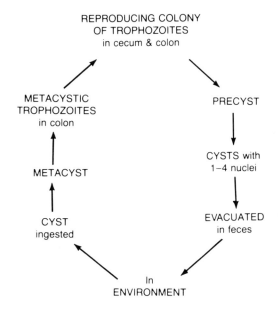

Fig. 4–1. *Entamoeba histolytica.* Diagram of the life cycle. (From Beaver, P.C., Jung, R.C., and Cupp, E.W. 1984. *Clinical Parasitology,* 9th ed. Philadelphia, Lea & Febiger, p. 104.)

agnosed in human feces. Some strains of *E. histolytica* are infected with viruses that appear to be pathogenic to the ameba, affecting either the nucleus or the cytoplasm. The significance of viral infections in amebae in relation to amebiasis prevalence rates in different geographic areas and to pathogenicity of different strains of *E. histolytica* is undetermined. In all species of intestinal amebae of man, parasitic fungi are occasionally seen that may be mistaken for normal parts of the ameba. *Sphaerita* lives in the cytoplasm and forms spherical masses of minute coccuslike refractile bodies that stain black in iron hematoxylin (Fig. 4–2). A second type, *Nucleophaga,* invades the nucleus of

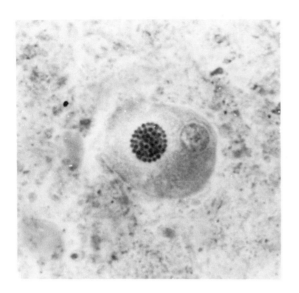

Fig. 4–2. *Sphaerita,* a parasitic fungus, in a trophozoite of *Entamoeba coli.* Celestine blue B. (× 1000.) (From Beaver, P.C., Jung, R.C., and Cupp, E.W. 1984. *Clinical Parasitology,* 9th ed. Philadelphia, Lea & Febiger, p. 109.)

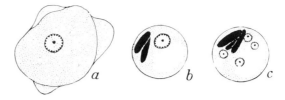

Fig. 4–3. *Entamoeba histolytica. a,* Trophozoite. *b,* Immature cyst. *c,* Ripe cyst. (× 1000.) (By E.C. Faust.)

the ameba. Presumably, these parasites and viruses affect the health of the amebic colony and thus the frequency and intensity of infection in the human population.

The Dysentery Ameba

Entamoeba histolytica
(Amebiasis)

Trophozoites of *Entamoeba histolytica* Schaudinn, 1903 were discovered and described by Lösch in 1875 from dysenteric stools of a patient in St. Petersburg (now Leningrad), U.S.S.R. Within the next two decades the pathogenicity of this organism was amply demonstrated, and it was clearly differentiated as a pathogen from *E. coli* and other harmless species.

Morphology, Biology, and Life Cycle. *E. histolytica* has four distinct stages in its life cycle, *viz.,* trophozoite, precyst, cyst, and metacyst (Fig. 4–1). The stages commonly recognized in the feces are trophozoites and cysts; only trophozoites are present in the tissues.

The *trophozoite* (Fig. 4–3a) in its natural habitat in the large intestine and in extraintestinal foci generally varies from 12 to 30 μm in diameter. However, trophozoites up to 90 μm in diameter have been observed in dysenteric stools.

The active trophozoite has a finely granular, somewhat viscous endoplasm and a clear ectoplasm

that has a grayish-green tinge when observed under the microscope. The pseudopodia are broadly fingerlike *(lobopodia).* During temporary progressive movement in one direction, a single pseudopodium characteristically takes the lead, drawing the entire organism after it. For attachment to cells or other surfaces, threadlike *filopodia* are formed and extend from the ectoplasm. These are evident in scanning electron micrographs (Martinez-Palomo, 1982).

The *nucleus* is spherical; its diameter is one fifth to one third that of the quiescent ameba. It is surrounded by a delicate nuclear membrane, which is studded on its inner surface with minute granules having a chromatin-staining reaction. In the center of the nucleus there is a single dense, beadlike chromatin body, the *karyosome.* Immediately around the karyosome there is an essentially clear halo, and extending radially between this and the nuclear membrane there are several to many delicate achromatic fibrils in the midst of a moderately dense nucleoplasm.

E. histolytica is unusual among eukaryotic organisms in that it lacks mitochondria, and it is anaerobic in its metabolism (Fahey *et al.,* 1984). In appropriate culture media it grows and multiplies best at a temperature of about 37°C, under reduced oxygen tension. Although its natural habitat is the lumen of the cecum and upper colon, as a tissue parasite it is able to develop normally in a bacteriologically sterile environment. Colonization occurs as a result of repeated binary fission.

Encystation occurs in the intestinal lumen. Usually during this process diffuse glycogen within the protoplasm of the trophozoite becomes concentrated in a mass that often has hazy margins; chromatic material is concentrated into bars, rods, or grapelike clusters *(chromatoidal bodies)* in the cytoplasm of the cyst (Fig. 4–3b). Either before the stool is passed or soon thereafter, the nucleus of the cyst divides into two, then each of the two daughter nuclei divides once again, so that the mature cyst typically has four nuclei (Fig. 4–3c).

Viable cysts of *E. histolytica* in the external environment are soon killed by drying, bacterial putrefaction of the medium, hypertonicity, direct sunlight, and heat. On being swallowed, viable cysts pass unchanged through the stomach into the small intestine. When they reach a level where conditions are suitable for colonization, excystation occurs and the amebae are ready to start a new cycle (see Fig. 4–1).

Pathogenesis. Infection with *Entamoeba histolytica* implies colonization. The speed with which this occurs and the depth of penetration of the intestinal wall depend on the pathogenic capacity of the particular strain of *E. histolytica* and host factors not yet identified. Isoenzyme patterns may differentiate pathogenic from nonpathogenic strains (Mathews *et al.*, 1983). The earliest colonization of *E. histolytica* in the intestine is at the cecal level. The characteristic lesion produced by invasive strains as the amebae enter the wall is a superficial minute cavity resulting from necrosis of the mucosal epithelium. The increasing colony usually proceeds to the base of the mucosa, where the lesion enlarges somewhat as the amebae reach the more resistant muscularis mucosae (Fig. 4–4). The amebae may then gradually erode a passage through the muscularis mucosae into the submucosa, where they spread out radially into the surrounding tissues. If this primary lesion is not complicated by accompanying bacteria, there is essentially no tissue reaction to the amebic invasion.

From the submucosa the amebae may proceed into the muscular coats and may even erode a passage into the serosa, in which case they are likely to cause perforation. They may effect an entry into the mesenteric venules or lymphatics and be carried into the liver and other extraintestinal sites. All soft tissues are subject to infection, although extraintestinal lesions develop most frequently in the liver. Wherever an amebic lesion develops outside the intestinal tract, it is secondary to lesions in the large intestine, except in cutaneous infection of the genitalia.

As the infection progresses, additional sites of invasion are likely to develop, although the cecal and then the sigmoidorectal areas are those in which a majority of the lesions are found.

The early uncomplicated amebic lesions are minute openings leading into a deeper enlargement

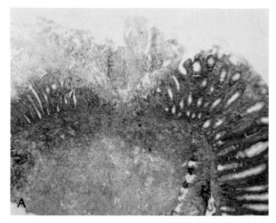

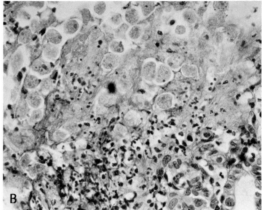

Fig. 4–4. *Entamoeba histolytica.* A, Shallow mucosal ulcer in section of rectal biopsy specimen. (× 20.) B, Higher magnification showing trophozoites at base of ulcer. (× 400.) (Adapted from Beaver, P.C., Jung, R.C., and Cupp, E.W. 1984. *Clinical Parasitology,* 9th ed. Philadelphia, Lea & Febiger, p. 111.)

in the submucosa, with tunneled connections between two or more lesions. They show no remarkable evidence of inflammatory reaction. Sooner or later the subsurface enlargement cuts off the blood supply to the overlying layers and the surface sloughs, leaving shaggy overhanging edges. As the lesion becomes chronic, round cell infiltration develops; the tissues then become infiltrated with neutrophilic leukocytes and fibroblasts, which tend to form a wall around the margin of the ulcer; and the overhanging edges become thickened (Fig. 4–5).

The extraintestinal amebic lesion at first consists of a small focus where one or more amebae have become lodged and have proceeded to colonize, producing necrosis of the surrounding host cells. In the liver, there is a tendency for these lesions to be multiple, but later one or at most a few may

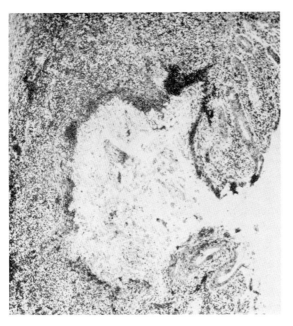

Fig. 4–5. *Entamoeba histolytica.* Chronic amebic ulcer of the colon involving the mucosa and submucosa. (× 56) (From Medical Museum Collection, Armed Forces Institute of Pathology in *Craig's Amebiasis and Amebic Dysentery,* Courtesy of Charles C Thomas, Springfield.)

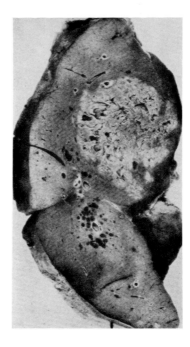

Fig. 4–6. *Entamoeba histolytica.* Amebic abscess of the liver, showing incomplete cytolysis of the tissues and absence of a well-defined abscess wall. (From Medical Museum Collection, Armed Forces Institute of Pathology in Faust, Russell and Jung's *Clinical Parasitology*, Philadelphia, Lea & Febiger.)

become enlarged to develop into the so-called "amebic liver abscess" (Fig. 4–6). Although these lesions are usually bacteriologically sterile, the amount of tissue necrosis produced by the amebae characteristically stimulates some local and systemic leukocytosis.

Symptomatology. The incubation period for infection has been reported as varying from a few days to 3 months or even a year. However, in most instances of very short incubation the presence of other types of enteric infection has not been adequately ruled out. In most cases it is impossible to determine the interval between exposure and the first symptoms. The onset may be insidious, with vague abdominal discomfort or soft stools for a variable period, or it may be sudden, with precipitate development of dysentery or acute abdominal pain. In hepatic amebiasis there frequently is no previous history of the primary infection in the colon.

Amebiasis may be classified clinically as intestinal, including both dysenteric and nondysenteric types, and extraintestinal, including both deep (hepatic, pulmonary, and cerebral) and cutaneous sites. Thus, amebiasis varies greatly with regard to both severity of disease and anatomic site involved. Nondysenteric intestinal amebiasis may be

completely asymptomatic or may present with abdominal pain and tenderness or diarrhea. Amebiasis may be only one of two or more concurrent disease processes, as, for example, amebic colitis associated with shigellosis, salmonellosis, carcinoma, appendicitis of bacterial etiology, cholecystitis, peptic ulcer, or idiopathic chronic ulcerative colitis. Furthermore, at times one or more amebic granulomas *(amebomas)* develop in the wall of the colon or rectum.

The patient with typical amebic dysentery will usually have tenesmus and sometimes abdominal cramps. Nevertheless, he ordinarily appears relatively well in spite of the gradual debilitation that occurs if the dysentery persists. He does not suffer the acute systemic intoxication seen in bacillary dysentery. The abdominal pain and tenderness in intestinal amebiasis, whether dysenteric or not, are mostly in the lower quadrants of the abdomen, especially on the right. Clinically, cecal amebiasis is sometimes mistaken for appendicitis.

Hepatic abscess usually presents with fever, an enlarged tender liver, bulging and fixation of the right leaf of the diaphragm, and frequently serous effusion of the right pleura.

Pulmonary amebiasis is usually a consequence

of rupture of a hepatic abscess into the chest cavity, the lung, and thence into a bronchus. The patient therefore presents with signs of pneumonia and expectoration of characteristic bitter, bile-flavored, liver-colored pus passing through the hepatobronchial fistula. Rarely amebic lung abscess occurs by hematogenous spread from the colon.

Amebiasis of the skin is invariably the result of damaged skin having been brought into contact with amebic trophozoites. It is thus seen most commonly in the perineum secondary to amebic dysentery, as a penile lesion acquired by anal intercourse, or on the abdomen at the mouth of a fistulous tract from the colon or from a hepatic abscess.

Diagnosis. Intestinal amebiasis cannot be reliably diagnosed on clinical grounds alone. Primary dependence is placed on direct microscopic examination of the feces or on recognition of the amebae in stained sections of tissue obtained at biopsy or autopsy. Distinguishing morphologic differences between *E. histolytica* and the other species of *Entamoeba* requires technical skill and experience (Table 4–1).

The typical stool in amebic dysentery consists of exudates, mucus, and blood and may contain little fecal material. On microscopic examination, in addition to motile amebae, Charcot-Leyden crystals are often seen. When formed, stools are negative for cysts; a specimen obtained by saline purgation may contain trophozoites. The main advantage of purgation, however, is that fresh specimens can be made available to the diagnostic laboratory.

Specimens should be examined promptly in unstained direct saline suspension preparations. Proctoscopic aspirates from ulcers of the colon invariably contain a variety of tissue cells that may be mistaken for amebae. When the specimen is obtained from a hepatic, pulmonary, or other extraintestinal abscess, recovery of amebae may be assisted by enzymatic digestion as described in the section on Technical Aids.

Culture techniques are unsuitable for routine diagnosis, since amebae usually cannot be grown in the test tube when they are not detected by direct microscopic examination.

If examination is to be made for amebae in tissues, the routinely stained sections should be superstained with Best's carmine. Amebic trophozoites in the tissues will be stained a strawberry pink.

The indirect hemagglutination test is a sensitive indicator of extraintestinal amebiasis. However, other serologic tests are used (Knoblock and Mannweiler, 1983), and several of them are available commercially as kits.

Treatment. The method of treating amebiasis varies with the clinical types (see Table 21–1). In severe amebic dysentery, the primary objective in treatment is to check the dysentery as rapidly as possible, not only to provide relief of discomfort but also to improve the chances of later eradicating the amebic infection. The drug of choice is metronidazole. Alcohol should be avoided during treatment with this drug. Emetine hydrochloride given intramuscularly for 4 to 5 days is effective in checking dysentery but frequently fails to eradicate the infection. Dehydroemetine is somewhat less toxic than emetine at comparable therapeutic doses. Antibiotics, including tetracyclines, erythromycin, and paromomycin are also effective.

If emetine is used, another amebicidal drug such as diiodohydroxyquin should be given to eradicate the amebic infection. If metronidazole or a tetracycline antibiotic is given, this alone may suffice, but parasitologic cure rate will be improved by concurrent administration of another drug such as diiodohydroxyquin. Several drugs provide high parasitologic cure rates in nondysenteric intestinal amebiasis. Among those commonly employed are diloxanide furoate and diiodohydroxyquin (see Table 21–1, p. 265). Although relatively safe, diiodohydroxyquin in therapeutic doses is known rarely to cause optic neuropathy.

In asymptomatic cases the first question is whether or not to treat the patient. While in the United States it is generally recommended that all cases of intestinal amebiasis be treated, this recommendation is not accepted in all parts of the world. In some countries the prevalence of intestinal amebiasis is high but the incidence of manifest disease is low. In such situations, routine treatment of all carriers would be impractical.

Drugs for treatment of amebic liver abscess are metronidazole, emetine (or dehydroemetine), or chloroquine, or all three together. Although emetine is more toxic than the other two, it is considered to be most effective. Metronidazole is nearly as effective and better tolerated. Alcohol should be avoided during the course of treatment. In the case of large abscesses, aspiration of pus in addition to drug therapy may be necessary for cure. Surgical incision and drainage are not recommended. Other

Table 4–1. Differential Characteristics of *Entamoeba histolytica,*
Entamoeba hartmanni, and *Entamoeba coli*

	Entamoeba histolytica	Entamoeba hartmanni	Entamoeba coli
TROPHOZOITE, UNSTAINED			
Size	8 to 30 μm	4 to 12 μm	15 to 50 μm
Motility	Active, progressive	Active, progressive	Rarely progressive
Pseudopodia	Digitiform; hyaline, rapidly extruded	Digitiform; rapidly extruded	Short, blunt; slowly extruded
Inclusions	Red blood cells; rarely bacteria	Bacteria, particles; no blood cells	Bacteria, particles; no blood cells
Nucleus	Usually invisible	Invisible	Rarely visible
TROPHOZOITE, IRON HEMATOXYLIN STAIN			
Nuclear membrane	Delicate; lined with fine chromatin dots	Thick; lined with coarse chromatin	Thick; lined with coarse chromatin
Karyosome	Minute; location central	Usually large; location variable	Large; location eccentric
CYST, IODINE-STAINED SALINE SMEAR			
Size	10 to 20 μm	5 to 10 μm	10 to 30 μm
Cytoplasm	Bright greenish-yellow	Yellowish-brown	Yellowish-brown
Glycogen mass	Diffuse, reddish-brown	Diffuse, brown	Brown, often discrete
Nuclei	1 to 4; karyosome central; chromatin beaded, refractive	1 to 4; chromatin *E. coli*-like	1 to 8; karyosome eccentric; chromatin coarse, refractive
CYST, IRON HEMATOXYLIN STAIN			
Size	10 to 20 μm	5 to 10 μm	10 to 30 μm
Cytoplasm	Finely granular	Coarsely granular	Coarsely granular
Chromatoidal bodies	Barlike or rodlike, with rounded ends	Often numerous; shape variable	Splinterlike, with angular ends
Nuclei	1 to 4; karyosome minute, central; chromatin beaded	1 to 4; karyosome variable; chromatin coarse	1 to 8; karyosome eccentric; chromatin coarse

forms of deep extraintestinal amebiasis are treated similarly.

Amebiasis cutis will respond to local therapy with topical antibiotics and treatment of the primary amebic disease, which is either amebic liver abscess or amebic dysentery.

Epidemiology. *E. histolytica* occurs in all areas of the world. Because of greater opportunity for exposure, the infection is usually more prevalent and produces more severe symptoms in warm climates, but the rates of infection are high in mental hospitals, prisons, children's homes, and other communities in cooler climates with poor personal and group hygiene compared with the rates for the general population of the same localities. People of all races and ages and of both sexes appear to be about equally susceptible to infection. Infants are not as commonly infected as older children, and young adults characteristically show a higher incidence than older persons.

Amebiasis usually is endemic, but outbreaks of serious proportions resulting from gross contamination of water with viable cysts of the ameba have been reported. Other modes of transmission include person-to-person contact, food handlers, and filth flies. Person-to-person contamination has been demonstrated to be the most likely method of spread in children's homes, mental hospitals, and rural populations in a temperate climate, while in tropical communities the most likely transmission is from food handlers, poor hygiene, and unpotable water supplies.

Many species of monkeys are natural hosts of *E. histolytica.* Dogs occasionally have been found to be infected, but the frequency of such infections is too low to affect the prevalence in man.

Control. Control of amebiasis must be undertaken as a public health measure. The cause for endemic, hyperendemic, or epidemic amebiasis in a population is to be found in its epidemiologic pattern, *viz.,* how the agent is maintained and propagated. Therefore, studies must be made to deter-

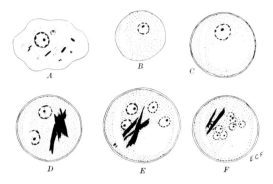

Fig. 4–7. *Entamoeba coli. A,* Trophozoite. *B,* Precyst. *C* to *F,* Cysts in progressive stages of maturity with 1 to 8 nuclei and chromatoidal bodies in *D, E,* and *F* and glycogen vacuoles in *C, E,* and *F.* Cysts with 4 nuclei are rarely seen. (× ca. 1000.) (By E.C. Faust.) (From Beaver, P.C., Jung, R.C., and Cupp, E.W. 1984. *Clinical Parasitology,* 9th ed. Philadelphia, Lea & Febiger, p. 126.)

mine whether water, food handlers, person-to-person contact, filth flies, or possibly reservoir hosts are the responsible factors. Then practical methods must be set up to control transmission.

Nonpathogenic Parasitic Amebae

Entamoeba gingivalis

Entamoeba gingivalis (Gros, 1849) Brumpt, 1913 is cosmopolitan in distribution. It is a parasite of the mouth of man and other mammals, including several species of monkeys and of dogs and cats, and it is most commonly found as a phagocyte in diseased gums and tonsils. Only the trophozoite stage has been described; the only plausible method of transmission is through droplet spraying of saliva or more intimate oral contact. *E. gingivalis* measures 5 to 35 μm in diameter. In most respects it closely resembles *E. histolytica,* with a few to several fingerlike pseudopodia, finely granular endoplasm, and clear ectoplasm. The nucleus contains a small karyosome that is central or slightly eccentric in position.

Entamoeba coli

Entamoeba coli (Grassi, 1879) Casagrandi and Barbagallo, 1895, with a worldwide distribution, is usually the most common amebic parasite of man. Although it is a harmless commensal in the lumen of the cecum and lower levels of the large intestine, its presence is evidence that the host has ingested fecal material. The differential characteristics of trophozoites and cysts are listed in Table 4–1. Bacteria and other enteric microbes, which are seen within food vacuoles, constitute the food of *E. coli,* although in a dysenteric menstruum this ameba will ingest red blood cells. Trophozoites of *E. coli* and other amebae are rarely seen in the stool except when it is frankly diarrheal. The cyst is usually larger than that of *E. histolytica.* When first formed the *cyst* has a single nucleus, but as it matures it passes through successive stages with 2 to 8 nuclei (Figs. 4–2, 4–7), occasionally reaching the extraordinary number of 16 to 32 or more. Frequently present are one or more dense masses of glycogen and sharp-ended chromatoidal bodies. There is no clinical indication for treatment, since *E. coli* is not pathogenic.

Entamoeba polecki

Entamoeba polecki von Prowazek, 1912, a cosmopolitan, nonpathogenic parasite of the colon of pigs and monkeys, is occasionally reported in humans. It doubtless is often mistaken for either *E. histolytica* or *E. coli.* The trophozoite resembles that of *E. coli* except for its smaller size (10 to 18 μm), and the cyst resembles that of *E. histolytica* in size (10 to 17 μm) and presence of ovoid chromatoidal bodies. Its most distinctive features are seen in the cyst, which has only one nucleus, generally resembling that of *E. histolytica,* and in a cytoplasmic mass that may be conspicuous in iron-hematoxylin or trichrome-stained smears. The chromatoidal bodies, generally bars with rounded ends, are only occasionally present.

Entamoeba hartmanni

Entamoeba hartmanni von Prowazek, 1912 is cosmopolitan in distribution, and in those localities where it has been accurately identified, its prevalence is approximately equal to that of *E. histolytica.* In older literature it was often recorded as "small race" *E. histolytica.* In size it resembles *Endolimax nana,* in number of nuclei in the mature cyst (4) it resembles *Entamoeba histolytica,* and in the nucleus and texture of the cytoplasm it resembles *E. coli* (Fig. 4–8). The trophozoites do not ingest red blood cells and generally do not show the vigorous motility that is characteristic of *E. histolytica.* In both cysts and trophozoites the nucleus is *histolytica*-like in that the karyosome generally (although not regularly) is centrally located, but it is *E. coli*-like in that it often has a relatively thick layer of peripheral chromatin irregularly distributed on the nuclear membrane (Table 4–1). The chromatoidal bodies characteristically are smaller, more numerous, and more tapered at the ends than are those of *E. histolytica,* although in the original species description the chromatoidals were characterized as thin bars and small granular bodies; these forms are commonly seen. Because the cysts of both species have four nuclei and both are so small that detailed features of their nuclear and cytoplasmic elements cannot be seen clearly in iodine-stained temporary mounts, *E. hartmanni* and *Endolimax nana* are often mistaken for each other. Even in iron-hematoxylin–stained permanent preparations identification is difficult, because the nucleus of *E. nana* in the trophozoite stage occasionally is *Entamoeba*-like. Fortunately, neither *E. nana* nor *E. hartmanni* is pathogenic.

Endolimax nana

Endolimax nana (Wenyon and O'Connor, 1917) Brug, 1918 is worldwide in distribution and often is found in as high a frequency in a population as *Entamoeba coli.* It is a commensal in the lumen of the cecum and lower levels of the large intestine and produces no lesions, but like *E. coli* its presence indicates that polluted material has been ingested. As the species name *nana* (i.e., dwarf) suggests, this ameba is small compared with *E. histolytica* and *E. coli.* In size and general appearance it resembles *Entamoeba hartmanni.* The trophozoite (Fig. 4–9) measures 8 to 10 μm or more in diameter. The endoplasm is finely granular with numerous minute vacuoles, so that it has a foggy appearance. In contrast, the ectoplasm, with one or more short fingerlike pseudopodia, is hyaline and almost transparent. The nucleus is ovoid or subspherical. A relatively large karyosome, consisting of a mass of one or more granules, is commonly eccentric in position, though the chromatin is variously arranged and may be concentrated at the nuclear membrane as it is in *Entamoeba* species. The mature cyst contains four nuclei. Chromatoidal bodies, if present, are coccoid or short curved rods.

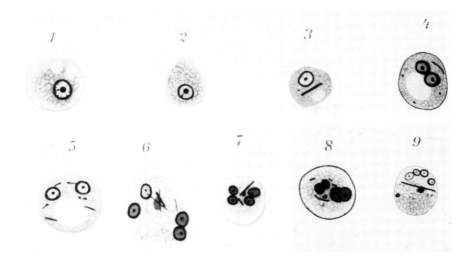

Fig. 4–8. *Entamoeba hartmanni.* Photocopies of 9 of the 11 original drawings by S.J.M. von Prowazek (1912, Arch. f. Protistenk. 22:241). The legends indicate that the diameters of the amebae, all drawn to the same scale, range from 7 to 13 μm.

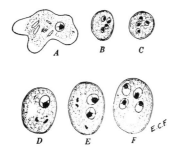

Fig. 4–9. *Endolimax nana. A,* Trophozoite. *B* through *F,* Cysts showing range in size and number of nuclei. (× 1000.) (By E.C. Faust.) (From Beaver, P.C., Jung, R.C., and Cupp, E.W. 1984. *Clinical Parasitology,* 9th ed. Philadelphia, Lea & Febiger, p. 128.)

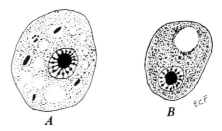

Fig. 4–10. *Iodamoeba buetschlii. A,* Trophozoite. *B,* Cyst. (× 1500.) (Adaptations by E.C. Faust.) (*A* From Wenrich, 1937. Studies on *Iodamoeba bütschlii* (Protozoa) with special reference to nuclear structure. Proceedings of the American Philosophical Society, 77:183–205, Plate I, fig. 13. *B* From Pan, C.-T., 1959. Nuclear division in the trophic stages of *Iodamoeba bütschlii* [Prowazek, 1912] Dobell, 1919. Parasitology, 49:543–551, Plate VIII, fig. 6.)

Iodamoeba buetschlii

Iodamoeba buetschlii (von Prowazek, 1911) Dobell, 1919 is probably cosmopolitan in distribution but it is seldom as common as *E. histolytica, E. coli,* or *Endolimax nana.* It is a harmless commensal living in the lumen of the large intestine. The trophozoite (Fig. 4–10) is sluggish, with little evidence of pseudopodial extension, and the thin layer of ectoplasm is not easily distinguished from the endoplasm. The trophozoite has a diameter of 8 to 20 μm. The nucleus is spherical and has a rather thick membrane and a large karyosome that is central or somewhat eccentric in position. This ameba is unique in its trophozoite stage in that it has one or two distinct rounded masses of glycogen in the cytoplasm. The cyst (Fig. 4–10) is variable in shape, usually irregularly rounded, measures 5 to 18 μm in diameter, and usually contains only one nucleus. The clearly outlined glycogen mass that stains a deep mahogany brown with iodine readily differentiates *I. buetschlii* from the other intestinal amebae.

Dientamoeba fragilis

Dientamoeba fragilis Jepps and Dobell, 1918 has been reported from many parts of the world but because of its minute size (usually 5 to 12 μm) and the fact that it exists only in the trophozoite stage, it is often overlooked in coprologic examinations unless it is stained with hematoxylin and searched for under the oil-immersion objective. This organism is an amebalike flagellate related to *Trichomonas,* not an ameba (see p. 16).

Pathogenic Free-Living Amebae

Free-living organisms that are capable of adapting to a parasitic existence are said to be *amphizoic.* Species of *Acanthamoeba* and *Naegleria* are among such organisms. In 1958, a colony of a free-living ameba, *Acanthamoeba,* was found growing in a culture of monkey kidney cells and was shown to be capable of invading the brain and meninges of mice and monkeys. In 1964 and 1965, similar amebae, thought to be *Acanthamoeba* but later classified as a species of the genus *Naegleria,* were identified in fatal cases of meningoencephalitis, two in Florida, and three in Australia. The victims had acquired the infection while swimming in freshwater lakes or ponds, and the portal of entry to the brain and meninges appeared to be the nasal mucosa and cribriform plate. In subsequent years similar cases, nearly all fatal, were reported from various parts of the United States, Europe, and Australia.

The two species of amphizoic amebae most frequently identified in human tissues are *Naegleria fowleri,* named after Dr. Malcolm Fowler who first recognized the disease caused by it, and *Acanthamoeba culbertsoni,* named after Dr. Clyde Gray Culbertson who first discovered colonization of the organisms in monkey kidney cell cultures. *Acanthamoeba* is classified in the family Acanthamoebidae, order Amoebida; this order also includes the family Endamoebidae, to which *Entamoeba histolytica* belongs. *Naegleria* is a member of the family Vahlkampfiidae, order Schizopyrenida. The two groups differ in their form of cell division and type of cysts, also in that there are transient flagellate forms in *Naegleria* but not in *Acanthamoeba.*

Naegleria fowleri
(Primary amebic meningoencephalitis)

Morphology, Biology, and Life Cycle. *Naegleria fowleri* Carter, 1970 lives in fresh water and moist soil and grows well in tissue cultures or other artificial media (John, 1982). Motile trophozoites from cultures or the cerebrospinal fluid are elongate, broad anteriorly, and vary in size around 7 by 20 μm, with a single broad pseudopod at the forward end; rounded forms generally are 15 μm or less in diameter. The nucleus is about 3 μm in diameter, with a relatively large central karyosome (endosome). When the species is transferred to water, contractile vacuoles become evident and flagellate forms with two flagella begin to appear among ameboid forms within one to several hours. The amebaflagellate forms are pyriform, with the flagella at the broad end; they may move rapidly forward or spin slowly in a circle. Cysts formed on agar cultures are spherical with a smooth, thick wall, uninucleate, and 7 to 10 μm in diameter. In tissue sections only trophozoites are seen, usually round in outline, with the nucleus a characteristic and distinctive feature (Fig. 4–11).

Pathogenesis and Symptomatology. The amebae colonize the nasal tissues and connected sinuses and extend the invasion along the olfactory nerves into the brain. Gross findings at necropsy

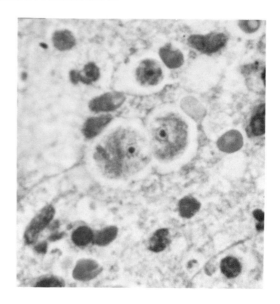

Fig. 4–11. *Naegleria.* Typical trophozoites in a brain impression smear from a 15-year-old girl who died 8 days after swimming in a lake in Virginia and 30 hours after admission to the hospital with chief complaints of severe frontal headache, diplopia, and reeling gait. (× 1300.) (By P.C. Beaver. Preparation courtesy of Dr. E.C. Nelson.)

resemble those of bacterial meningitis. Invaded areas of the brain are soft, and the meninges are congested and purulent. In tissue sections the amebae are most evident in the perivascular tissues, where inflammatory cells are few or absent. A distinctive feature of the ameba is its characteristic nucleus with a large, dense, central endosome. The symptoms of the disease are essentially those of a fulminant bacterial meningitis.

Diagnosis. A history of exposure to stagnant or thermal water 3 to 6 days before the onset of symptoms of meningitis or meningoencephalitis should suggest the possibility of *Naegleria* infection. The amebae are most readily recognized by their motility in unstained wet preparations; they are recognized with difficulty in Gram- or Wright-stained smears. Culture isolation from cerebrospinal fluid or tissues should be attempted on a plate of 1.5% non-nutrient agar seeded with living *Escherichia coli,* grown separately and added.

Treatment. Among the more than 100 reported cases of primary amebic meningoencephalitis, few with *Naegleria* infection have survived. One such case was that of a 9-year-old girl in California who had been swimming in hot springs. She was given amphotericin B and miconazole intravenously and intrathecally, rifampin orally, and sulfisoxazole intravenously (Seidel *et al.,* 1982). In an earlier case, successful treatment with intravenous and intraventricular amphotericin B was reported.

Epidemiology. Numerous cases of primary amebic meningoencephalitis have been reported in the United States, mainly in the southeastern states and California. Elsewhere, case reports have been most numerous from Australia, New Zealand, Belgium, and Czechoslovakia. The ameba in some cases has not been reliably identified as *Naegleria* as distinct from *Acanthamoeba*. In firmly diagnosed cases, *Naegleria* infections usually were acquired while swimming, diving, skiing, or other contact with freshwater lakes, ponds, streams warmed by industrial effluent, or natural thermal springs or streams. *N. fowleri* grows well at high temperatures and tolerates temperatures up to about 45°C. Although cysts in air-borne dust are a theoretical source of infection, the flagellate stage taken into the nose in water is the usual infective source (Dorsch *et al.*, 1983).

Prevention. Although chlorinated water has been implicated in a high proportion of cases elsewhere, no *Naegleria* infection is known to have been acquired in a standard swimming pool in the United States. *N. fowleri* will generally not be found in pools with a free chlorine residual of 1.0 mg per liter and a pH range of 7.0 to 7.6 (Esterman *et al.*, 1984). The best protective measure is to avoid exposure in warm natural water, especially thermal springs and streams. Infection probably is not acquired from cysts in air-borne dust (Dorsch *et al.*, 1983).

Acanthamoeba Species
(Granulomatous amebic encephalitis, uveitis, and corneal ulceration)

Unlike *Naegleria fowleri*, which causes fulminating, rapidly fatal (usually less than 1 week) primary amebic meningoencephalitis, the pathogenic species of *Acanthamoeba* cause a granulomatous amebic encephalitis that is insidious in onset, follows a chronic course leading to death, or produces chronic uveitis or ulceration of the cornea. Species invading the brain are *A. castellanii* (Douglas, 1930) Page, 1967, *A. culbertsoni* (Singh and Das, 1970) Sawyer and Griffin, 1975, *A. astronyxis* (Ray and Hayes, 1954) Page, 1967, and *A. polyphaga* (Puschkarew, 1913) Page, 1967. *A. castellanii* and *A. polyphaga* also have been identified as causing ulceration of the cornea and lesions of the iris and ciliary body. Different strains of these

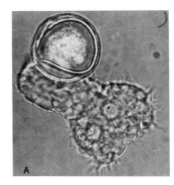

Fig. 4–12. *Acanthamoeba culbertsoni.* Culture forms in wet preparations. *A,* Trophozoite with numerous acanthopodia, a nucleus, and a contractile vacuole and attached to a cyst with an atypical endocyst wall. *B,* Cyst with typical polyhedral endocyst wall and spherical ectocyst. (Unstained, × 700.) (Adapted from Beaver, P.C., Jung, R.C., and Cupp, E.W. 1984. *Clinical Parasitology,* 9th ed. Philadelphia, Lea & Febiger, p. 141.)

species differ widely in pathogenicity (Visvesvara *et al.*, 1983).

Morphology, Biology, and Life Cycle. The only life cycle stages of *Acanthamoeba* species are trophozoites and cysts. There is no flagellate form. The active trophozoite of all *Acanthamoeba* species has an irregular shape with spinelike pseudopodia *(acanthopodia)* arising from lobopodia and other areas of the body (Fig. 4–12). Forward movement generally is not perceptible. Because trophozoites of the various species are morphologically similar and the size ranges are relatively great and overlapping (the usual size being more than 20 μm in greatest diameter), specific identification of trophozoites is not feasible. Cysts, on the other hand, display differences that can be recognized by specialists. All are spherical, with a double wall forming a smooth or slightly wrinkled ectocyst and a roughly polyhedral or stellate endocyst. Specific identification in individual cases requires the application of immunoperoxidase or immunofluorescent staining techniques.

Pathogenesis and Symptomatology. Invasion of the brain occurs in chronically ill and immunosuppressed patients. When the primary site of invasion is the skin, the onset of central nervous system symptoms comes several months to a year later. In some cases the initial symptoms have been sore throat and fever; the time from onset of symptoms to death was less than 3 weeks in only one case. Reported autopsy findings include necrotizing granulomatous lesions in various parts of the brain, not including the olfactory lobes. Sections have shown focal hemorrhage, multinucleated giant cells, and cysts as well as trophozoites. In other parts of the body chronic granulomatous or exudative lesions caused by *Acanthamoeba* have been described in skin, kidneys, liver, adrenal and thyroid glands, lymph nodes, breast, ear, prostate, and eye. In some cases the eye lesions followed trauma (Samples *et al.*, 1984).

Diagnosis. Amebae may be detected in cerebrospinal fluid, teased tissues, or scrapings from corneal or skin lesions. Attempts to isolate *Acanthamoeba* in culture from cerebrospinal fluid or brain tissue generally have not been successful, although isolation from other tissues has been reported (Visvesvara *et al.*, 1983). Amebae with the characteristic nucleus, especially when cysts also are present, can be identified in tissue sections. Special (immunoenzymatic) staining of formalin-fixed tissues may be useful in the detection and identification of the amebae.

Treatment. For all forms of *Acanthamoeba* infection, treatment remains problematic. Experience in cases of amebic ulceration of the cornea and laboratory studies suggest the possible effectiveness of sulfonamides. No effective preventive measures are known.

Epidemiology and Control. *Acanthamoeba* infection of the brain has been reported in 15 or more cases in England, India, Zambia, Korea, Peru, Venezuela, and the United States. In at least 10 cases invasion of the eye was recorded, and in 4 cases the amebae were found in vaginal exudate. In some cases invasion of the brain followed initial colonization of the skin or eye. The source of infection was presumed to be dust or water in some cases, but in most instances there had been no contact with natural bodies of water. Effective control measures have not been established.

Coprozoic Amebae

Free-living, coprozoic amebae have been reported from time to time in specimens of human feces submitted for examination.

SUMMARY

1. All amebae have an active trophozoite stage in which they multiply by binary fission. The parasitic amebae form cysts, which serve as the transfer stage to a new host; infection is acquired when cysts are swallowed.
2. Man is parasitized by *Entamoeba histolytica, E. gingivalis, E. hartmanni, E. coli, E. polecki, Endolimax nana,* and *Iodamoeba buetschlii.* All these species except *E. gingivalis* have a cystic stage. *E. gingivalis* lives in the mouth, the others in the colon.
3. The only tissue-invading intestinal ameba of man is *Entamoeba histolytica,* which is worldwide in distribution. Infection usually is asymptomatic, but some strains have the capacity to invade and cause ulceration of the colon, especially in the cecal and sigmoidorectal areas. Secondary to lesions in the colon, *E. histolytica* may also invade and produce lesions in extraintestinal foci, especially the liver.
4. The symptoms in amebiasis are remarkably variable, including, on the one hand, acute fulminating dysentery, exhausting diarrhea, appendicitis syndrome, and abscess of the liver, lungs or brain, and, on the other hand, asymptomatic infection.
5. Diagnosis of amebiasis by clinical procedures is tentative and requires laboratory confirmation.
6. Treatment usually is satisfactory with several relatively specific antiamebic drugs.
7. *Naegleria fowleri,* a free-living ameba, can invade the central nervous system through the nasal mucosa, causing rapidly fatal meningoencephalitis. The infection usually is acquired while swimming in stagnant freshwater lakes or ponds. Species of *Acanthamoeba,* also free-living, produce chronic primary lesions in the skin or cornea and secondarily invade deeper organs including the brain, causing a fatal granulomatous encephalitis. No satisfactory treatment is known.

REFERENCES

Dorsch, M.M., Cameron, A.S., and Robinson, B.S. 1983. The epidemiology and control of primary amoebic meningoencephalitis with particular reference to South Australia. Trans. R. Soc. Trop. Med. Hyg., *77*:372–377.

Esterman, A., Roder, D.M., Cameron, A.S., Robinson, B.S., Walters, R.P., Lake, J.A., and Christy, P.E. 1984. Determinants of the microbiological characteristics of South Australian swimming pools. Appl. Environ. Microbiol., *47*:325–328.

Fahey, R.C., Newton, G.L., Arrick, B., Overdank-Bogart, T., and Aley, S.B. 1984. *Entamoeba histolytica:* A eukaryote without glutathione metabolism. Science, *224*:70–72.

John, D.T. 1982. Primary amebic meningoencephalitis and the biology of *Naegleria fowleri.* Annu. Rev. Microbiol., *36*:101–123.

Knobloch, J., and Mannweiler, E. 1983. Development and persistence of antibodies to *Entamoeba histolytica* in patients with amebic liver abscess. Analysis of 216 cases. Am. J. Trop. Med. Hyg., *32*:727–732.

Martinez-Palomo, A. 1982. The Biology of *Entamoeba histolytica.* New York, Research Studies Press, 161 pp.

Mathews, H.M., Moss, D.M., Healy, G.R., and Visvesvara, G.S. 1983. Polyacrylamide gel electrophoresis of isoenzymes from *Entamoeba* species. J. Clin. Microbiol., *17*:1009–1012.

Samples, J.R., Binder, P.S., Luibel, F.J., Font, R.L., Visvesvara, G.S., and Peter, C.R. 1984. *Acanthamoeba* keratitis possibly acquired from a hot tub. Arch. Ophthalmol., *102*:707–710.

Seidel, J.S., Harmatz, P., Visvesvara, G.S., Cohen, A., Edwards, J., and Turner, J. 1982. Successful treatment of primary amebic meningoencephalitis. N. Engl. J. Med., *306*:346–348.

Visvesvara, G.S., Mirra, S.S., Brandt, F.H., Moss, D.M., Mathews, H.M., and Martinez, A.J. 1983. Isolation of two strains of *Acanthamoeba castellanii* from human tissue and their pathogenicity and isoenzyme profiles. J. Clin. Microbiol., *18*:1405–1412.

Chapter 5

Ciliate Protozoa

The ciliate protozoa (Ciliophora) constitute a large group characterized by numerous cilia. Many ciliates are free-living and possibly an even larger number are parasites in the digestive tract of termites, wood roaches, and herbivorous mammals. Near the anterior end of the body there is a conical mouth, the *cytostome* (Fig. 5–1A), and at the opposite end an anal opening, the *cytopyge* (Fig. 5–1B). Ciliates have two types of nuclei, a large macronucleus and nearby a small micronucleus (or at times more than one). Multiplication is by transverse binary fission, with division of the cytoplasm following that of the nuclei. Many species undergo conjugation, during which exchange of nuclear material occurs. The only ciliate that is a parasite of man is *Balantidium coli*.

Balantidium coli
(Balantidiasis)

Balantidium coli (Malmsten, 1857) Stein, 1862 has a cosmopolitan distribution in hogs and is a common parasite of several species of monkeys. In man, it is found mostly in warm climates.

Morphology, Biology, and Life Cycle. The organism has two stages, trophozoite and cyst. The trophozoite (Fig. 5–1A) is the largest of the protozoa that parasitize man. It is ovoid, covered with short cilia that are constantly in motion during life, and has a vigorous forward movement as it plows through even relatively dense suspensions of feces. It varies considerably in size (50 to 100 μm in length by 40 to 70 μm in width). The anterior end is somewhat conical, and the posterior end is broadly rounded. To one side of the anterior tip there is a funnel-shaped *peristome*, which leads into the *cytostome*. A minute cytopyge is situated at the opposite end. One, and at times two, large, slowly pulsating *contractile vacuoles* lie within the cytoplasm (Fig. 5–1B). The body is covered with a relatively tough pellicle. Lying somewhat posterior to the equator of the organism is a large kidney-shaped *macronucleus*, and lying along the lesser curvature of the macronucleus is a minute *micronucleus*.

The natural habitat of *Balantidium coli* is the cecal level of the large intestine, but it also inhabits lower levels. It feeds on host cells, bacteria, and other substances in the lumen of the bowel.

Asexual reproduction consists of transverse binary fission, in which the micronucleus first divides mitotically, then the macronucleus amitotically, followed by the cytoplasm, resulting in two daughter organisms. Although conjugation has been observed in *B. coli*, this is not a common occurrence and apparently is not essential for its propagation.

The cyst, spherical and about 50 μm in diameter, is the transfer stage. On encystation the cilia are soon lost, although the markings on the cell surface remain (Fig. 5–2).

Pathogenesis and Symptomatology. In the hog, there is little if any evidence that *Balantidium coli* invades the intestinal wall. In monkeys and humans the mucosal layer may be penetrated, with extensive submucosal destruction. Once established in the tissues, the parasite may move through the muscularis mucosae into the submucosa, where it spreads out radially, causing rapid destruction of the tissues (Fig. 5–3). However, unlike *E. histolytica*, it rarely invades the muscular coats and it has seldom been found in extraintestinal tissues. While balantidial lesions may develop at any level of the large intestine, they occur most commonly in the cecal and sigmoid-rectal regions.

The symptoms in balantidiasis vary from fulminating dysentery or acute diarrhea to an essentially asymptomatic carrier state. In this respect they parallel the broad spectrum of symptoms in amebic colitis.

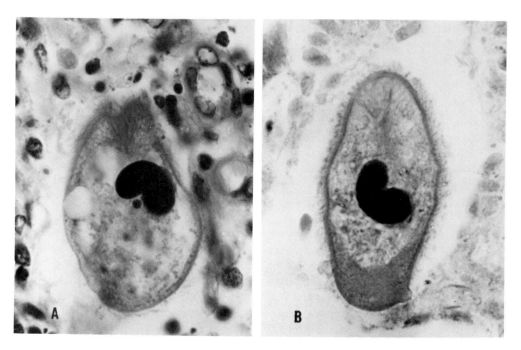

Fig. 5–1. *Balantidium coli*. Trophozoites in hematoxylin-eosin stained section of ulcerated colon of man in Costa Rica. *A*, Showing cytostome, macronucleus, micronucleus and contractile vacuole. *B*, Showing cilia, macronucleus, margin of cytostome, and cytopyge (protruding at bottom right). (× 1000.) (From Beaver, P.C., Jung, R.C., and Cupp, E.W. 1984. *Clinical Parasitology*, 9th ed. Philadelphia, Lea & Febiger, p. 214.)

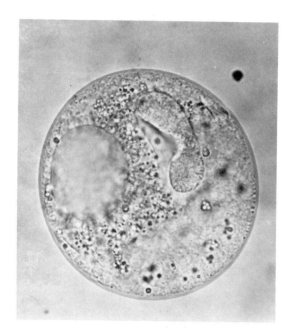

Fig. 5–2. *Balantidium coli*. Cyst from zinc sulfate concentrate of fresh feces of chimpanzee, unstained, showing macronucleus and contractile vacuole. The vacuole usually disappears in older cysts. (× 625.) (By P.C. Beaver.)

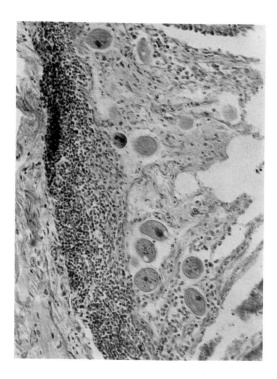

Fig. 5–3. *Balantidium coli*. Trophozoites in section of ulcerated colon of a 4-year-old child in Puerto Rico. (× 160.) (By P.C. Beaver.)

Diagnosis and Treatment. Diagnosis is made on recovery of the characteristic trophozoites or cysts in the feces. Care must be taken to ensure that the stool specimen and reagents used in making fecal films for microscopic diagnosis are not contaminated by free-living infusoria; otherwise, these ciliates may be mistaken for *B. coli*.

Clinical and experimental tests with diiodohydroxyquin, tetracycline drugs, and metronidazole have demonstrated that these drugs are effective in relieving the symptoms, and in some cases they produce eradication of the infection (Garcia-Laverde and de Bonilla, 1975).

Frequently balantidiasis may coexist with a debilitating disease such as malnutrition or trichuriasis that is injurious to the colon. The balantidial infection may disappear spontaneously following the correction of such contributory conditions.

Epidemiology. Infection is acquired by swallowing viable cysts of *B. coli*. The number of human infections with this parasite is small indeed compared with the opportunities for acquiring the infection from animal reservoirs. Apparently humans are relatively refractory, since infection develops only occasionally from this type of exposure. In contrast, once an infection has become established in man, it can be more easily transmitted from person to person, particularly in tropical communities and mental hospitals where personal and group hygiene is poor. Outbreaks of up to 110 cases have been reported from the Seychelles Islands, Papua New Guinea, and the Pacific Island of Truk (Walzer *et al.*, 1973).

Control. Since balantidiasis is common in hogs and lower primates and human infection from such sources is infrequent, protection from exposure to animal sources is not primarily indicated. In contrast, protection from exposure to human sources requires attention.

SUMMARY

Infection with *Balantidium coli*, a large ciliate protozoan, is acquired from ingesting cysts passed in feces. Man appears to be relatively refractory to infection with *B. coli* from monkeys, pigs, or other animal reservoirs, but once the infection becomes established it may produce extensive ulcers in the mucosa and submucosa of the large intestine. The symptoms in human balantidiasis range from fulminating dysentery or diarrhea to an essentially asymptomatic condition. Treatment with tetracycline or metronidazole usually is effective.

REFERENCES

1. Garcia-Laverde, A., and de Bonilla, L. 1975. Clinical trials with metronidazole in human balantidiasis. Am. J. Trop. Med. Hyg., *24*:781–783.
2. Walzer, P.D., Judson, F.M., Murphy, K.B., Healy, G.R., English, D.K., and Schultz, M.G. 1973. Balantidiasis outbreak in Truk. Am. J. Trop. Med. Hyg., *22*:33–41.

Chapter 6

Coccidia, Malarial Parasites, *Babesia,* and *Pneumocystis*

R. G. Yaeger

The coccidia are members of the class Sporozoea, an exclusively parasitic group that typically requires alternation of sexual and asexual reproduction in the life cycle. The piroplasmas belong to the same class. *Pneumocystis carinii* has been grouped with the Sporozoea by some workers, but others believe it is a yeast; however, until its taxonomic position and life cycle are more completely known, it can be regarded as a protozoan.

THE COCCIDIA

The species of coccidia, suborder Eimeriina, that commonly parasitize man belong to four genera: *Cryptosporidium, Isospora, Sarcocystis,* and *Toxoplasma.* Like other closely related genera, these coccidians have similar, independent gametocytes, the male or microgametocyte and the female or macrogametocyte. The female gametocyte produces a single macrogamete, and the male gametocyte produces multiple gametes, following which an oocyst is formed after fertilization of a female by a male gamete. The oocyst in species of *Isospora* and *Sarcocystis* produces two internal sporocysts, each with four sporozoites; in *Cryptosporidium* the sporocyst stage is omitted. Only two species of coccidia are known to undergo schizogony and gametogony in man, *viz., Isospora belli* and *Cryptosporidium muris.*

In the life cycle of *Isospora* species, the infective stage is the *sporozoite,* produced in units of four within each of the two sporocysts developed in the oocyst, the stage evacuated in the host's feces. When ripe oocysts are swallowed and reach the small intestine, the sporozoites, on becoming free

of the oocyst and sporocyst membranes, enter the intestinal epithelium and transform into trophozoites. These develop into *schizonts,* and each schizont produces several merozoites internally. These asexual merozoites enter other epithelial cells, with repetition of asexual multiplication. Eventually some of the merozoites transform into *male* and *female gametocytes.* Each male gametocyte produces a number of *male gametes,* and each female gametocyte transforms into a single *female gamete.* Male and female gametes unite to produce the zygote. A resistant cell wall is secreted around the spherical zygote, which then becomes the *oocyst.* The enclosed cell divides into two equal units, the *sporocysts.* Within each sporocyst four curved sausage-shaped sporozoites are developed (Fig. 6–1).

Cryptosporidium muris
(Cryptosporidiosis)

The genus *Cryptosporidium* was first described by Tyzzer in 1907 as a minute coccidian parasite in the gastric crypts of a laboratory mouse. He named it *Cryptosporidium muris.* Since that time various other species have been described from mammals, birds, reptiles, and fish. All of the forms found in mammals are now regarded as the same species, *Cryptosporidium muris* (Tyzzer, 1907), and there is only one valid species for each of the other three groups of vertebrates (Levine, 1984).

Morphology, Biology, and Life Cycle. In experimentally infected mammals, all known stages of this parasite are found in the brush border of the mucosal epithelium of the stomach and intestine.

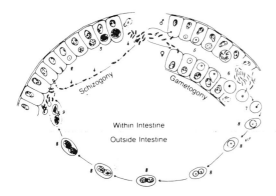

Fig. 6–1. *Isospora belli.* Diagram of life cycle. *1,* Sporozoites entering intestinal mucosa. *2.* Young trophozoite in mucosal cell. *3,* Development of a schizont. *4,* Merozoites shed from ruptured cell. *5,* Gametocytes, male *(above)* and female *(below),* developed from merozoites. *6,* Microgametes. *7,* Union of gametes to form zygote. *8,* Maturing stages of sporoblasts and sporocysts in oocyst. *9,* Sporocysts shed from oocyst. (By E.C. Faust.)

Trophozoites and schizonts, 2 to 5 μm in diameter, are within the microvillous border attached to the surface of the epithelial cells (Fig. 6–2). Schizonts produce eight crescent-shaped merozoites that are released to repeat the schizogonic cycle or to form macro- and microgametocytes that mature and by fertilization produce a zygote. The zygote develops a protective outer wall to become an oocyst 4 to 5 μm in diameter (see Fig. 18–2, p. 250). Within the oocyst four sporozoites are formed; these are the infective stages. Oocysts in fresh feces are infective. Infection occurs when sporozoites released from ingested ripe oocysts enter the brush border of the mucosal epithelium.

Pathogenesis and Symptomatology. The minute round or ovoid bodies may be very numerous on the surface of mucosal epithelial cells. Although they may appear to be extracellular, the cytoplasm of the parasite is in contact with the host cell cytoplasm. Whether damage to the mucosa is mechanical or otherwise is unclear (Tzipori, 1983). Electron micrographs have revealed some areas showing degenerate and degenerating cells (Bird and Smith, 1980). Most studies, however, suggest that minimal histopathologic changes occur in individuals whose immunity has not been compromised. An increased incidence of *Cryptosporidium* infection has been reported in people with acquired immune deficiency syndrome, and in some cases the organisms have been present in biliary (Pitlik *et al.,* 1983) and bronchial (Forgacs *et al.,* 1983) as well as intestinal mucosal epithelium. However, healthy people also are susceptible to infection (Current *et al.,* 1983). The incubation period ranges from one to several weeks. Onset of illness may be accompanied by fever, malaise, nausea, and vomiting; this is followed by abdominal cramping and diarrhea. Stools may be watery or semiliquid, and the diarrhea usually clears in 1 or 2 weeks unless an immune deficiency state exists. Malabsorption may occur when symptoms are prolonged. Signs and symptoms are similar to those of giardiasis.

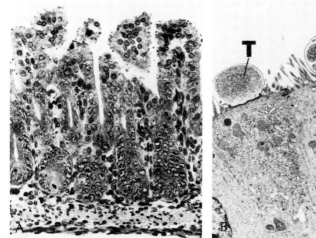
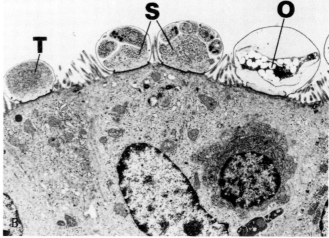

Fig. 6–2. *Cryptosporidium muris.* Developmental stages of a human isolate after 6 days in a suckling mouse. *A,* Section of ileum showing numerous parasites in brush border of villi. (× 270.) *B,* Electron micrograph of a trophozoite (T), two schizonts (S), and an oocyst (O) in the microvillous portion of the host cells. (× 4400.) (From Reese, N.C., Current, W.L., Ernst, J.V., and Bailey, W.S. 1982. Cryptosporidiosis of man and calf: A case report and results of experimental infections in mice and rats. Am. J. Trop. Med. Hyg., *31:*226–229, p. 228.)

Diagnosis. Most infections may be diagnosed by finding the oocysts in the feces. These stages frequently are in numbers sufficient to be seen in a direct fecal smear, stained or unstained. More often the oocysts are seen in concentrates prepared by centrifugal flotation with either the zinc sulfate or sucrose method. Fecal smears stained by a modified acid-fast technique enable the differentiation between yeasts and the oocysts (see Technical Methods section). The oocysts may also be visualized with the Giemsa stain, but the results are variable. Phase-contrast microscopy may also be used to identify the oocysts. Biopsy specimens of intestinal mucosa have also been used to detect the organisms (see Fig. 18–2, p. 250).

Treatment. No safe and effective chemotherapeutic agent has been identified. Occasional successes have been reported but since spontaneous cure occurs in immunologically normal individuals, only supportive treatment is necessary.

Epidemiology. *Cryptosporidium* infection is found in many mammals, including man. Infections are acquired through ingestion of oocysts from human or animal feces. Oocysts are infective when passed, and they are resistant to ordinary disinfectants. Surveys have detected *Cryptosporidium* oocysts in 4% of 884 patients with gastroenteritis in Australia (Tzipori *et al.*, 1983), and 4% of 278 preschool children in Costa Rica (Mata *et al.*, 1984).

Control. As cryptosporidiosis is a fecal-borne infection, control measures taken for similarly transmitted organisms should be effective.

Isospora belli
(Coccidiosis, coccidiosis belli)

Isospora belli Wenyon, 1923 is widely distributed but is more prevalent in warmer climates. Isolated cases have been reported from many countries, and reports suggest that infection is evenly distributed in all regions around the equator.

Morphology, Biology, and Life Cycle. The enteroepithelial cycle, consisting of schizogonic and sporogonic stages in the epithelial cells of the small intestine, was described from biopsy specimens by Brandborg *et al.* (1970). In freshly passed stools the oocysts of *Isospora belli* are found typically in an unsegmented condition; they ripen after their discharge from the host's intestine. They measure from 20 to 33 μm in length by 10 to 19 μm in breadth. Within the wall of this early stage oocyst there is a single spherical granular mass of proto-plasm, with a central dense nuclear mass. When the fecal specimen is kept at 25 to 30°C for several hours, the protoplasmic mass divides into two equal masses, the immature sporocysts. Within 18 to 36 hours four falciform sporozoites, each with a minute central nucleus, are formed inside each sporocyst (Fig. 6–3).

Pathogenicity and Symptomatology. The invasion with destruction of intestinal mucosa by the coccidia is responsible for mucous diarrhea, low-grade fever, chills, anorexia, and nausea. These symptoms may be mild and transient, lasting for less than a month, or severe and exhausting; less frequently they may become chronic, with periodic exacerbation of acute symptoms. The infection may persist for more than a year.

Diagnosis. A diagnosis is based upon finding the immature oocyst in freshly discharged feces, often of a diarrheal type. These oocysts are transparent and are likely to be overlooked in direct fecal films, especially since only a few are present in the average infection. They are best seen at a reduced light level and can be concentrated by either the formalin-ether sedimentation or zinc sulfate centrifugal flotation technique.

Treatment. In the average case, rest and a bland diet are sufficient to allow spontaneous elimination of the parasites. Cotrimoxazole (trimethoprim, 80 mg and sulfamethoxazole, 400 mg) in a dosage of 2 tablets every 6 hours for 10 days, then 2 tablets twice daily for 3 weeks, has provided cure (Westerman and Christensen, 1979). In a chronic case of 10 months' duration, cure was obtained with pyrimethamine 75 mg plus sulfadiazine 4 g 4 times a day for 21 days, followed by pyrimethamine 37.5 mg plus sulfadiazine 2 g twice daily for an additional 28 days.

Epidemiology. In general, these infections appear sporadically, are of short duration, are more common in children than in adults, may be familial in occurrence, and occasionally appear epidemically in groups subject to gross exposure from contaminated persons, soil, food, or drink. Poor environmental sanitation and poor personal hygiene provide abundant opportunity for human exposure from the infested *milieu* containing the highly resistant oocysts.

Control. Improvement in sanitary and hygienic conditions is indicated.

Sarcocystis hominis
(Coccidiosis hominis)

Sarcocystis hominis (Railliet and Lucet, 1891) Levine, 1977 is a parasite of the human intestine. For many years small mature

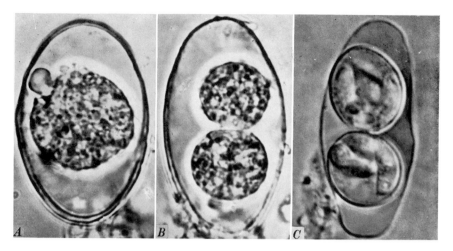

Fig. 6–3. *Isospora belli.* A, Oocyst from fresh feces. B, Maturing oocyst with two sporoblasts. C, Mature oocyst with four sporozoites in each of two sporocysts. (× ca. 2000.) (By J.E. Gullberg from material furnished by E.K. Markell.) (From Beaver, P.C., Jung, R.C., and Cupp, E.W. 1984. *Clinical Parasitology,* 9th ed. Philadelphia, Lea & Febiger, p. 153.)

sporocysts, free or within an intact oocyst wall, were regarded as *Isospora* when seen in human feces; these are now presumed to have been either *S. hominis* or *S. suihominis.* Owing to the confusion in differentiating this species from similar species found in man, data from past reports may not be reliable with respect to geographic distribution (Levine and Tadros, 1980). However, it can be presumed that *S. hominis* has been present in many areas where rare beef is eaten.

Morphology, Biology, and Life Cycle. Although intact oocysts with sporocysts are occasionally seen, the sporocysts are usually mature, free, and infective when passed in the feces. They are ovoid, about 9 by 15 μm, with a transparent wall, and contain four elongate, crescent-shaped sporozoites. When cattle ingest the infective sporocysts, the sporozoites are released and, presumably, make their way to endothelial cells of the viscera, where asexual multiplication (schizogony) takes place. Merozoites released by rupture of the infected host cell eventually enter the skeletal muscle where elongate cysts known as sarcocysts are formed. When mature, these cysts contain many elongate merozoites and may remain viable in muscle for many months. When a sarcocyst is ingested by man, the merozoites are liberated and invade the lamina propria of the intestinal mucosa, where male and female gametes are formed. Fertilization produces a zygote which then, still within the host cell, becomes surrounded by a wall and is now an oocyst. This is followed by maturation, resulting in two sporocysts each containing four sporozoites. After liberation from the intestinal mucosa into the feces, the oocyst ruptures and releases the mature sporocysts (Fig. 6–5B).

Pathogenesis and Symptomatology. In most cases infection is self-limited and symptoms are mild or absent, and hence many infections probably are undetected. One report described six patients in a Bangkok hospital with acute abdominal symptoms and who had large numbers of sporogonic stages of what was believed to be *Sarcocystis hominis* in the lamina propria of resected segments of ileum or jejunum (Bunyaratvej *et al.,* 1982).

Diagnosis. Infection is detected by finding the characteristic sporocysts and occasionally oocysts in the feces; reducing the intensity of the light increases the probability of recognizing these stages. Concentration techniques facilitate detection.

Treatment. As observed infections have been asymptomatic and self-limited, no chemotherapy has been necessary.

Epidemiology. A study in southern Germany revealed that almost 100% of 1,007 slaughtered cattle of various age groups and both sexes had sarcocysts in their muscle, and about two thirds were *S. hominis* acquired through fecal contamination of food or water by infected people. Prevalence of this infection in the human population, acquired by eating rare beef, is unknown.

Control. Human infection can be prevented by cooking beef, and *S. hominis* infection in cattle can be avoided by proper disposal of human feces.

Sarcocystis suihominis
(Coccidiosis suihominis)

Sarcocystis suihominis Heydorn, 1977, originally considered to belong to the genus *Isospora,* is now known to be a species of *Sarcocystis* that infects man and is distinct from *S. hominis* and *S. miescheriana;* the latter is another species occurring in pigs. Although the Netherlands and Central Europe are included in its area of endemicity, *S. suihominis* probably occurs in other areas, including the United States. However, it has been confused with other coccidia whose sporocysts are similar.

Morphology, Biology, and Life Cycle. The life cycle is similar to that of *S. hominis* except that the pig is the intermediate host (Fig. 6–4). The stage usually seen in feces is the sporocyst, which is ovoid, about 10 by 13 μm, and contains four elongate, crescent-shaped sporozoites (Fig. 6–5A). The intact oocyst, containing two sporocysts, may occur in freshly passed feces (Fig. 6–4); these stages are slightly smaller than the corresponding stages of *S. hominis.* After ingestion by a pig, sporocysts liberate sporozoites, which penetrate the intestinal mucosa and undergo two cycles of schizogony in the vascular endothelium. Merozoites that escape from schizonts enter skeletal and cardiac muscle, where sarcocysts develop. When ingested by man, the zoites escape from the sarcocysts and initiate the sexual cycle; in 11 to 13 days, sporocysts appear in the feces and may continue for 2 months or longer.

Pathogenesis and Symptomatology. Mild fever and diarrhea were observed in 1 of 3 infected volunteers, while in another group of 8 all experienced acute diarrhea and vomiting with chills and perspiration 6 to 24 hours after eating raw pork from an experimentally infected pig; within 12 to 24 hours, their symptoms decreased.

Diagnosis. Infection is detected by finding the sporocysts,

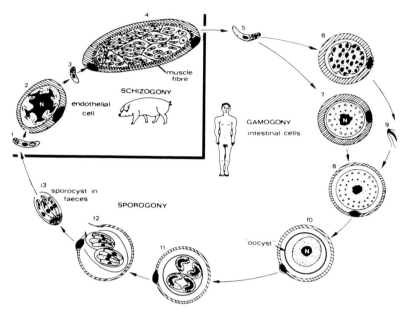

Fig. 6–4. *Sarcocystis suihominis.* Diagram of life cycle. *1,* Sporozoite. *2,* Schizont formed from sporozoite within endothelial cell of the pig, giving rise to one or more generations of merozoites by multiple simultaneous division of the nucleus. *3,* Merozoite, which enters a muscle fiber. *4,* Cyst formed by merozoite within the muscle fiber with production of large round metrocytes and elongate merozoites (also called bradyzoites, or zoites). *5,* When man eats raw pork containing cysts, merozoites are set free in the intestine. *6 and 7,* Micro- and macrogamonts formed from merozoites develop in a parasitophorous vacuole within cells of the lamina propria. *8 and 9,* The nonmotile macrogamete *(8)* is fertilized by a motile microgamete *(9)* and becomes a zygote. *10,* The zygote is surrounded by a wall and becomes an oocyst. *11,* Two sporocysts are formed, each developing four sporozoites while still in the oocyst in the host cell. *12,* The oocyst wall is broken and the two sporocysts, each containing four sporozoites, are set free and discharged into the feces. *13,* When ingested by a pig, the sporocyst liberates its four sporozoites *(1),* which then find their way to cells of the vascular endothelium *(2).* (Adapted by P.C. Beaver from Frenkel, J.K., *et al.* 1979. Sarcocystinae: *Nomina dubia* and available names. Z. Parasitenk., *58:*115–139. In Beaver, P.C., Jung, R.C., and Cupp, E.W. 1984. *Clinical Parasitology,* 9th ed. Philadelphia, Lea & Febiger, p. 156.)

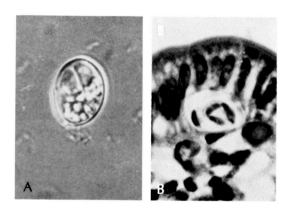

Fig. 6–5. *Sarcocystis* sporocysts. *A, S. suihominis* sporocyst in suspension of fresh feces. (× 1200.) *B, S. hominis.* Section of resected ileum from a man in Thailand, showing portions of sporocysts containing mature sporozoites in an oocyst. (× ca. 1000.) *A,* Courtesy of R. Fayer. From Beaver, P.C., Jung, R.C., and Cupp, E.W. 1984. *Clinical Parasitology,* 9th ed. Philadelphia, Lea & Febiger, p. 158. *B,* From Bunyaratvej, S., Bunyawongwiroj, P., and Nitiyanant, P. 1982. Human intestinal sarcosporidiosis. Report of six cases. Am. J. Trop. Med. Hyg., *31:*36–41, p. 38.)

and occasionally oocysts, in the feces. The zinc sulfate centrifugal flotation method enhances the probability of detection.

Treatment. No specific treatment is known.

Epidemiology. Although natural infections with this species are known to occur in pigs and man from various regions, the prevalence in either host is unknown. Reports from earlier studies, before the existence of more than one species was known, are probably inaccurate. Persistence of sarcocysts in pig muscle for months to years and the shedding of sporocysts for at least 2 months by infected persons assure the endemicity of this species in some areas.

Control. Infection of pigs can be avoided by the proper disposal of human feces, and human infection can be prevented by the proper cooking of pork.

Sarcocystis "lindemanni"
(Sarcocystosis)

The organisms for which the name *Sarcocystis lindemanni* was established were nonprotozoan organisms having no relationship to Sarcosporidia. Sarcocysts seen in man are morphologically similar to species of *Sarcocystis* occurring in other mammals, birds, and reptiles. For species developing sarcocysts in muscle tissue, man is an incidental intermediate host. Final hosts are unknown in all cases. The designation *Sarcocystis "lindemanni"* is now used merely as a convenience to cover all the numerous unidentified species of sarcocysts observed in human skeletal and cardiac muscle (Beaver *et al.,* 1979).

Of the 40 or more reported cases of human sarcocystosis, 13 of the infections probably were acquired in Southeast Asia, 8

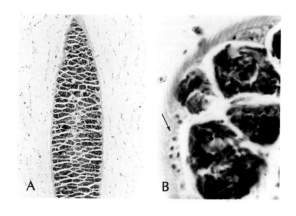

Fig. 6–6. *Sarcocystis.* Cyst in section of leg muscle of a man in Uganda, East Africa. *A,* Longitudinal, slightly oblique section showing a thick cyst wall and many compartments filled with zoites. (× 50.) *B,* Portion of transverse section of cyst showing villi on the outer surface, metrocytes *(arrow)* adjacent to the wall, and zoites in compartments formed by septa. (× 500.) (From Beaver, P.C., Gadgill, R.K., and Morera, P. 1979. *Sarcocystis* in man: A review and report of five cases. Am. J. Trop. Med. Hyg., 28:819–844.)

in India, 5 in Central or South America, 4 each in Africa and Europe, 3 in the United States, 1 in China, and 2 in unknown localities. Sarcocysts were seen in either cardiac or skeletal muscle but not in both. Four different types of sarcocysts were described from skeletal muscle and 3 distinct types from cardiac muscle. Those in skeletal muscle were spindle-shaped or cylindrical and up to several millimeters in length, with diameters ranging from 100 μm to more than 200 μm (Fig. 6–6A). Cysts in cardiac muscle were smaller, with diameters less than 70 μm and with rounded ends. The cyst wall may have a covering of thickly set villi, giving a striated appearance (Fig. 6–6B), or it may be thin and smooth. Septa may divide the cyst into compartments containing the banana-shaped zoites that in the different species fall into large, medium, or small sizes with diameters of 2 to 3, 1.5, or 1 μm, respectively.

There have been no reports of inflammation or other evidence of pathogenicity caused by mature sarcocysts. However, experimental infections in animals indicate that massive destruction of the vascular endothelium occurs during the earlier schizogonic stage prior to muscle invasion. Sarcocysts are usually found incidentally during examination of biopsy or autopsy specimens. They can be differentiated from *Toxoplasma* cysts, which have a thinner wall without villi and smaller zoites that stain much more intensely by the PAS method. There is no known specific treatment for the muscle stage; moreover, in view of the lack of evidence of pathogenicity of the muscle stage and the excellent prognosis, treatment is probably unnecessary. Since infection is presumed to be acquired by ingesting mature sporocysts, protection of food and drink from the feces of carnivorous animals is indicated as a preventive measure.

Toxoplasma gondii
(Toxoplasmosis)

Toxoplasma gondii Nicolle and Manceaux, 1908, discovered in a small North African rodent, *Ctendodactylus gundi,* is found in a large number of mammals including man, and in birds. Although

infection is cosmopolitan, surveys indicate that prevalence is highest in hot, humid climates and lowest in dry, cold climates.

Morphology. Five stages occur in the life cycle of *Toxoplasma gondii*. Although all five occur in cats, only two stages are found in man, other mammals, and in birds. These two stages are (1) the intracellular trophozoite or proliferative form (tachyzoite) usually seen during acute infection (Fig. 6–7), and (2) the encysted form (bradyzoite) that is found during chronic or latent infection (Fig. 6–8A). Reproduction is by *endodyogeny,* a process of division wherein two daughter zoites are formed within the parent parasite, which is destroyed when the young zoites are released. The trophozoites are crescent-shaped, 4 to 8 μm in length, 2 to 3 μm in width, and with one end more pointed than the other. Evident in Giemsa-stained preparations of various types of smears are a delicate azure cytoplasm and a reddish spherical or ovoidal nucleus that is usually nearer the blunter end of the parasite (Fig. 6–7A). Electron micrographs reveal a complex system of organelles that clearly demonstrate the taxonomic relationship of this organism to the class Sporozoea. One of these structures is a rather short, truncate, hollow conoid, located at the more pointed anterior end. In histologic sections the trophozoites often appear to be ovoid. The cysts that occur in chronic infection are formed when the parasites multiply and produce a wall within a host cell (Fig. 6–8A). The cyst wall is eosinophilic, argyrophilic, and weakly PAS-positive; the organisms within the cyst are strongly PAS-positive. During acute infection, groups of proliferative stages may be seen in a wide range of host cell types. These have been termed "pseudocysts" and "terminal colonies" and can be differentiated from the true cysts in that the organisms are at most only slightly PAS-positive, and the cyst membrane is neither argyrophilic nor PAS-positive.

Biology and Life Cycle. The life cycle of *T. gondii* eluded investigators for more than 6 decades. Congenital transmission in man was known as early as 1939, and infection following ingestion of improperly cooked meat was later recognized. It is now known that *T. gondii* is a coccidian parasite of the domestic cat. Other members of the cat family Felidae develop infection and are responsible for maintenance of the disease in areas where the domestic cat is absent.

During primary infection, for periods up to 2 weeks, the cat sheds unsporulated oocysts that

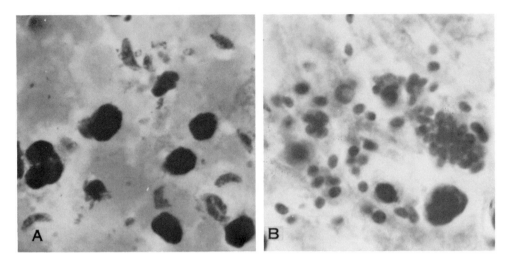

Fig. 6–7. *Toxoplasma gondii,* proliferative forms. *A,* Crescent-shaped organisms in an impression smear. Giemsa stain. (× 1200.) *B,* Rounded forms, free and in a pseudocyst (intracellular) in a section of brain of a congenitally infected infant. (× 1200.) (By R.G. Yaeger.)

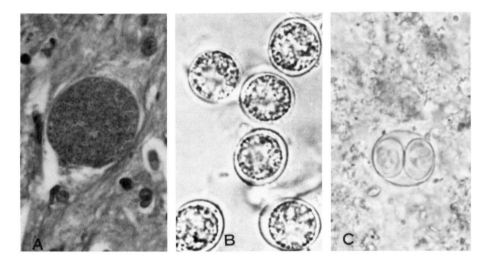

Fig. 6–8. *Toxoplasma gondii. A,* Cyst in the brain of a chronically infected mouse (× 480.) *B,* Oocysts recovered from fresh feces of a cat during the 4th day after eating a chronically infected mouse bearing cyst forms in the brain and other tissues; the oocysts are approximately 10 × 12 μm. (× 1200.) *C,* Oocyst containing two sporocysts, each containing four sporozoites after 7 days of development in a culture of washed feces from an infected cat. (× 1200.) (By R.G. Yaeger).

PLATE I

Plasmodium vivax. Stages in erythrocytes in Giemsa-stained thin-film preparations. *1,* Normal-sized red cell with marginal ring form trophozoite. *2,* Young signet ring form trophozoite in a red cell. *3,* Slightly older ring form trophozoite in red cell showing basophilic stippling. *4,* Polychromatophilic red cell containing young tertian parasite with pseudopodia. *5,* Ring form trophozoite showing pigment in cytoplasm in an enlarged cell containing Schüffner's stippling.* *6* and *7,* Tenuous medium trophozoite forms. *8,* Three ameboid trophozoites with fused cytoplasm. *9, 11, 12,* and *13,* Older ameboid trophozoites in the process of development. *10,* Two ameboid trophozoites in one cell. *14,* Mature trophozoite. *15,* Mature trophozoite with chromatin, apparently in the process of division. *16, 17, 18,* and *19,* Schizonts showing progressive steps in division (presegmenting schizonts). *20,* Mature schizont. *21, 22,* Developing gametocytes. *23,* Mature microgametocyte. *24,* Mature macrogametocyte. (From Wilcox, A.: *Manual for the Microscopical Diagnosis of Malaria in Man.* 1960 ed. Washington, D.C., U.S. Department of Health, Education, and Welfare, Public Health Service Publication No. 796, 1960, Plate I.)

---

*Schüffner's stippling does not appear in every infected cell, as would be indicated by these drawings, but it can be found with any stage from the fairly young ring form onward.

PLATE I

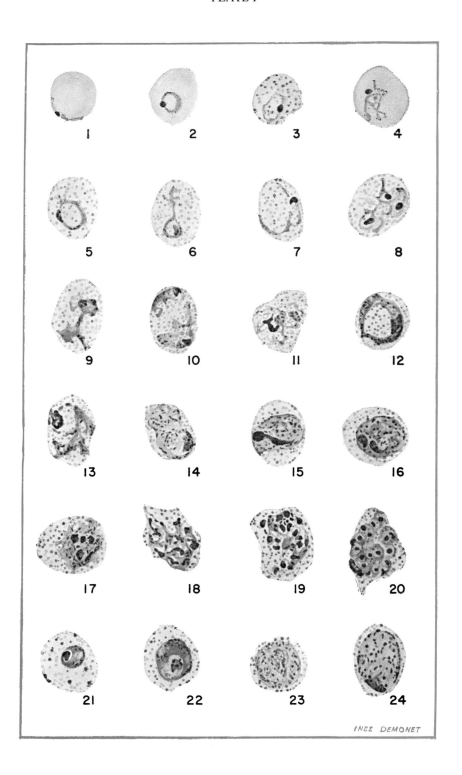

INEZ DEMONET

PLATE II

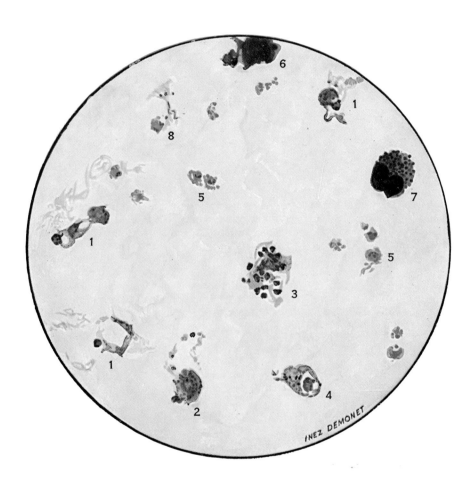

Plasmodium vivax. Giemsa-stained thick-film preparation. The film contains three developing trophozoites, an immature and mature schizont, a microgametocyte, clumps of blood platelets, an eosinophil, and a neutrophil. *1,* Ameboid trophozoites. *2,* Schizont—two divisions of chromatin. *3,* Mature schizont. *4,* Microgametocyte. *5,* Blood platelets. *6,* Nucleus of neutrophil. *7,* Eosinophil. *8,* Blood platelet associated with cellular remains of young erythrocytes. (From Wilcox, A.: *Manual for the Microscopical Diagnosis of Malaria in Man.* 1960 ed. Washington, D.C., U.S. Department of Health, Education, and Welfare, Public Health Service Publication No. 796, 1960, Plate V.)

Plasmodium falciparum stages. Human erythrocytes in Giemsa-stained thin-blood preparation. *1*, Young ring form trophozoite. *2*, Double infection of single cell with young trophozoites, one a "marginal form," the other a "signet ring" form. *3* and *4*, Young trophozoites showing double chromatin dots. *5* to *7*, Developing trophozoite forms. *8*, Three trophozoites in one cell. *9*, Trophozoite showing pigment in a cell containing Maurer's clefts. *10* and *11*, Two trophozoites in each of two cells showing variation of forms. *12*, Almost mature trophozoite showing haze of pigment throughout cytoplasm and Maurer's clefts in the cell. *13*, Estivo-autumnal slender forms. *14*, Mature trophozoite, showing clumped pigment. *15*, Parasite in the process of initial chromatin division. *16* to *19*, Various phases of the development of the schizont ("presegmenting schizonts"). *20*, Mature schizont. *21* to *24*, Successive forms in development of the gametocyte, usually not found in the peripheral circulation. *25*, Immature macrogametocyte. *26*, Mature macrogametocyte. *27*, Immature microgametocyte. *28*, Mature microgametocyte. (From Wilcox, A.: *Manual for the Microscopical Diagnosis of Malaria in Man.* 1960 ed. Washington, D.C., U.S. Department of Health, Education, and Welfare, Public Health Service Publication No. 796, 1960, Plate III.)

PLATE III

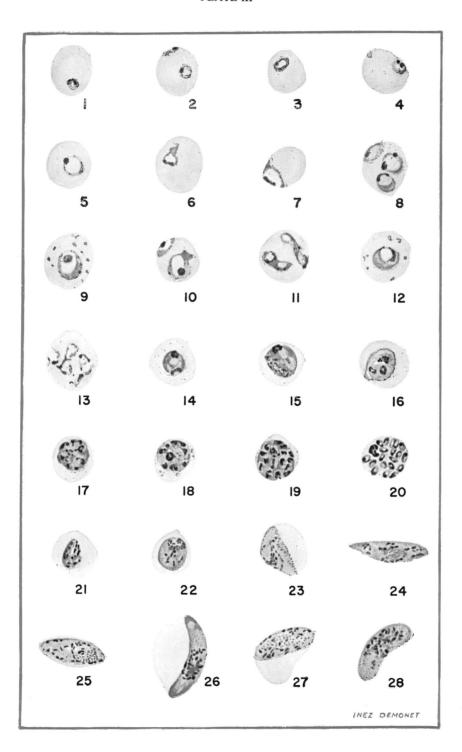

INEZ DEMONET

PLATE IV

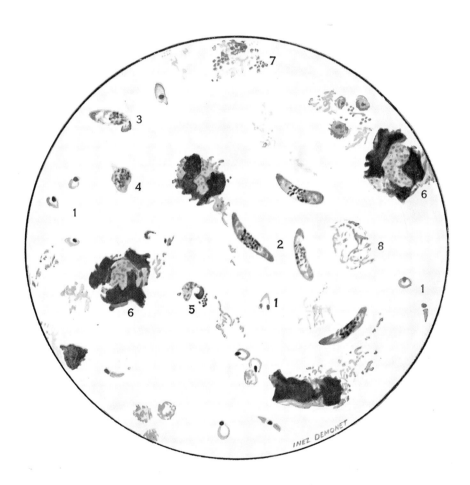

Plasmodium falciparum. Giemsa-stained thick-film preparation. The film contains numerous ring stage tropho-zoites, five normal gametocytes, one "rounded-up" and one degenerate gametocyte, leukocytes, blood platelets, and remains of red cell stroma. *1,* Small trophozoites. *2,* Gametocytes—normal. *3,* Slightly distorted gametocyte. *4,* Rounded-up gametocyte. *5,* Disintegrated gametocyte. *6,* Nucleus of leukocyte. *7,* Blood platelets. *8,* Cellular remains of young erythrocyte. (From Wilcox, A.: *Manual of Microscopical Diagnosis of Malaria in Man.* 1960 ed. Washington, D.C., U.S. Department of Health, Education, and Welfare, Public Health Service Publication No. 796, 1960, Plate VII.)

Plasmodium malariae. Stages in human erythrocytes in Giemsa-stained thin-film preparation. *1*, Young ring form trophozoite. *2* to *4*, Young trophozoite forms showing gradual increase of chromatin and cytoplasm. *5*, Developing ring form trophozoite showing pigment granule. *6*, Early band form with elongated chromatin, some pigment apparent. *7* to *12*, Forms that developing trophozoite may take. *13* and *14*, Mature trophozoites, one a band form. *15* to *19*, Phases in development of the schizont ("presegmenting schizonts"). *20*, Mature schizont. *21*, Immature microgametocyte. *22*, Immature macrogametocyte. *23*, Mature microgametocyte. *24*, Mature macrogametocyte. (From Wilcox, A.: *Manual for the Microscopical Diagnosis of Malaria in Man*. 1960 ed. Washington, D.C., U.S. Department of Health, Education, and Welfare, Public Health Service Publication No. 796, 1960, Plate II.)

PLATE V

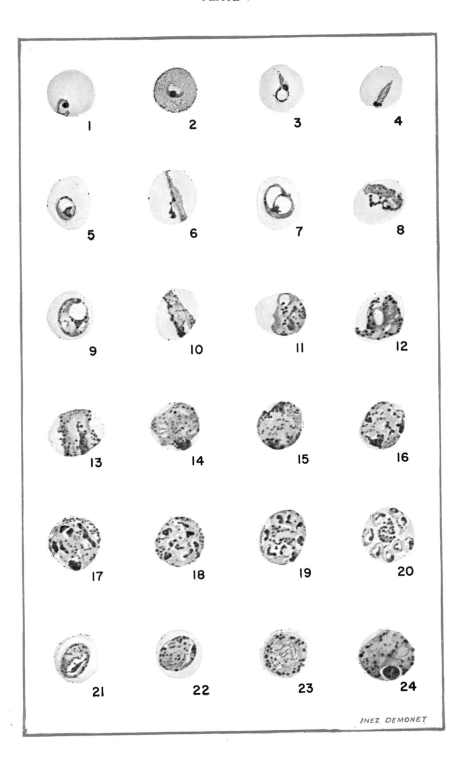

INEZ DEMONET

PLATE VI

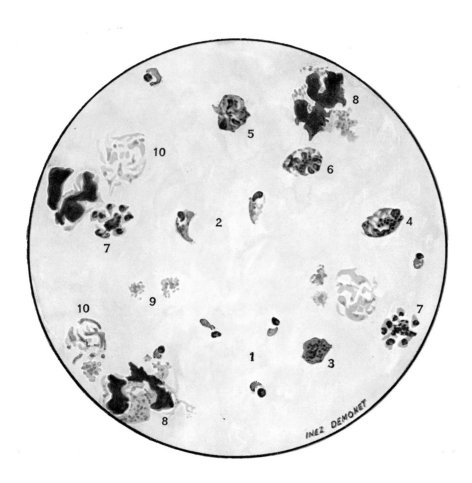

Plasmodium malariae. Giemsa-stained thick-film preparation. The film contains young and developing trophozoites, mature trophozoites, young and mature schizonts, neutrophilic leukocytes, blood platelets, and remains of red cell stroma. *1*, Small trophozoites. *2*, Growing trophozoites. *3*, Mature trophozoites. *4* to *6*, Schizonts (presegmenting) with varying numbers of divisions of the chromatin. *7*, Mature schizonts. *8*, Nucleus of leukocyte. *9*, Blood platelets. *10*, Cellular remains of young erythrocytes. (From Wilcox, A.: *Manual of Microscopical Diagnosis of Malaria in Man*. 1960 ed. Washington, D.C., U.S. Department of Health, Education, and Welfare, Public Health Service Publication No. 796, 1960, Plate VI.)

measure approximately 10 by 12 μm and contain a sporoblast but are not infective (Fig. 6–8*B*). Sporulation at room temperature (20 to 22°C) requires 3 to 4 days; during this time the zygote divides into two sporoblasts, and four sporozoites are formed within each of these. The ripe, infective oocyst thus contains two sporocysts, each with four sporozoites (Fig. 6–8*C*). These oocysts are relatively resistant to a variety of chemicals and will remain infective in the soil for at least 1 year. Ingestion of the infective oocyst by a susceptible bird or mammal may lead to an acute infection that usually subsides to a chronic infection, or the initial infection may be relatively mild and unrecognized. During the acute stage proliferative forms occur in various tissues (Fig. 6–7*B*), but in the chronic phase of the disease it is the cyst form that is found, most frequently in the central nervous system (Fig. 6–8*A*) and muscle, occasionally in other tissues.

The enteroepithelial cycle that occurs in cats includes both asexual multiplication (schizogony) and sexual reproduction (gametogony) within the mucosal epithelium of the small intestine (Fig. 6–9). The final product of the sexual phase of the cycle in the cat is the fertilized macrogamete or zygote, which then protects itself with a thin but remarkably resistant wall before elimination in the feces as the unsporulated oocysts (Fig. 6–8*B*). If a susceptible cat ingests sporulated oocysts and develops intestinal infection, the animal will pass oocysts in 21 to 24 days. However, if a cat is fed an acutely ill mouse with proliferative forms of *T. gondii* in its tissues, oocysts will appear in the cat's feces in 9 to 11 days. Finally, when a chronically ill mouse with cysts in its tissues is fed to a cat, oocysts are shed in the cat's feces after only 3 to 5 days. These observations suggest that reproduction in the proliferative stage and in the cyst stage in the tissues of nonfelines that ingest oocysts fulfills an essential part of the life cycle of the parasite; hence, when a cat ingests tissues infected with one or the other of these, the cycle is completed in a much shorter time. The cat possibly may also have an extraintestinal infection, *i.e.,* proliferative or cyst forms in various tissues that are infective to animals eating the cat.

Pathogenesis and Symptomatology. The large number of humans and animals with serum antibodies to *Toxoplasma* suggests that most infections are relatively asymptomatic. The most seriously affected among humans are the newborn, who acquire infection transplacentally, often during the

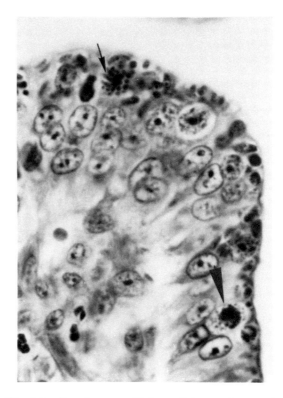

Fig. 6–9. *Toxoplasma gondii*. Intracellular enteric stages in the mucosal epithelium of an experimentally infected cat showing merozoites in mature schizont *(small arrow)*, microgametocyte *(large arrow)*, and macrogametocytes in various stages of development near luminal surface of the host cell. (× 1000.) (By P.C. Beaver. Preparation courtesy of R.G. Yaeger.) (From Beaver, P.C., Jung, R.C., and Cupp, E.W. 1984. *Clinical Parasitology*, 9th ed. Philadelpia, Lea & Febiger, p. 165.)

second or third trimester of fetal development, usually from a symptomless mother. At birth or shortly thereafter, these infants commonly have evidence of retinochoroiditis, cerebral calcification, and occasionally hydrocephalus or microcephaly (Sabin's tetrad). Psychomotor disturbances also may be detected at this time. Occasionally, complications of central nervous system involvement appear several years later. The most common form of toxoplasmosis acquired postnatally is manifested by lymphadenitis, fever, headache, and myalgia; also, during the first week or two, splenomegaly and a fleeting erythematous rash may be present. There is a typhuslike exanthematous form of the disease, which may produce myocarditis, meningoencephalitis, and an atypical pneumonia; death often occurs in such cases. A third, rare form primarily involves the central nervous system, usually with a fatal outcome, and a fourth type of noncongenital infection is retinochoroiditis, in which ocular lesions originate in the retina and spread to the choroid; severe cases may require enucleation.

Diagnosis. Occasionally *Toxoplasma* can be detected and identified in smears of lymph node, bone marrow, spleen, brain, or other material. The organisms are readily identified in impression smears or smears of fluid material, but in histologic preparations of fixed tissues they may not have the typical morphologic appearance. Body fluids or ground tissues may be inoculated intraperitoneally into young laboratory mice from a *Toxoplasma*-free colony, and after 7 to 10 days the peritoneal fluid and smears of lung, spleen, and liver are examined for the proliferative forms. Serum from the inoculated animals may also be tested for the presence of antibodies. Serologic tests should be done in all cases of suspected toxoplasmosis, and a variety of good tests are now available—the Sabin-Feldman dye test, the indirect fluorescent antibody test, the ELISA test, the indirect hemagglutination test, and the complement fixation test. Serum titers for the dye, indirect fluorescent antibody, ELISA, and indirect hemagglutination tests appear earlier, reach much higher levels, and drop much later than do those obtained with the complement fixation test. A high IgM indirect fluorescent antibody titer or a serial 2-tube rise in titer to a high level in any standard test establishes the diagnosis of acute infection. Tests of serum taken at intervals of several weeks can be useful in determining the course of infection.

Treatment. As a rule patients with acute toxoplasmosis who are otherwise normal do not require treatment, but treatment is indicated for those with severe symptoms or active retinochoroiditis and for immunologically compromised patients. Clindamycin plus sulfadiazine has been recommended for the treatment of ocular toxoplasmosis (Lakhanpal *et al.*, 1983), but the potential side-effects of clindamycin (such as pseudomembranous colitis) must be weighed against those of pyrimethamine. In pregnant women diagnosed as having acute toxoplasmosis, the possibility of acute congenital infection must be considered; in some cases chemotherapy with its inherent side-effects or a therapeutic abortion may be recommended.

Epidemiology. Evidence accumulated during recent years helps to explain the prevalence of *Toxoplasma* infection. It has been estimated that approximately half of the population in the United States has the chronic asymptomatic form of toxoplasmosis. The prevalence also increases with age,

a reflection of continued exposure to the risk of infection either by eating raw or undercooked meat or through ingestion of oocysts introduced into the environment by cats. Congenital transmission of toxoplasmosis accounts for relatively few of the many infections seen in man, even though such infections probably account for the majority of acute, fatal infections. Toxoplasmosis acquired by the mother during pregnancy (2 to 6 cases per 1000 pregnancies in the United States) may result in severe and often fatal damage to the fetus. In contrast, a chronically infected woman will rarely, if ever, have an infected child (Krick and Remington, 1978). Organ transplants or transfusions of whole blood or cellular fractions from donors who are asymptomatic but who may have latent forms of the parasite in their tissues may transmit infection, especially if the recipients are on immunosuppressive drugs. However, it is just as likely that the recipient would already have a latent infection, and immunosuppressive therapy would thus produce a relapse of toxoplasmosis.

Control. Proper cooking of meat is essential in view of various reports of isolation of *Toxoplasma* from sheep, swine, and cattle. Although freezing may kill the more resistant cyst forms, it is not as dependable as adequate heating to destroy the infectivity. Although outbreaks of toxoplasmosis caused by the ingestion of raw or undercooked meat have been reported, the principal mode of transmission of *Toxoplasma*, worldwide, is by ingestion of oocysts shed into the environment in the feces of cats. These stages are known to remain viable in the soil for at least a year and are a source of infection for mice, rats, birds, and other prey, which then return the infection to cats (Frenkel and Ruiz, 1981). An outbreak of acute toxoplasmosis among American soldiers in Panama provided epidemiologic evidence that the infections were acquired through drinking water from a jungle stream (Beneson *et al.*, 1982). Freshly passed oocysts are not infective; hence, there is no danger if the feces of cats are safely disposed of before sporulation. The usual practice of permitting cats to run outdoors ensures sporulation of the oocysts because of the animal's habit of burying its feces in soil. Cats may become infected more than once, but in subsequent infections oocysts may not be shed. Kittens can become infected by ingesting oocysts shed by the parent animals or by kittens from a previous litter. Protection of children's sand boxes is advisable, as cats generally have access to play

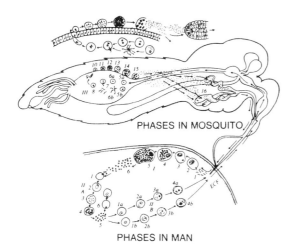

Fig. 6–10. Life cycle of the malaria parasite. *I*, Pre-erythrocytic phase. Sporozoites *(1)* introduced into man by the infected mosquito enter cells of the liver and, by asexual multiplication or schizogony *(2 to 5)*, produce merozoites *(6)*. *II*, Erythrocytic phases. Merozoites from pre-erythrocytic schizonts invade red blood cells, producing trophozoites *(1 to 5)*, leading to replicative schizogony *(6)* and formation of female *(1a to 4a)* and male *(1b to 4b)* gametocytes. *III*, Mosquito phases. Gametocytes, taken up with the peripheral blood of man, reach the mosquito's midgut *(5a, 5b)*, where they mature into female and male gametes *(6a, 6b)*. One male gamete enters a female gamete *(7)*, producing a zygote *(8)*, which becomes the motile ookinete *(9)* and migrates to the outer stomach wall, where it forms the oocyst. The oocyst grows *(10 to 14)*, producing a large number of sporozoites. When mature, the oocyst bursts *(15)*, releasing the sporozoites, which reach the salivary glands *(16)* and pass down the salivary ducts to the hypopharynx, to be introduced into man when the mosquito takes its next blood meal. (Adapted from original of E.C. Faust.)

areas. In view of the various routes of transmission, the possibilities for control are limited. Attempts at artificial immunization of cats have been only partially successful (Frenkel and Smith, 1982a,b).

THE MALARIAL PARASITES

Malarial Parasites As A Group

The malarial parasites are species of the phylum Apicomplexa, class Sporozoea, suborder Haemosporina (see p. 11). The life cycle, like that of other coccidia, includes an asexual phase *(schizogony)* alternating with a sexual one *(gametogony* followed by *sporogony)*. However, the malarial parasites require two hosts: (1) a vertebrate host in which the asexual phase develops and *gametocytes* are produced, and (2) a vector host in which the gametocytes become mature *gametes* (Fig. 6–10). Following maturation, the *microgamete* unites with the *macrogamete* to form a *zygote,* which then becomes the *oocyst* that produces *sporozoites.* When the numerous sporozoites are introduced into the

vertebrate host, they develop into the asexual stage. There are two separate transfer stages, the gametocyte and the sporozoite. The asexual phase *(schizogony)* is found only in the vertebrate host, while maturation and union of sex cells followed by production of sporozoites take place only in bloodsucking invertebrates, mostly arthropods and predominantly mosquitoes.

In many species of malarial parasites of birds the earliest asexual stages occur in the fixed cells of the reticuloendothelial system and the endothelial lining cells of the blood capillaries, after which some of the asexual daughter cells *(merozoites)* invade red blood cells and initiate erythrocytic infection. The malarial parasites in monkeys and man establish their first foci exclusively in the nonphagocytic cells of the liver before the parasites are released into circulating blood to parasitize red blood cells.

All malarial parasites belong to the genus *Plasmodium,* in which much of the asexual development takes place in red blood cells, with the production of pigment, deposited within the body of the parasite. The growing asexual parasite *(trophozoite)* incompletely utilizes hemoglobin, leaving residues of globin and an iron porphyrin hematin; the latter is the malaria pigment, a compound of hematin and protein.

Historical Notes. Although the clinical manifestations of malaria were recorded in ancient medical classics and the ravages of malaria were severe during the later days of the Roman Empire, it was not until 1880 that Alphonse Laveran, in Algeria, first demonstrated the parasites microscopically within red blood cells in fresh wet films.

By 1894 Patrick Manson was firmly convinced that malaria was mosquito-transmitted, and he persuaded Ronald Ross of the Indian Medical Service to test this theory experimentally. Ross first completed the mosquito phase of the cycle in 1898 by employing the parasites of avian malaria in *Culex fatigans.* Later in West Africa he demonstrated similar development of the human parasites in *Anopheles gambiae* and *A. funestus.* During 1898–1899 Bignami, Bastianelli, and Grassi in Italy worked out the complete mosquito phase of human plasmodia in *Anopheles maculipennis.* A field test by British investigators demonstrated conclusively that malaria is transmitted by mosquitoes.

Meanwhile Golgi (1886) first accurately described the tertian parasite and Grassi and Feletti (1890, 1892) assigned the names *vivax* to this species and *malariae* to the quartan parasite, while Welch (1897), in Baltimore, named the species with crescent-shaped gametocytes *falciparum*. Stephens (1922) described and named the fourth malarial parasite of man, *P. ovale*. In a comprehensive text, Bruce-Chwatt (1980) has presented information on the malarial parasites, the vectors, the disease, the epidemiology, and the rationale and technique of malaria control.

Geographical Distribution. The species of plasmodia adapted to man are relatively host-specific and occur where *Anopheles* mosquitoes are abundant and humans with gametocytes in their blood are present. Malaria has been reported from areas as far apart as the Dvina River, near Archangel, in the U.S.S.R. (64°N) and Cordova, in Argentina (32°S). It has occurred at heights of 9,086 feet in the Cochabamba region of Bolivia and at 9,348 feet in Tadzhik, U.S.S.R. Factors that influence the effectiveness of a particular species of *Anopheles* in the transmission of malaria are (1) susceptibility to infection by the parasite, (2) survival long enough for development and transmission of the sporozoites, (3) a preference for human blood, and (4) presence in sufficient numbers.

The world distribution of malaria is shown in Fig. 6–11A.

Biology and Life Cycle. Asexual development occurs in fixed tissue cells and in erythrocytes, followed by gametogony.

PRE-ERYTHROCYTIC DEVELOPMENT. Inoculation occurs when an infected female *Anopheles* mosquito injects saliva containing sporozoites into cutaneous blood vessels preparatory to taking a blood meal. The sporozoites circulate in the bloodstream, but within a half hour they have disappeared. The first colonization takes place in parenchymal cells of the liver.

Following the inoculation of large numbers of sporozoites of *Plasmodium vivax, P. falciparum,* and *P. ovale* in human volunteers and *P. malariae* in chimpanzees, the first evidence of infection was seen 48 hours to 7 days later in the parenchymal cells of the liver, where young schizonts in active nuclear division were observed. These are termed primary exoerythrocytic (EE) schizonts or pre-erythrocytic schizonts. The schizonts grow remarkably in size and produce thousands of merozoites by the 7th or 8th day after inoculation (Fig. 6–12). Krotoski *et al.* (1982) reported the discovery of small, persistent, postsporozoite stages in parenchymal cells of the liver of a rhesus monkey

infected with *Plasmodium cynomolgi bastianellii,* a simian malarial species similar to *P. vivax.* These small uninucleate forms, named *hypnozoites,* are believed to undergo schizogony months or years later, resulting in the production of merozoites that reinfect the host's blood. These investigators believe that this phenomenon occurs in man with the relapsing species *P. vivax* and *P. ovale.*

Following sporozoite-induced infection, the prepatent period for *P. vivax* is 8 days, for *P. falciparum* 6 days, for *P. ovale* 9 days, and for *P. malariae* 13 days. The average incubation period, *i.e.,* the time between inoculation of sporozoites and the first appearance of clinical signs, of which fever is the most common, is 12 days for *P. falciparum,* 13 to 17 days for *P. vivax* and *P. ovale,* and 28 to 30 days for *P. malariae.*

ASEXUAL DEVELOPMENT IN RED BLOOD CELLS. When merozoites that have developed in pre-erythrocytic foci enter the red blood cells, they transform into trophozoites, which grow and develop into schizonts, each producing the number of merozoites characteristic of the species of *Plasmodium.* When fully matured, the merozoites break out of the parasitized red cell and soon actively enter other red cells to repeat the asexual cycle.

The time required to complete one asexual multiplication in red blood cells varies with the different species: for *P. vivax* and *P. ovale* it is 48 hours, for *P. malariae,* 72 hours, and for *P. falciparum,* 36 to 48 hours but with less regularity than in the other species. Moreover, in *P. falciparum* only the young trophozoites are typically seen in circulating erythrocytes, occasionally with older gametocytes, while the more mature trophozoites, young gametocytes, and schizonts tend to be sequestered in the deeper circulation.

EARLY GAMETOGONY. In individuals bitten by infected *Anopheles* mosquitoes, gametocytes begin to appear in circulating erythrocytes after a few to several asexual multiplications, those of *P. falciparum* usually appearing relatively late. These cells do not multiply or develop further unless taken up by a suitable mosquito host.

MOSQUITO PHASE OF LIFE CYCLE. Once the ripe gametocytes are ingested by a female *Anopheles* in a blood meal and reach the midgut, they transform into mature gametes. One *macrogametocyte* develops a single *macrogamete* (oocyte or unfertilized ovum), and one *microgametocyte* produces several flagellated *microgametes.* A microgamete

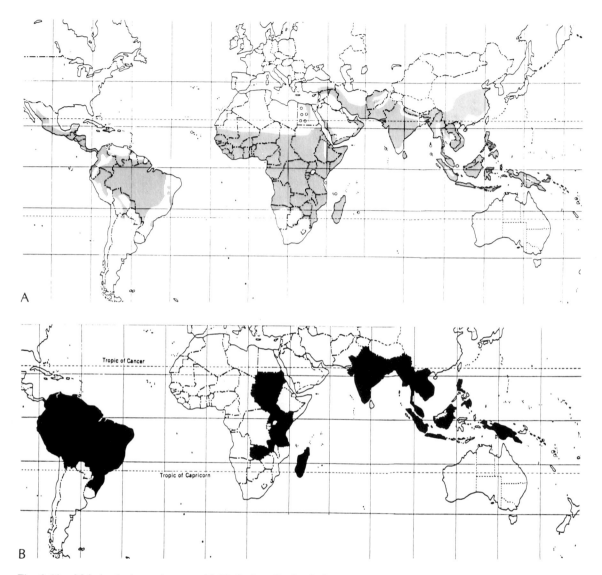

Fig. 6–11. Malaria, *A*, Approximate world distribution. Shading indicates areas where malaria transmission occurs or the risk of infection is significant. Small circles indicate isolated sites of malaria transmission, including oases (in Egypt), Cape Verde, Zanzibar, Mauritius and the Comoros, the Maldives, Vanuatu, the Andaman and Nicobar Islands, Hong Kong, Macao, and Singapore. *B*, Areas of the world where chloroquine-resistant *Plasmodium falciparum* is known to occur. (Adapted by R.C. Jung. *A*, From map in WHO Weekly Epidemiologic Record, July 1983. *B*, From map in WHO Report of the Steering Committee of the Scientific Working Groups on Malaria, June 1980–June 1983.)

then enters a macrogamete, resulting in a *zygote* that becomes a motile *ookinete*, migrates through the stomach wall, and becomes an *oocyst* just under the outer membrane of the stomach.

The oocyst grows rapidly and develops internal nuclear centers. Each center then produces a large number of delicate, spindle-shaped *sporozoites*. By the time the sporozoites become mature, the wall of the greatly enlarged oocyst bursts, releasing the sporozoites into the hemocele of the mosquito. The sporozoites then migrate to the salivary glands,

which they enter, and from there they pass down through the salivary ducts into the median tube (hypopharyngeal tube) of the mosquito's proboscis. When the mosquito next takes a blood meal, sporozoites are injected into the cutaneous blood vessels of the victim and initiate a new infection.

The optimal temperature and corresponding time for complete development of the sexual phases in the mosquito differ in the three common species of human malarial parasites: for *Plasmodium vivax*, 25°C and about 11 days; for *P. falciparum*, 30°C

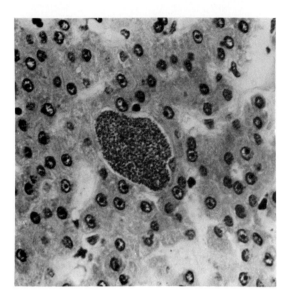

Fig. 6–12. *Plasmodium cynomolgi.* Mature pre-erythrocytic schizont at 8 days of infection. Giemsa stain. (× 500.) (Courtesy of W.A. Krotoski.) (From Beaver, P.C., Jung, R.C., and Cupp, E.W. 1984. *Clinical Parasitology,* 9th ed. Philadelphia, Lea & Febiger, p. 177.)

and 10 to 11 days, and for *P. malariae,* 22°C and 18 to 21 days.

Plasmodia Producing Human Malaria

Plasmodium vivax
(Benign tertian malaria)

Plasmodium vivax (Grassi and Feletti, 1890) is the most widely distributed of the malarial parasites of man, and in cooler climates it is the only indigenous species.

Stages of *P. vivax* in the Human Host. Stages in man are (1) sporozoite introduced into the skin by the infected mosquito, (2) pre-erythrocytic schizonts, and (3) asexual forms and gametocytes in erythrocytes.

Sporozoite. Sporozoites are minute, motile, and spindle-shaped, about 14 μm long with rather blunt ends.

Pre-Erythrocytic Development. The sporozoite enters a parenchymal cell of the liver, where it transforms into a trophozoite. By the 8th day it has grown to 42 μm in diameter and has produced more than 10,000 merozoites (Fig. 6–11). On rupture of the parasitized host cell, the freed merozoites gain access to the bloodstream and enter red blood cells to initiate erythrocytic infection. In *vivax* and *ovale* infections, parasites may persist in the liver for several years, but whether these are the hypnozoites described by Krotoski *et al.* (1982) or are stages derived from exoerythrocytic schizogony remains to be determined; it is also possible that both mechanism are involved.

Infection in the Red Blood Cells (Plate I). Once the merozoite has entered a red blood cell, it transforms into a young trophozoite containing a large vacuole and a distinct nuclear mass on one margin, the so-called "signet ring" stage. The ring rapidly enlarges; its cytoplasm develops ameboid movement and grows at the expense of the red cell. Meanwhile, the red blood cell swells and becomes paler, and in Giemsa- or Wright-stained thin blood films, minute reddish-orange dots, called Schüffner's granules, become evident in the stroma of the red cell. The ameboid outline of the growing parasite becomes its most conspicuous feature, and pigment within it increases with size and age of the parasite. Soon the nucleus begins to divide.

By the 36th hour, practically all of the swollen red blood cell is occupied by the parasite, which becomes irregularly rounded and as a maturing schizont forms 12 to 24 merozoites arranged rather irregularly in a rosette pattern around a central mass of pigment.

Shortly before the 48th hour, the merozoites break out of the host cell and are temporarily free in the plasma. Soon they enter uninfected red blood cells and initiate a replication of the asexual cycle. Repeated asexual production of the parasites builds up the parasitemia, with corresponding reduction in the number of circulating red blood cells. Typically, however, there is host response to parasite activity, consisting of phagocytosis of the free merozoites and even some of the parasitized red cells (Fig. 6–13), so that decreased destruction of erythrocytes results eventually, and after several asexual cycles the primary parasitemia disappears. After a period of weeks in tropical strain infections or months in temperate-zone strains, parasitemia again develops, caused by a new supply of merozoites released from exoerythrocytic foci.

Gametocyte Production (Plate I). After one or more cycles of asexual reproduction in the blood, gametocytes appear as solid rounded parasites within swollen, pale red blood cells. Schüffner's granules are already present in the stroma of the red cell. As the gametocytes grow, they retain a rounded contour and do not exhibit ameboid activity. When fully developed, the microgametocyte has a diffuse cytoplasm and a rather loose skein of nuclear chromatin typically lying within a hyaline

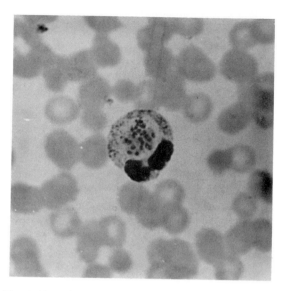

Fig. 6–13. *Plasmodium vivax.* Schizont in a neutrophil granulocyte. Giemsa stain. (× 1000.) (By P.C. Beaver. Preparation by R.G. Yaeger.) (From Beaver, P.C., Jung, R.C., and Cupp, E.W. 1984. *Clinical Parasitology,* 9th ed. Philadelphia, Lea & Febiger, p. 195.)

vacuole; the hematin pigment is scattered throughout the cytoplasm. The mature macrogametocyte has denser cytoplasm, a smaller solid nucleus, and little if any hyaline area around it. The malarial pigment is arranged in small agglomerations or in a wreathlike configuration near the margin of the cytoplasm. These mature gametocytes constitute the stage of transfer to the mosquito host.

Thick Blood Films. In well-stained, thick films prepared by Giemsa's or Field's technique, malarial parasites are condensed or shrunken. As the films have been dehemoglobinized, red-cell boundaries are not apparent (Plate II). Special training is therefore required for thick blood film diagnosis, especially if the type of malaria is to be identified.

Plasmodium falciparum
(Malignant tertian malaria)

Plasmodium falciparum (Welch, 1897) Schaudinn, 1902 is most prevalent in the tropics and subtropics. Stages of *P. falciparum* in the human host are (1) entering sporozoite; (2) pre-erythrocytic schizont; (3) asexual forms in the red blood cells, and (4) gametocytes developing in the red blood cells.

Sporozoite. The *P. falciparum* sporozoite resembles that of *P. vivax,* although it is more slender and more pointed at the ends.

Pre-Erythrocytic Development. In approximately 30 minutes after inoculation, the sporozoites disappear from circulating blood. In human volunteers given sporozoite inoculations, the trophozoite had grown to a schizont 60 μm in diameter by the 6th day and produced about 40,000 merozoites. Except for the somewhat shorter time required for development and ripening of the trophozoite into a mature schizont, pre-erythrocytic development in *falciparum* infection closely parallels that of *P. vivax* infection. There appears to be only one brood of merozoites from exoerythrocytic schizonts, after which residual infection is maintained by erythrocytic parasites.

Infection in Red Blood Cells (Plate III). The first appearance of *P. falciparum* in circulating blood is on the 7th day following sporozoite inoculation. The earliest stage of the red cell parasite is a very minute oval or circular ring with a distinct nuclear dot on one side and a very delicate rim of cytoplasm surrounding a vacuolated center. Frequently the young *falciparum* parasite is found on the margin of the red blood cell just under the cell membrane, with the nuclear dot producing a bulge at the surface. Various stages of binary nuclear division in the ring stage of the trophozoite can often be observed, followed by binary fission of the cytoplasm to form two-ring stage parasites.

Later stages of the *falciparum* trophozoite, the stages of schizogony and the early stages of gametocytes, typically develop only in visceral blood. This is attributable to changes on the surface of the infected erythrocyte resulting in adherence to the walls of deeper blood vessels. With some stains there are reddish granules (Maurer's clefts) in the uninfected portion of the parasitized red cell (Plate III, Fig. 9).

Schizogony usually begins about 24 hours after infection of the red cell and continues during the next 12 to 24 hours, with a total production of 8 to 36 (usually 18 to 24) small merozoites arranged in a rosette pattern around a hematin pigment center.

Escape of the merozoites from a ruptured cell, the short time they are free in the blood plasma, and their entry into uninfected red cells typically occur in visceral blood. One asexual erythrocytic cycle commonly requires 36 to 48 hours.

Gametocyte Production (Plate III). Gametocytes in the immature stages are seldom seen in peripheral blood. They are rounded or oval, with distinct cell membranes. Somewhat later, when they appear in the circulation, they are bluntly falciform; then, as they mature, they become crescentic, tending to occupy one side of a considerably distended red blood cell. Finally, the red cell membrane becomes only a thin, almost transparent veil that can be observed clearly on the concave side of the parasite; when fully ripe, the gametocyte may slip out of this envelope. Immature gametocytes of *P. falciparum* are sexually indistinguishable, but the mature cells are readily differentiated.

Thick Blood Films. The asexual stages of *Plasmodium falciparum* are the shortest of the three common species of malarial parasites and can be readily recognized and diagnosed in thick films (Plate IV). The young trophozoite is a complete or partial azure-stained ring, and the chromatin dot takes an intensely deep-red stain. The schizonts consist of dense masses of purplish-red chromatin surrounded by a common or individual cytoplasmic envelope. The hematin pigment is readily recognized as a few grains or one small mass of dark metallic material. The mature gametocytes ("crescents") are frequently as characteristic as in thin films. All have a wealth of hematin pigment, which is either dispersed (microgametocyte) or a single mass (macrogametocyte).

Plasmodium malariae
(Quartan malaria)

Plasmodium malariae (Grassi and Feletti, 1892) is probably the species that Laveran first observed and studied. It is seen less frequently than *P. vivax* and *P. falciparum* and is rarely dominant in a malarious region.

Stages of *P. malariae* in the human host are (1) entering sporozoite, (2) pre-erythrocytic schizont, (3) erythrocytic schizonts, and (4) gametocytes in red blood cells.

Sporozoite. The sporozoite resembles that of *P. vivax* and *P. falciparum* but is coarser in appearance.

Pre-Erythrocytic Development. Development of trophozoites into mature schizonts in parenchymal cells of the liver requires about 13 days, with production of about 2,000 primary merozoites.

Infection in Red Blood Cells (Plate V). The erythrocytic asexual development of *P. malariae* is synchronized, with replication every 72 hours. The earliest trophozoite is small, ovoid or ringlike, with little ameboid activity. It is smaller, more compact, and utilizes less hemoglobin than does *P. vivax*. As it enlarges, it ranges in shape from broadly oval to delicate or broad band form ex-

tending across the entire diameter of the host cell, frequently with a vacuole. The fully developed trophozoite never quite fills the unswollen red blood cell, which may have a slightly dusky hue. The hematin pigment is dark and usually coarse, and it gradually accumulates in a dark greenish-black mass in the center of the trophozoite.

Schizogony results in 8 (6 to 12) nuclear masses, around each of which there is a small oval envelope of cytoplasm. These merozoites are arranged symmetrically around a mass of hematin granules. On maturity the merozoites break out of the parasitized red blood cells, and after a short, free interval in the blood plasma they invade other red cells.

Gametocyte Production (Plate V). The immature gametocytes of *P. malariae* bear a general resemblance to those of *P. vivax*, but they are smaller and more compact. When they reach maturity, their size is never equal to that of the normal erythrocyte and the parasitized cell is not enlarged. The ripe microgametocyte has denser cytoplasm, frequently more concentrated coarse hematin granules, and a smaller subspherical nucleus.

Thick Blood Films. On the whole, thick films of *Plasmodium malariae* are more readily diagnosed than are those of *P. vivax*, because the plasmodia have more continuous cytoplasm and appear less shrunken (Plate VI). Early trophozoites usually have a relatively regular subspherical cytoplasm in which the chromatin mass lies to one side. More mature trophozoites are solid, with a few distinct dots of hematin pigment and an identifiable eccentric chromatin mass. Young schizonts are difficult to identify as such because their chromatin masses are poorly defined. The ripe schizonts usually appear as distinct merozoites massed in a neat rosette around a hematin center. The gametocytes are characterized as small compact bodies, with undivided chromatin masses in the macrogametocytes, granular dispersed chromatin in the microgametocytes, and a wealth of dark hematin pigment.

Plasmodium ovale
(Ovale tertian malaria)

Plasmodium ovale was named and described as a distinct species on the basis of the enlarged, irregularly oval distortion of many of the red cells parasitized by it. *Plasmodium ovale* infection continues to be contracted at a low level among people in endemic areas. It is most common in West Africa, where higher percentages of Duffy blood group–negative people are found, because such individuals are refractory to infection with *P. vivax* but not with *P. ovale* (Mathews and Armstrong, 1981). Cases diagnosed in recent years among individuals foreign to endemic zones provide clinical and parasitologic evidence that this infection may be characterized by prolonged latent periods (15 months up to 4 years) before manifesting the primary paroxysm of chills and fever.

The long interval between development of *P. ovale* in parenchymal cells of the liver and patent infection is believed to be due to quiescence of the parasite following inoculation of a few sporozoites, with slow development in two or more pre-erythrocytic cycles and finally erythrocytic schizogony after months, or even years.

Most *P. ovale* infections are acquired in African areas south of the Sahara, *viz.,* Guinea, Liberia, Ghana, Togo, Nigeria, and Cameroon, where *Anopheles gambiae* breeds in moist and often forested areas.

All the stages that develop in the exoerythrocytic foci and red blood cells in *P. vivax* are also found in *P. ovale*.

Sporozoite. The sporozoites are slightly more plump than usual, elongate, blunter at one end, and measure 11 to 12 μm in length.

Pre-Erythrocytic Development. Pre-erythrocytic schizonts were demonstrated in the parenchymal cells of the liver of a human volunteer 9 days after *P. ovale*-infected mosquitoes had fed on the subject.

Infection in Red Blood Cells. In certain respects the erythrocytic cycle of *P. ovale* resembles that of *P. vivax;* in others it is more like *P. malariae*. The cycle requires 48 hours. The unparasitized portion of the infected red blood cell (Fig. 6–14) exhibits Schüffner's stippling to a more marked degree than it does in *P. vivax*. The young trophozoite is ring-formed, with a condensed nuclear mass, but the cytoplasm is more compact than that of *P. vivax*, and it usually stains a deeper blue. The vacuole is frequently less conspicuous, and there is no ameboid movement. Occasionally two plasmodia develop in the same red blood cell.

As the trophozoite grows, it continues to be relatively condensed, like that of *P. malariae*; it is frequently rounded, at times distinctly oval or elongated, but not typically band form. Many of the parasitized red cells become oval or pyriform if the blood smear is made very thin and dried rapidly; otherwise, the infected erythrocyte is essentially normal in shape. It may be normal in size or some-

what swollen, but it is not appreciably paler than normal. The malarial pigment is relatively scant and of a light brown color. When schizogony is initiated, the nucleus divides until a relatively small number of chromatin masses (6 to 12, usually 8) are produced, as in *P. malariae*. The mature schizont is rounded or oval and nearly fills the infected red blood cell. The hematin granules are concentrated in a single central mass, around which merozoites are irregularly arranged. The ripe merozoites are irregularly oval, relatively large, and their nuclei have a tendency to be lenticular or vacuolated.

Gametocyte Production. The gametocytes in the red cells are much more like those of *P. malariae* and *P. vivax*, are rounded in outline, are compact, and have a similar staining reaction (Fig. 6–14). Differentiation from the same stage of *P. vivax* has to be made on the smaller, more compact character of *P. ovale* and the number of merozoites in the mature schizont.

Thick Blood Films. Although thick films effectively concentrate *P. ovale*, they make it difficult to differentiate these organisms from *P. malariae* and *P. vivax*, since the shapes of the parasitized cell and Schüffner's granules are not evident.

Pathogenesis and Symptomatology

Pathogenesis

As far as is known, the pathogenicity of malaria is related to the erythrocytic infection; the small amount of tissue destruction in exoerythrocytic foci appears not to produce signs or symptoms. The plasmodia in red blood cells grow and segment at the expense of the host cells. As the number of parasites increases, with each successive schizogony the number of erythrocytes is decreased, owing not only to rupture of the parasitized cells but to lysis of nonparasitized cells. When the debris of the ruptured cells, together with the merozoites and their metabolic by-products, is set free into the bloodstream, it stimulates chemoreceptors of the temperature-regulating mechanism of the host to conserve heat. The amount of pyrogen released initially is not enough to produce a marked reaction, although it may cause prodromal symptoms *(vide infra)*. As the number of invaded red blood cells increases and the asexual cycle of the parasites becomes more synchronized, the quantity of pyrogen becomes sufficient to produce the characteristic chills and fever of a malarial attack. The speed with which this process develops depends on the

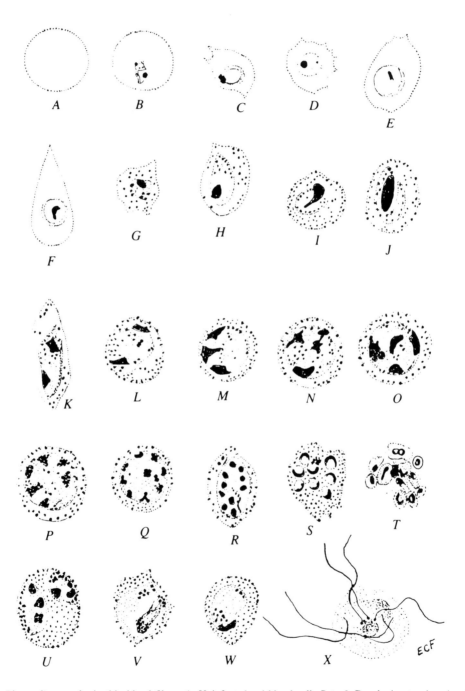

Fig. 6–14. *Plasmodium ovale,* in thin blood films. *A,* Uninfected red blood cell. *B* to *J,* Developing trophozoites in oval and otherwise misshapen cells. *K* to *S,* Developing schizonts. *T,* Merozoites from ruptured cell. *U,* Two schizonts in one red cell. *V,* Microgametocyte. *W,* Macrogametocyte. *X,* Exflagellation of microgametocyte, producing 6 microgametes. Schüffner's granules are shown in *G* through *W.* (Adaptations by E.C. Faust. *B* to *R* and *T* from Stephens, J.W.W., and Owen, D.U. 1927. *Plasmodium ovale.* Ann. Trop. Med. Parasitol., *21:*293–302. Plate xix, figs. 1, 3–6, 9–12, 14. *S* and *U* to *X* from James, S.P., Nicol, W.D., and Shute, P.G. 1933. *Plasmodium ovale* Stephens 1922. Parasitology, *25:*87–95, Plate xi, figs. 3, 4, 8–10.)

species of *Plasmodium* and on the host's immunologic reaction to the invader. *P. vivax* and *P. ovale* prefer the youngest erythrocytes, whereas *P. malariae* prefers the oldest, thus limiting the maximum parasitemias of these species. *P. vivax* infection builds up rapidly, *P. ovale* about half as fast, and *P. malariae* only about a third as rapidly as *P. vivax*.

Infection with *P. falciparum* differs from the other types in a number of respects, and with few exceptions it is the species responsible for fatal malaria. It invades erythrocytes of all ages and is thus capable of producing very extensive parasitemias. The schizogonic cycle in the bloodstream requires not more than 48 hours but is frequently less synchronized. Moreover, in *P. falciparum* infection there is a tendency for more than one parasite, frequently several, to develop in a single red blood cell. Thus, in two or three asexual cycles, the number of infected red cells frequently reaches a dangerous threshold, often without the production of a typical chill followed by fever. Likewise, erythrocytes containing *P. falciparum* parasites tend to adhere to one another and to the lining of blood vessels, causing blockage of blood capillaries in vital areas such as brain, lungs, and kidneys, and toxic products interfere with oxygen utilization by the host cells. With each successive escape of merozoites from ruptured red blood cells and discharge of necrotic red cell debris into the plasma, there is new stimulus to humoral and cellular systemic reactions.

Destruction of red blood corpuscles by the plasmodia produces an anemia that may be normocytic and normochromic or, in chronic and relapsing cases, may resemble pernicious anemia. In severe infections the number of erythrocytes may be reduced to one fifth of normal. Moreover, agglutination of the parasitized red blood cells in *P. falciparum* infection and loss of plasma from the blood vessels in all types of malaria are responsible for so-called "sludging" of the corpuscular elements in the vessels. Thus a progressive decrease in the number and quality of circulating erythrocytes, with corresponding reduction in oxygen conveyance (hence oxygen starvation of the tissue), is followed by multiple thrombosis in the smaller blood vessels and progressive decrease in circulating blood volume.

The *spleen* is typically enlarged, congested, and soft and hemorrhagic in the acute primary stage and hard in the chronic stage. Its color darkens as

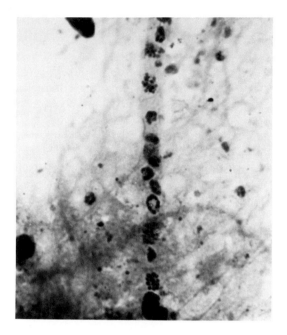

Fig. 6–15. *Plasmodium falciparum.* Brain smear showing numerous schizonts in blood capillary. Giemsa stain. (× 1000.) (By P.C. Beaver. Preparation courtesy of R.G. Yaeger.) (From Beaver, P.C., Jung, R.C., and Cupp, E.W. 1984 *Clinical Parasitology*, 9th ed. Philadelphia, Lea & Febiger, p. 196.)

the amount of pigment increases. The *liver* is hypertrophic and congested in acute malaria and contains deposits of pigment. The *bone marrow* undergoes the same changes as the spleen, but to a lesser degree. The *kidneys* are congested, as the glomerular capillaries become thrombotic with accumulation of parasitized red cells, free hematin, and wandering macrophages. Quartan malaria may cause a focal, proliferative, and membranous glomerulonephritis. The *pulmonary capillaries* share the same congestive process. In cerebral malaria, the *brain* is edematous and may have a grayish color owing to malarial pigment, and there may be extensive plugging of the capillaries by parasitized erythrocytes (Fig. 6–15). All *mucous membranes* may exhibit petechial hemorrhage. The *heart* may show fatty degeneration and be mottled with pericardial and endocardial petechiae, and the capillaries usually are congested and often occluded by the parasitized erythrocytes. In *P. falciparum* malaria the *placenta* manifests a remarkable concentration of plasmodia in all stages of development in the maternal blood sinuses.

Symptomatology

The *biological incubation period* for each of the 4 species of human plasmodia is provided earlier in this chapter. Some *P. vivax* infections are reported to have protracted incubation periods of 9 months or longer, and *P. ovale* of several years. When parasites first enter the erythrocytes (*i.e.,* parasitemia), there are no clinical manifestations of the disease. After one or more asexual erythrocytic multiplications, malaise and a slightly elevated temperature may occur. Synchronization of schizogony frequently occurs during this prodromal period. When a sufficient number of mature schizonts rupture simultaneously, depending on the immune status of the individual, a definite febrile episode ensues.

The Malarial Paroxysm. Primary overt *P. vivax, P. ovale,* or quartan malaria characteristically develops suddenly with a shaking chill, followed by a fever of 40° to 40.6°C (104° to 105°F), accompanied by evidences of an acute febrile disease, such as headache, muscular pains, malaise, nausea and vomiting, abdominal pain, and increased pulse and respiration rates. After several hours, the fever terminates by crisis and is followed by a drenching sweat, especially in *P. vivax* malaria. Afterward the patient is exhausted but feels marked relief. Pernicious symptoms such as coma, convulsions, or cardiac failure rarely occur in *P. vivax, P. ovale,* or quartan malaria. In *P. falciparum* infection the initial chill is usually less pronounced and the fever more prolonged. Much more frequently than in the other species, *P. falciparum* malaria is accompanied by pernicious manifestations variously referred to as comatose, bilious, algid, cardialgic, choleraic, pneumonic, or other. Because of its protean manifestations, malaria may at times mimic virtually any disease syndrome; there may be no remarkable rise in temperature.

Following an essentially symptomless remission which varies with the species, there is a second paroxysm of essentially equal intensity, followed by several additional ones of somewhat lesser magnitude extending over a period of up to 3 weeks or more before the symptoms are terminated. *This series of paroxysms constitutes the primary attack.*

Relapse. Following the termination of the primary attack, either naturally or following treatment, parasites are depressed or may completely disappear from the blood. In *P. falciparum* and quartan malaria this constitutes cure, since in these infections exoerythrocytic development does not persist. In the other two types of malaria, one to several more attacks, *i.e.,* true *relapses,* characteristically occur. Relapses of *P. vivax* malaria usu-

ally continue over a period of 2 to 3 years before the infection is terminated; those of *P. ovale* malaria occur infrequently and rarely persist longer than 1 year.

Recrudescence. In *P. falciparum* and quartan malaria a renewal of clinical manifestations after weeks, months, or years without re-exposure is attributed to the persistence of parasites in the blood at levels too low to be detected or to produce symptoms. Such parasitemias may persist for up to one year in *P. falciparum* infections and for many years in quartan infections.

Complications in Malaria. *P. vivax, P. ovale,* and quartan malaria are relatively benign. *P. falciparum* malaria, on the other hand, is prone to produce serious complications. The signs and symptoms vary depending on the organs most affected by tissue anoxia, *i.e.,* they may be cerebral, gastrointestinal, hyperpyretic, or algid. In cerebral malaria due to *P. falciparum* infection, there may be a sudden primary onset with hyperpyrexia, convulsions, deepening coma, and often death resulting from shock and anoxia. Gastrointestinal malaria results principally in vomiting and diarrhea. Hyperpyrexia in *P. falciparum* infection mimics that of heat stroke. Algid malaria is characterized by vascular collapse and shock. Nephrosis is more likely to occur with quartan malaria than with the other kinds.

Malaria in Hyperendemic Areas. In populations living in highly malarious areas and subject to periodic re-exposure throughout life, typical overt manifestations are usually observed only in the young. Malaria is a major cause of death in children, and they are the subjects from whom the true malarial index of the community should be obtained on the basis of parasitemia and the degree of splenic enlargement. Older children and adults who have survived earlier attacks have developed considerable tolerance to the disease.

Blackwater Fever (Hemoglobinuric Fever). A clinical episode complicating *P. falciparum* malaria is blackwater fever, a manifestation of repeated attacks that have been inadequately treated with quinine. Occasionally resumption of quinine therapy or quinine treatment of a new attack is followed by massive destruction of uninfected erythrocytes. Typically, within a few days of onset there are severe chills with rigor, high fever, jaundice, vomiting, rapidly progressive anemia, and the passage of dark red or black urine. Hemoglobinuria occurs only in persons who have lived in areas where *P. falciparum* infection abounds; likewise this disease is most common during the *P. falciparum* season. It is believed that the hemolysis is caused by erythrocytic autoantibodies derived from previous infections and reacting with autoantigens initiated by fresh erythrocytic infection with the same *P. falciparum* strain. The quininized and parasitized red blood cell acts as an antigen against which hemolysins are formed. Blackwater fever has become uncommon as other antimalarial drugs have replaced quinine (Bruce-Chwatt, 1980).

Diagnosis and Treatment

Diagnosis

Malaria is frequently confused with other diseases that simulate it in the production of chills and fever. On the other hand, the typical paroxysm may be lacking in malaria. In susceptible individuals exposed to *P. falciparum* malaria, the occurrence of chills and fever and other symptoms may warrant a clinical diagnosis of *P. falciparum* malaria and start of treatment pending laboratory confirmation. This should be the case only if rapid laboratory diagnosis is not available.

Since malarial paroxysms are caused by the release of plasmodial merozoites at the end of each period of schizogony, blood films taken just before or at the height of the malarial paroxysm will contain a detectable number of the parasites. If the films are made during afebrile intervals, there may be fewer or no parasites in the red blood cells, especially in cases of *P. falciparum* malaria. However, once the infection becomes chronic, both trophozoites and gametocytes may at times be found in the blood of persons presenting no suggestive symptoms. Parasites are not likely to be circulating in the blood during suppressive therapy, immediately following curative treatment, or soon after self-medication with antimalarial drugs.

Mixed Infections. When two species of malaria are present, there appears to be an antagonism between them. *P. falciparum* is dominant over *P. vivax* which, in turn, predominates over *P. ovale* and *P. malariae*. Thus in a mixed infection with *P. falciparum* and *P. vivax*, the latter would be initially suppressed and not diagnosed. Later, the exoerythrocytic stages of *P. vivax* could produce a relapse.

Thick blood films are frequently necessary to detect the parasites. The thick film allows rapid examination of a large volume of blood in a small area on the slide, thus saving valuable time. Staining of thick blood films is carried out according to the Giemsa technique (see Technical Aids). Although thick films provide concentration of the parasites, it is also essential that thin films be prepared because the malarial species can be more readily identified on these, especially by less experienced examiners. Comparative information on the differential diagnostic characters of the malarial parasites of man is found in Table 6–1.

Treatment

Antimalarial drugs may be used for the following purposes: (1) treatment of malarial attacks, (2) suppression, (3) prophylaxis, and (4) interference with transmission. Drugs that are capable of destroying some stages of one species of *Plasmodium* may be ineffective against other stages or other species. The efficacy of a drug in accomplishing the above objectives depends on its spectrum of activity.

The Malarial Attack. In treating the patient who is suffering from an attack of malaria, the goal is to provide as rapid and certain relief as possible from the miseries and perils that accompany the erythrocytic infection. At present chloroquine and amodiaquine are the most effective drugs available for this purpose. These drugs are usually given orally, but parenteral preparations are available for use in comatose or vomiting patients. Pyrimethamine and chlorguanide eradicate the parasites, but since they act primarily against the schizont, their action may be delayed. Chloroquine and amodiaquine have no effect against the exoerythrocytic parasites. For resistant malaria, see below.

Suppression. Malaria suppression is the administration of a drug for the purpose of preventing or postponing attacks of malaria, although infection is not prevented. Drugs that destroy the erythrocytic parasites are used, including chloroquine, amodiaquine, pyrimethamine, and chlorguanide. After a variable period following the termination of suppression of *P. vivax* or *P. ovale* malaria, a delayed primary attack may occur. In the case of *P. falciparum* malaria which is resistant to chloroquine, other suppressives must be used, including diaminodiphenylsulfone (DDS), pyrimethamine, sulfa drugs, and tetracycline antibiotics. In all situations suppressive medication should be continued for 6 weeks after the subject leaves the endemic area.

Prophylaxis. True causal prophylaxis of malaria

Table 6–1. Differential Characters of Malarial Parasites of Man in Giemsa-Stained Thin Blood Films

	P. vivax*	P. malariae	P. falciparum
Stages in blood	Trophozoites, schizonts, gametocytes	Trophozoites, schizonts, gametocytes	Early trophozoites, mature gametocytes
Schizogony cycle	48 hours	72 hours	36 to 48 hours
Pigment (hematin)	Pale brown, in fine grains and minute rods, scattered	Dark brown or black, in coarse grains, rods, or clumps	Dark brown or black, in coarse grains or small masses
Multiple infection of red blood cell	Uncommon	Rare	Common
Host cell of mature schizont	Enlarged, pale; Schüffner's dots	Normal size, often has dusky hue; Ziemann's dots	Normal size; Maurer's clefts
Trophozoites, ring forms with vacuole	Small and large; usually one chromatin dot	Small and large; usually one chromatin dot, or band forms, compact	Small, two chromatin dots and appliqué forms common
Segmenting schizonts	Irregular; chromatin in fine grains or irregular clumps	Oval or round; chromatin in coarse grains or irregular clumps; band forms	Rarely present; ovoid with chromatin in large granules and small clumps
Segmented schizonts	Fill greatly enlarged cell; 12 to 24 merozoites (usually 18 to 20), irregularly arranged around pigment	Almost fill normal-sized cell; 6 to 12 merozoites (usually 8 to 10) arranged around pigment	Rarely present, fill two thirds of cell; 8 to 36 merozoites (usually 18 to 24) arranged around pigment
Gametocytes	Round	Round	Crescentic

*P. ovale is similar to P. vivax. Depending upon the stages present in a smear, it is difficult to differentiate between them. P. ovale trophozoites are less ameboid, the cytoplasm stains a richer blue, the pigment granules are a darker brown, and the mature schizont has fewer merozoites. In the thinner areas of a smear the infected erythrocyte may be oval or fimbriated in shape; however, this is not a consistent feature.

would imply the destruction of sporozoites as they enter the body. Although no drug yet available is capable of this objective, primaquine destroys the exoerythrocytic forms of *P. vivax, P. ovale,* and quartan infections and so may be used for prophylaxis, but it is not useful in the treatment of the attack. Primaquine has the disadvantage of causing hemolysis, especially in blacks with glucose-6-phosphate dehydrogenase deficit. It should not be used concurrently with atabrine. Because *P. vivax* parasites develop resistance to primaquine administered in suboptimal amounts, tolerated doses may fail to control the parasitism or fever.

Dosages. For *clinical attacks of malaria* (all species of *Plasmodium* that parasitize man), the recommendations for treatment are as follows: (a) *chloroquine phosphate,* orally, 1 g (600 mg base) immediately, then 500 mg (300 mg base) in 6 hours, and 500 mg on the 2nd and 3rd days; or (b) *amodiaquine hydrochloride,* orally, 780 mg (600 mg base) immediately, followed by 520 mg (400 mg base) on the 2nd and 3rd days.

For *suppressive treatment,* (a) *chloroquine phosphate,* orally, 500 mg (300 mg base) weekly during period of exposure; or (b) *amodiaquine hydrochlo-*

ride, orally 520 mg (400 mg base) every week during period of exposure; or *pyrimethamine,* orally, 25 mg (base) weekly during period of exposure.

For *radical cure and interference with transmission, give primaquine phosphate,* orally, 26.3 mg (15 mg base) daily, for 14 days, to be administered following clinical treatment or beginning 1 to 2 weeks before completion of suppressive treatment. Primaquine eliminates *P. falciparum* gametocytes from the blood and thus interferes with the transmission of infection. (See Table 21–1, page 265.)

Resistant Malaria. Increasing numbers of cases of drug-resistant *P. falciparum* malaria have been noted in various parts of the world, especially Southeast Asia. A summary of the occurrence of chloroquine-resistant *P. falciparum* malaria is shown in Fig. 6–11B.

When *P. falciparum* malaria does not respond to treatment with chloroquine or amodiaquine as described above, or if recrudescence occurs following such treatment, quinine alone or in combination with other drugs must be used. If the patient is severely ill and it is not known whether the strain of malaria is resistant to chloroquine, quinine should be used as well. The dosage is quinine sulfate 650 mg every 8 hours for 7 to 10 days. Patients should be kept in bed during the treatment. If oliguria occurs, the drug should be temporarily discontinued.

Quinine may be given intravenously. This is definitely hazardous and should be done only if the drug cannot be given in any other way. A 0.1% solution of quinine dihydrochloride in normal saline solution is given by slow intravenous drip, with continuous observation of blood pressure and pulse to detect adverse cardiovascular reaction. The dose is 10 mg/kg over a period of 2 hours. It may be repeated in 8 hours, but only if absolutely necessary. The total in 24 hours should not exceed 20 mg/kg body weight. It is preferable to give other drugs concurrently with the quinine, such as sulfadoxine, 1.0 g, plus pyrimethamine, 50 mg, in a single dose, or tetracycline, 250 mg, 4 times daily for 7 days.

Suppression of resistant *P. falciparum* malaria may be achieved by administration of pyrimethamine, 25 mg base, plus sulfadoxine, 500 mg, once weekly or double these doses every 2 weeks, or by diphenylsulfone, 25 mg daily, plus pyrimethamine, 25 mg base once weekly.

Although dexamethasone has been recommended for cerebral malaria, a study by Warrell *et al.* (1982) suggests that it is deleterious and should not be used. Corticosteroids may be useful in malarial hemoglobinuria (blackwater fever). Intravenous administration of low molecular dextran is of value to improve capillary blood flow in patients who are critically ill with *P. falciparum* malaria.

Epidemiology

The epidemiology of human malaria rests on basic information on the etiologic agents in man and *Anopheles* mosquitoes. Occasionally malaria is transmitted by transfusion of whole blood from an infected donor or from one drug addict to another through use of a common contaminated hypodermic needle. It also has been transmitted congenitally and through organ transplant, but such instances are rare.

Malaria acquired locally by mosquito bite is termed *autochthonous,* and when contracted outside the area and brought in, it is called *imported.* If malaria is acquired from an imported case it is termed *introduced,* and when contracted by parenteral inoculation (*e.g.,* by blood transfusion), it is called *induced.*

The disease is *endemic* where there is a constant measurable incidence of cases and natural transmission over a succession of years. If there is a rapid rise in the incidence that is well above the usual level or if a significant number of cases suddenly occurs in a previously nonmalarious area, it is termed an *epidemic* unless the rise is seasonal. Malaria that occurs naturally in an area is said to be *indigenous.*

Different strains of the same species of malaria differ in virulence and in their relationship to relapse time. Tropical strains of *Plasmodium vivax* are likely to produce relapse much earlier than those originating in temperate regions; they also have a tendency to produce more relapses. In contrast, *P. falciparum,* the most dangerous of all the malarial parasites of man, does not cause relapse, and except in the case of resistant strains, it is eradicable by use of modern drugs that destroy only the erythrocytic parasites of *P. vivax* and *P. ovale. P. malariae* does not relapse, but parasites may persist in the blood at very low levels for many years.

All species of human malarial parasites are capable of producing infection in all species of *Anopheles* mosquitoes that are satisfactory hosts of any of these plasmodia. No race of mankind is naturally immune to infection with any of the four species of malarial parasites, but some races have considerable tolerance to the parasite to which the population has been exposed. However, sickle cell hemoglobin appears to offer partial protection against *P. falciparum* malaria, and there is evidence that glucose-6-phosphate dehydrogenase (G6PD) deficiency may also protect against this infection to a lesser degree. Absence of the Duffy blood group determinants (Fy[a] and Fy[b]) results in relative insusceptibility of these individuals to *P. vivax* infection. Infants and other young children in endemic areas are highly susceptible. However, the transfer of protective substances from an immune mother to the fetus via the placenta decreases susceptibility of infants during the postnatal period. Pregnancy is accompanied by decreased levels of protective immunity in the expectant mother, and this may aggravate anemia of pregnancy. There is no difference in susceptibility with respect to sex.

Transmission requires gametocytes of both sexes in the proper stage of ripeness in the circulating blood, and in sufficient numbers. The vitality of the gametocytes is also critical, and this will vary from individual to individual patient, at different times during the infection, and probably also with the virulence of the strain of *Plasmodium*.

People in whom gametocytes are commonly circulating in peripheral blood over a considerable period of time are *carriers* who constitute a continuing danger to the community. Malaria is frequently introduced into a nonmalarious community by one or more gametocyte carriers who have acquired the infection in an endemic area. *Anopheles* mosquitoes acquire the infection from the carrier and pass it on to susceptible members of the population.

Factors Relating to the Mosquito Host. The site chosen for oviposition by different species of *Anopheles* may be densely shaded or sunny, and it may be related to particular types of aquatic vegetation or plankton. It is not uncommon for several species of *Anopheles* to occur in the same area. Usually one species is the more important transmitter in a particular area. A susceptible species of mosquito that breeds near human habitations, prefers human blood, and feeds indoors at night is likely to be a dangerous vector. The most notorious transmitter is *Anopheles gambiae*, a native of tropical Africa.

Control

Control of malaria has as its main objective reduction of *Anopheles* below the transmission level. The complementary line of attack is to prevent transmission of the plasmodia from man to mosquito by treatment of infected people, prophylactic chemotherapy, and protection of infected and uninfected populations from anopheline vectors. To effect control, the following measures are essential: (1) protection of the human population from exposure to bites of *Anopheles*, (2) carrying out programs to prevent breeding of *Anopheles* mosquitoes, (3) treatment of human infections with antimalarial drugs wherever practical, (4) establishment of malaria surveillance programs, and (5) institution of programs to dispense practical advice to the public on preventive measures.

BABESIA AND PNEUMOCYSTIS

Babesia Species
(Babesiosis)

Biology and Life Cycle. *Babesia* species produce fulminating hemolytic malarialike disease known as babesiosis, piroplasmosis, or redwater fever. These parasites occur in most parts of the world where there are vector ticks. Babesiosis is an important disease of cattle, especially in the tropics, but *Babesia* species occur in other mammals, including dogs and cats. Human cases have been attributed to species of *Babesia* from cattle, rodents, and horses, but species from other hosts are probably infective to man. In the mammalian host, *Babesia* occurs only in the trophozoite stage—which may be pear-shaped, spherical, ovoid, spindle-shaped, or ameboid—and only in erythrocytes. It undergoes asexual reproduction, forming pairs or tetrad groups within the cell; organisms rupture the cell and infect other erythrocytes. Ticks become infected by ingesting infected erythrocytes but do not themselves transmit the infection later during feeding. Instead, the organisms penetrate the developing ova of the tick, thus infecting the young which eventually hatch from the eggs; subsequently, the parasites penetrate the salivary glands of the young ticks, where they continue reproduction and are available for transmission to the mammalian host when the tick feeds.

The first three reported human cases of babesiosis occurred in individuals whose spleens had been removed, indicating that man is not normally susceptible to infection with *Babesia*. However, more recent cases observed in residents of the United States occurred in patients with intact spleens and no history of blood transfusion or parenteral drug use; one of these patients had found a tick deeply embedded in her skin some weeks earlier. One of the cases was first reported as possible introduced *P. falciparum* malaria and another was at first thought to be Rocky Mountain spotted fever, but both were correctly diagnosed when the pretreatment blood smears were reviewed at a reference laboratory. It is probable that in most cases the infections go unrecognized and the patients are either treated for malaria or recover spontaneously.

Pathogenesis and Symptomatology. In clinically manifest babesiosis, there may be an acute onset of shaking chills, headache, fever of 104°F (40°C), and pain in the abdomen, muscles, and back. Onset of anemia may be rapid, and jaundice may be detectable.

Diagnosis. The parasites are best observed in Giemsa-stained thin blood films, and although distinct signet rings such as are seen in malarial parasites do not occur, pale areas that represent a vacuole may be present (Fig. 6–16). As only tro-

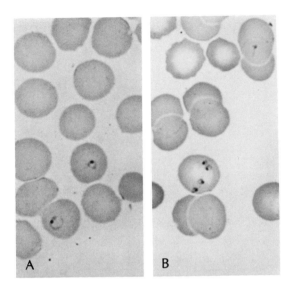

Fig. 6–16. *Babesia microti.* Ring stages in human blood smears. Two single parasites are in the left field, and two pairs are in a single erythrocyte in the right field. Giemsa stain. (× ca. 1200.) (Photomicrographs by Centers for Disease Control, Atlanta, Ga. Courtesy of G. Healy.) (Adapted from Beaver, P.C., Jung, R.C., and Cupp, E.W. 1984. *Clinical Parasitology,* 9th ed. Philadelphia, Lea & Febiger, p. 207.)

phozoites occur in the erythrocytes, *Babesia* infection is more likely to be confused with *Plasmodium falciparum* infection than with the other kinds of human malaria.

Treatment. Pentamidine isethionate is effective against babesiosis in animals and should be considered for use in severe human infections. It is available from the Parasitic Diseases Division, Centers for Disease Control, Atlanta, Georgia.

Epidemiology and Control. The epizootiology of babesiosis involves transmission from mammal to mammal by ixodid ticks. Transmission to people usually occurs in rural areas where infected ticks and mammals are found. Human infection can be prevented by avoiding exposure to tick bites. Splenectomized individuals are very susceptible to babesiosis and have a significantly higher fatality rate; hence, such persons should take special precautions against exposure.

Pneumocystis carinii
(Pneumocystosis)

Historical. In 1909 Carlos Chagas observed an organism in the lungs of guinea pigs infected with *Trypanosoma cruzi;* he later observed these parasites in the lungs of cats, dogs, and in a man who was also infected with *T. cruzi.* Initially he interpreted the organisms as a schizogonic stage of *T. cruzi,* but upon further observation he realized that this was a distinctly different parasite. A similar role in the reproduction of trypanosomes was ascribed to these pneumocysts by Carini in 1910, after he had observed them in the lungs of rats infected with *Trypanosoma lewisi.* Although *Pneumocystis* parasites have been considered as fungi by some workers and as protozoa by others, their characteristics suggest that they belong to the Sporozoea. Yoneda *et al.* (1982) concluded that *Pneumocystis* is a protozoan, presumably in the superclass Rhizopoda. These parasites have been found in many species of mammals, including man.

Although *Pneumocystis* pneumonia, or interstitial plasma cell pneumonia as it is sometimes called, was first described as a clinical and pathologic entity in 1938, it was not until 1951 that Vanek identified *P. carinii* as the etiologic agent. The majority of cases described earlier were in infants who were premature, malnourished, or had had frequent bacterial infections. As more cases were reported, it became apparent that *Pneumocystis* is a ubiquitous, opportunistic parasite that can produce pulmonary disease in individuals whose immunity is naturally low or suppressed either by an infection or by chemotherapy. In recent years *Pneumocystis* has become well known because of its association with acquired immune deficiency syndrome (AIDS).

Morphology, Biology, and Life Cycle. *Pneumocystis carinii* is seen in two forms that may be in the alveolar walls as well as in the alveoli. The trophozoites range from 1 to 5 μm and consist of a small nucleus surrounded by a mass of protoplasm that is variable in size; these forms are best seen in Giemsa-stained impression smears of lung but can also be identified in Giemsa or hematoxylin-stained tissue sections. Electron microscopy shows filopodia or pili projecting from the amebalike trophozoites. The cysts are about 5 μm in diameter and are usually present among the uninucleate forms. In Giemsa-stained touch imprints of lung or smears prepared from bronchial washings, the cysts appear as round masses of unstained cytoplasm containing 2 to 8 purple-stained nuclei (Fig. 6–17*D*). Presumably, the life cycle consists of asexual multiplication in the trophozoite stage and also in the cyst stage. However, the proposed life cycles are based primarily upon observations of material obtained from experimentally induced

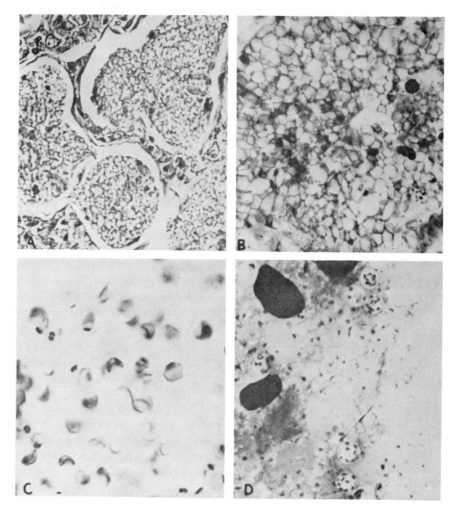

Fig. 6–17. *Pneumocystis carinii* in human lung. *A*, Section showing characteristic honeycomb pattern of alveolar exudate; hematoxylin and eosin stain. (× ca. 400.) *B*, Section prepared with Warthin-Starry stain to emphasize honeycomb pattern of material in alveoli. (× 1200.) *C*, Section stained with Gomori's methenamine-silver stain to show characteristic comma-shaped thickening in cyst wall of parasite. (× 1200.) *D*, Impression smear of lung showing several parasites with eight nuclei and numerous small uninucleate forms. Giemsa stain. (× 1200.) (By R.G. Yaeger.)

disease in immunosuppressed rats, and further work is needed to complete details of the life cycle. It is not known whether transmission occurs during close contact between hosts or by means of a stage capable of surviving in the outside environment for a significant period. Experimental infections in rats are not initiated by introducing *Pneumocystis;* it is either already present in the lungs or enters from the environment during immunosuppressive treatment.

Pathogenesis and Symptomatology. The presence of large numbers of *Pneumocystis* in the lungs results in intra-alveolar aggregates of serous exudate, various stages of the parasite, histiocytes, lymphocytes, plasma cells, and cellular or microbial debris. In advanced cases, most of the alveoli

are partially or completely filled and the septa are thickened (Fig. 6–17A). The material in the alveoli persists, with little phagocytosis or other inflammation, and there is deficient expectoration. At autopsy the lungs are dense in areas where the parasites are most numerous and the alveoli are mostly filled; grossly, such areas look and feel like pancreas. Microscopically, the alveoli have a honeycomb appearance, especially in tissue sections stained by the PAS or Warthin-Starry method (Fig. 6–17B). The septa are thickened by an infiltrate of lymphocytes, histiocytes, and also by plasma cells, unless there has been a deficiency of immunoglobulin production. Parasites may not be numerous in the thickened septa, even though many are in the alveoli.

The incubation period of pneumocystosis is at least 6 weeks but may be much longer, depending upon the factors affecting the individual's resistance. Patients on high doses of corticosteroids or other immunosuppressive drugs develop symptoms in 6 to 8 weeks. The infection may be suspected in any patient with a diffuse or nodular bilateral pulmonary infiltrate that is disproportionate with the minimal physical findings, consisting of malaise, anorexia, slight fever, dyspnea, or nonproductive cough, and with lungs usually clear to percussion and auscultation except for scattered rales. Chest roentgenograms reveal a fairly uniform reticulonodular infiltration. The white blood cell count may be normal or slightly elevated, and occasionally there is an eosinophilia. As the disease progresses, there is increased dyspnea and cyanosis until death occurs by asphyxia.

Diagnosis. Although some diagnoses have been made on the basis of clinical observations, every effort should be made to demonstrate *Pneumocystis* in material from the patient. Bronchial aspirates, transbronchial biopsy, and open lung biopsy and percutaneous pulmonary needle biopsy have been successfully employed. Ordinary cough specimens are usually unsatisfactory. Open biopsy has the advantage of allowing selection of the area most likely to contain numerous parasites. Animal inoculation is not useful because natural infection is almost universal and it requires 6 to 8 weeks. Although *Pneumocystis* has been cultured, the technique is primarily maturation of the uninucleate forms present in the inoculum and not analogous to bacterial cultures, in which large numbers of organisms are derived from a few; therefore it is impractical.

Giemsa staining of impression smears of tissue or smears of the sediment from bronchial aspirates reveals the uninucleate trophozoites as well as the organisms within cysts (Fig. 6–17*D*). Gomori's methenamine silver stain of impression smears as well as of tissue sections will stain the cyst wall and the distinctive crescent-shaped thickenings in the cyst wall, which resemble a pair of parentheses. Reducing the time in the methenamine silver solution results in a better preparation, and the cysts are more clearly differentiated from the yeast forms of fungi. The cysts may also be stained with toluidine blue, Gridley's method for fungi, and the Papanicolaou stain.

Although an immunofluoresence test for *Pneumocystis* has been described, it is not generally used because of low immunoglobulin production in immunosuppressed patients and positive findings in subjects with no obvious disease; in fact, it appears that a very high percentage of normal individuals have detectable levels of antibody to this parasite. Detection of antigenemia is a promising immunologic test, even though it can be detected in individuals without apparent pulmonary disease (Pifer, 1983); on the basis of antigen titer, it might be possible to decide which individuals should receive chemotherapy.

Treatment. The treatment of choice is a combination of trimethoprim, 20 mg/kg body weight per day, and sulfamethoxazole, 100 mg/kg body weight per day, which is administered orally in 4 divided doses for 14 days. An alternative drug is pentamidine, 4 mg/kg body weight per day, which is administered intramuscularly for 12 to 14 days; however, physicians using this drug should watch for hematologic changes. Pentamidine therapy is recommended for patients who have not responded to trimethoprim-sulfamethoxazole treatment. Antibiotics are not effective against this parasite. Supportive measures are usually necessary in advanced cases; these include administration of oxygen by intubation and continuous negative pressure–assisted ventilation.

Prognosis. When the disease has reached an advanced stage, the prognosis is poor, especially in individuals whose immunity is suppressed. Also, recurrent infection can occur. If the disease is suspected and diagnosed early and proper treatment is given, the mortality rate may be 10% or lower.

Epidemiology. Investigations in various areas of the world have revealed that infection with *Pneumocystis* is relatively common in man as well as other species. Overt disease, in contrast, is rare except in immunocompromised individuals. The organisms can be found in the lungs of healthy individuals. No vector has been identified, and although *Pneumocystis* has been reported from numerous species of mammals, transmission to humans from other animal species has not been demonstrated. Congenital infection in rats has been reported (Pifer, 1983), and this mode of transmission may be responsible for some human infections.

Control. At the present time no preventive measures are available. Serious infection should be anticipated in individuals whose immunity is compromised so that treatment can be given early.

SUMMARY

1. Four species of the coccidia, *Cryptosporidium muris, Isospora belli, Sarcocystis hominis,* and *S. suihominis* produce gastroenteritis in man. *Cryptosporidium* and *Isospora* undergo asexual and sexual reproduction within a single host, *S. hominis* reproduces asexually in cattle and sexually in man, and *S. suihominis* reproduces asexually in swine and sexually in man. Infections usually terminate spontaneously in immunocompetent individuals.

2. *Sarcocystis "lindemanni"* is a complex of species that occurs in the cyst form in skeletal and heart muscle of man; the definitive hosts in which sexual reproduction occurs are unknown. Essentially no pathology is associated with the sarcocysts, which are primarily incidental findings in autopsy or biopsy specimens.

3. *Toxoplasma gondii* is a common coccidian parasite of birds and mammals, including man. The domestic cat and other felines are natural hosts in which sexual reproduction generates oocysts that are shed into the environment. Infection can be transmitted congenitally, by ingestion of raw meat containing tissue cysts or tachyzoites, or by ingestion of food or drink contaminated with ripe oocysts that may remain infective in soil for at least a year. Most human infections are essentially symptomless, but acute disease may result from immune deficiency conditions. Congenitally acquired toxoplasmosis may be fatal.

4. The malarial parasites *(Plasmodium vivax, P. ovale, P. malariae,* and *P. falciparum)* reproduce asexually in man and sexually in *Anopheles* mosquitoes. The infected mosquito injects sporozoites that enter liver parenchymal cells and undergo pre-erythrocytic schizogony to produce numerous merozoites. Merozoites released into the bloodstream enter erythrocytes and undergo schizogony to produce more merozoites. The asexual reproductive cycle in erythrocytes usually requires 48 hours in *P. vivax* and *P. ovale,* 72 hours in *P. malariae,* and 36 to 48 hours in *P. falciparum.* Some merozoites that enter erythrocytes develop into macro- and microgametocytes that will initiate the sexual cycle if ingested by a susceptible mosquito. Malarial infection can be acquired by blood transfusion, congenitally, by organ transplant, and by the shared use of contaminated needles by intravenous drug users.

Pathology is primarily due to the erythrocytic stages and involves not only the red blood cells but also the spleen, liver, and other visceral organs; in *P. falciparum* malaria changes in the surface of the infected erythrocyte lead to hemostasis in the blood sinuses and capillaries, particularly in the brain, lungs, coronary vessels, and kidneys.

A malarial paroxysm is caused by pyrogenic substances released by the simultaneous rupture of erythrocytic schizonts. It consists of a shaking chill, then burning fever followed by sweating. A series of paroxysms constitutes an attack, after which there is a remission lasting from a few weeks to several months. In *P. vivax* and *P. ovale* there may be relapses due to exoerythrocytic foci, whereas in *P. falciparum* and *P. malariae* there may be recrudescences due to persistent low parasitemia. Diagnosis of malaria is usually made by the microscopic examination of stained blood films.

Chloroquine and amodiaquine are used to treat a malarial attack; these are not effective in eradicating exoerythrocytic forms. If *P. falciparum* malaria does not respond to these drugs or if recrudescence occurs following such treatment, quinine alone or preferably quinine in combination with sulfadoxine plus pyrethamine or in combination with tetracycline should be used. Drugs used for suppression of malaria include chloroquine, amodiaquine, and pyrimethamine. In areas of chloroquine-resistant *P. falciparum* malaria, other suppressives such as diaminodiphenylsulfone, pyrethamine plus sulfadoxine, and tetracycline antibiotics must be used. Primaquine is used to eradicate exoerythrocytic foci in *P. vivax* and *P. ovale* infection.

Control of malaria involves protection of individuals from mosquitoes, treatment of gametocyte carriers, reduction of the *Anopheles* mosquito population, education of the people, and maintenance of an adequate malaria surveillance program.

5. *Pneumocystis carinii* usually causes disease only in patients with immunologic suppression. Organisms proliferate rapidly when resistance fails, and soon the alveoli fill with organisms and exudate. Minute uninucleate forms and cysts containing 2 to 8 uninucleate forms can be found in appropriately stained biopsies and bronchial washings. *Babesia* infections, transmitted by ixodid ticks from rodents, cattle, and other mammals, cause a severe malaria-like disease in humans.

REFERENCES

Beaver, P.C., Gadgil, R.K., and Morera, P. 1979. *Sarcocystis* in man: A review and report of five cases. Am. J. Trop. Med. Hyg., 28:819–844.

Benenson, M.W., Takafuji, E.T., Lemon, S.M., Greenup, R.L., and Sulzer, A.J. 1982. Oocyst-transmitted toxoplasmosis associated with ingestion of contaminated water. N. Engl. J. Med., *307*:666–669.

Bird, R.G., and Smith, M.D. 1980. Cryptosporidiosis in man: Parasite life cycle and fine structural pathology. J. Pathol., *132*:217–233.

Brandborg, L.L., Goldberg, S.B., and Breidenbach, W.C. 1970. Human coccidiosis—a possible cause of malabsorption. The life cycle in small-bowel mucosal biopsies as a diagnostic feature. N. Engl. J. Med., *283*:1306–1313.

Bruce-Chwatt, L.J. 1980. *Essential Malariology.* London, William Heinemann Medical Books Ltd., 354 pp.

Bunyaratvej, S., Bunyawongwiroj, P., and Nitiyanant, P. 1982. Human intestinal sarcosporidiosis: Report of six cases. Am. J. Trop. Med. Hyg., *31*:36–41.

Current, W.L., Reese, N.C., Ernst, J.V., Bailey, W.S., Heyman, M.B., and Weinstein, W.M. 1983. Human cryptosporidiosis in immunocompetent and immunodeficient persons. Studies of an outbreak and experimental transmission. N. Engl. J. Med., *21*:1252–1257.

Forgacs, P., Tarshis, A., Ma, P., Federman, M., Mele, L., Silverman, M.L., and Shea, J.A. 1983. Intestinal and bronchial cryptosporidiosis in an immunodeficient homosexual man. Ann. Intern. Med., *99*:793–794.

Frenkel, J.K., and Ruiz, A. 1981. Endemicity of toxoplasmosis in Costa Rica. Transmission between cats, soil, intermediate hosts and humans. Am. J. Epidemiol., *113*:254–269.

Frenkel, J.K., and Smith, D.D. 1982a. Immunization of cats against shedding of *Toxoplasma* oocysts. J. Parasitol., *68*:744–748.

———. 1982b. Inhibitory effects of monensin on shedding of *Toxoplasma* oocysts by cats. J. Parasitol., *68*:851–855.

Krick, J.A., and Remington, J.S. 1978. Toxoplasmosis in the adult—an overview. N. Engl. J. Med., *298*:550–553.

Krotoski, W.A., Garnham, P.C.C., Bray, R.S., Krotoski, D.M., Killick-Kendrick, R., Draper, C.C., Targett, G.A.T., and Guy, M.W. 1982. Observations on early and late post-sporozoite tissue stages in primate malaria. I.

Discovery of a new latent form of *Plasmodium cynomolgi* (the hypnozoite), and failure to detect hepatic forms within the first 24 hours after infection. Am. J. Trop. Med. Hyg., *31*:24–35.

Lakhanpal, V., Schocket, S.S., and Nirankari, V.S. 1983. Clindamycin in the treatment of toxoplasmic retinochoroiditis. Am. J. Ophthalmol., *95*:605–613.

Levine, N.D., 1984. Taxonomy and review of the coccidian genus *Cryptosporidium* (Protozoa, Apicomplexa). J. Protozool., *31*:94–98.

———, and Tadros, W. 1980. Named species and hosts of *Sarcocystis* (Protozoa: Apicomplexa: Sarcocystidae). System. Parasitol., *2*:41–59.

Mata, L., Bolanos, H., Pizarro, D., and Vives, M. 1984. Cryptosporidiosis in children from some highland Costa Rican rural and urban areas. Am. J. Trop. Med. Hyg., *33*:24–29.

Mathews, H.M., and Armstrong, J.C. 1981. Duffy blood groups and vivax malaria in Ethiopia. Am. J. Trop Med. Hyg., *30*:299–303.

Pifer, L.L. 1983. *Pneumocystis carinii:* A diagnostic dilemma. Pediatr. Infect. Dis., *2*:177–183.

Pitlik, S.D., Fainstein, V., Garza, D., Guarda, L., Bolivar, R., Rios, A., Hopfer, R.L., and Mansell, P.A. 1983. Human cryptosporidiosis: Spectrum of disease. Report of six cases and review of the literature. Arch. Intern. Med., *143*:2269–2275.

Tzipori, S. 1983. Cryptosporidiosis in animals and humans. Microbiol. Rev., *47*:84–96.

———, Smith, M., Birch, C., Barnes, G., and Bishop, R. 1983. Cryptosporidiosis in hospital patients with gastroenteritis. Am. J. Trop. Med. Hyg., *32*:931–934.

Warrell, D.A., Looareesuwan, S., Warrell, M.J., Kasemsarn, P., Intaraprasert, R., Bunnag, D., and Harinasuta, T. 1982. Dexamethasone proves deleterious in cerebral malaria. A double-blind trial in 100 comatose patients. N. Engl. J. Med., *306*:313–319.

Westerman, E.L., and Christensen, R.P. 1979. Chronic *Isopora belli* infection treated with co-trimoxazole. Ann. Intern. Med., *91*:413–414.

Yoneda, K., Walzer, P.D., Richey, C.S., and Birk, M.G. 1982. *Pneumocystis carinii:* Freeze-fracture study of stages of the organism. Exp. Parasitol., *53*:68–76.

Helminths and Helminthic Infection

Chapter 7

Introduction to the Helminths

The designation "helminth" means "worm." Broadly interpreted, it refers to any worm or worm-like animal; in a more restricted sense, it refers to a parasitic worm. It comprises two large phyla, the Platyhelminthes (flatworms) and the Nematoda (true roundworms), as well as two smaller ones, the Nematomorpha (hair snakes) and Acanthocephala (thorny-headed worms), and one class group of the Annelida, the Hirudinea (leeches).

Classes

The two classes of Platyhelminthes to be considered, the Trematoda (flukes) and Cestoidea (tapeworms), are parasitic in all or most of their life cycle stages. Many species of the phylum Nematoda are free-living; possibly about an equal number are parasitic, either throughout life or during an essential part of the cycle. The Nematomorpha are parasitic in the hemocele of certain insects during development to near maturity, at which time they escape into fresh water to complete their development, mate, and oviposit. The Acanthocephala are exclusively endoparasitic. The Hirudinea are free-living worms that can be considered parasites only when they attach themselves to victims in order to engorge on their blood. They usually are not regarded as helminths, but as ectoparasites that occasionally take blood from internal as well as external sites; they are of sufficient medical importance to merit inclusion here.

Adaptations

Special adaptations for the parasitic mode of life and for species survival are more apparent in the helminths than in the protozoa. The complete or partial loss of the digestive tract in certain parasitic helminths is presumed to be because of their location in the host's intestine or tissues, where predigested nutrients are abundant. The alimentary tract of ancestral forms has entirely disappeared from all stages of the tapeworms and Acanthocephala; it is greatly reduced or nearly absent in many of the trematodes, and although present and complete in most nematodes, it is much reduced in some. A related adaptation in the trematodes and cestodes is evident in the tegument, which on its outer surface has a coat of microvilli morphologically not unlike that of the intestinal mucosa of vertebrates.

Worm Population

Size. While most of the vital systems of parasitic helminths have been modified toward simplification in proportion to reduced demands, the reproductive system has been modified toward increased capacity. However, with few exceptions, reproduction to increase the parasite population within the same host (internal autoinfection) does not occur among helminths; as a general rule, the number of individuals in a worm population living within a given host does not exceed the number of infective eggs or larvae that entered from the outside. Moreover, under usual conditions of host and environment, the number of worms that reach maturity in any given host is limited to levels that are tolerable to both host and parasite. Thus most of the people who are infected with helminths are asymptomatic carriers, and the diseased individuals among the infected group are those with the heaviest worm burdens. The terms "light," "moderate," and "heavy" as applied to worm burdens are of course relative and differ for the various species of helminths and in people of different ages and physical status.

Assessment. In general, although there are important exceptions, the number of eggs or larvae being eliminated in the feces, urine, or sputum is roughly proportional to the number of worms generating them. However, a common error in the interpretation of egg output is to overlook the fact that the individual "egg-count" is actually an *estimate* based on a small sample and therefore represents a wide statistical plus or minus range (Greenberg and Beck, 1984). Another common error is to accept estimates of egg output per worm as applicable to all infections with that species, irrespective of the worm burden or such host variables as age and diet. When worms are crowded, the collective egg output is great, but the output per worm is relatively low, depending on the degree of crowding. The basic principle to be considered in the assessment of helminth infections is that while essentially all species of worms or their larvae are pathogenic when present in large numbers, light infections, defined specifically for each species and for different geographic regions, generally are well tolerated.

Factors. Some of the factors that determine the prevalence of helminthic infections and the incidence of diseases caused by them are well understood. The basic life cycles of nearly all common worm parasites of man and domestic animals have been described, though details are lacking in some. These will be discussed in relation to particular parasites. The factors that determine helminth populations, in a more general way, are those associated with the host-parasite relationship, i.e., the immune factors derived from the host responses and the complex role of existing infection in the prevention or modulation of additional infection and of reinfection. The effect of an existing population of mature worms on young forms entering the same host to occupy the same niche is difficult to assess apart from host factors. Massive infection of course depends initially on massive inoculation of infective larvae or eggs, an event that can be explained; the factors that permit development of some individual worms and bar the development of others are poorly understood.

The presence of one species of helminth apparently has little influence on the entry and development of other species in the same host. The coexistence of several species of helminth in the same individual, i.e., polyhelminthism, is widely prevalent (Buck *et al.*, 1978). Infection with one parasite may appear to increase a host's susceptibility to infection with another (Keita *et al.*, 1981). On the other hand, low endemicity or absence of certain helminths has been noted in regions where their presence was expected, and in experimental animals a prior or existing infection with one species may have a partial immunizing effect against another (Mimori *et al.*, 1983).

Types of Life Cycle

In some helminths the life cycle is direct and relatively simple, involving only one host species and a brief period of development of an infective transfer stage. An example is the pinworm, *Enterobius vermicularis*. In a group referred to as soil-transmitted helminths the life cycle involves only one host, man, but the infective transfer stage (larvae remaining in the eggs, as in *Ascaris lumbricoides* and *Trichuris trichiura*, or free in the soil, as in the hookworm species) requires a period of development in soil, i.e., the soil functions as an intermediate host. In others the man-to-man cycle involves essential development in one intermediate host, as in the filarial worms and most tapeworms, or two intermediate hosts, as in most trematodes, the first being a snail or other mollusc, the second an animal or plant that is eaten by people (such as larval lung flukes in crabs and certain larval liver flukes in fish or others on aquatic vegetation). In addition, certain nematodes, cestodes, and trematodes include in their life cycles a special kind of transmission known as *paratenesis,* involving *paratenic* hosts. Intermediate hosts provide the parasite with sustenance for essential development, protection, and availability to its final host. In a prey-predator relationship paratenic hosts acquire the larval stage after it has developed to the infective stage in soil or an intermediate host and provide for its protection, support, and availability to its final host. By predation or cannibalism, the larval parasite can pass through a series of paratenic hosts. The example for which the term paratenesis was coined is seen in the enzootic cycle of *Toxocara canis,* a cause of visceral larva migrans (see p. 165).

Evidences of Helminthic Infection

Worms and larvae that migrate through or reside in tissues generally produce eosinophilia, focally in the tissues, in the blood, or in both. Persistent hypereosinophilia is the most widely recognized general sign of a helminthic infection (Weller, 1984). Helminthic infections frequently are *occult* or *cryptic,* either because they are *prepatent* or *nonpatent.* Infections with helminths that are natural parasites of man are prepatent in the early stages before eggs or larvae are produced. Certain helminths of animals develop in man but do not produce eggs or larvae and therefore the infections are not patent. Such infections are referred to as nonpatent. In addition to eosinophilia, common signals of occult helminthic infections, somewhat in order of their significance or frequency, are hepatomegaly, pneumonitis, bronchial asthma, urticaria, subcutaneous cysts or swellings, neurologic disturbances, and deviations in behavior.

REFERENCES

Buck, A.A., Anderson, R., MacRae, A.A., and Fain, A. 1978. Epidemiology of poly-parasitism. I. Occurrence, frequency and distribution of multiple infections in rural communities in Chad, Peru, Afghanistan, and Zaire. Tropenmed. Parasitol., 29:61–70.

Greenberg, E.R., and Beck, J.R. 1983. The effects of sample size on reticulocyte counting and stool examination. The binomial and Poisson distributions in laboratory medicine. Arch. Pathol. Lab. Med., 108:396–398.

Keita, M.F., Prost, A., Balique, H., and Ranque, P. 1981. Associations of filarial infections in man in the savanna zones of Mali and Upper Volta. Am. J. Trop. Med. Hyg., 30:590–592.

Mimori, T., Nawa, Y., Korenaga, M., and Tada, I. 1983. *Nippostrongylus brasiliensis* and *Strongyloides ratti:* Concurrent infection in normal and immunized rats. Aust. J. Exp. Biol. Med. Sci., 61:435–437.

Weller, P. 1984. Eosinophilia. J. Allergy Clin. Immunol., 73:1–10.

Chapter 8

Intestinal, Hepatic, and Pulmonary Flukes (Trematodes)

E.A. Malek

TREMATODES AS A GROUP

Trematodes (class Trematoda) constitute a major subdivision of the phylum Platyhelminthes, which also includes the Turbellaria and the Cestoidea. Of the three recognized subclasses, *viz.*, Monogenea, Aspidogastrea, and Digenea, only the Digenea (digenetic trematodes) produce infections in man.

Life Cycle. Digenetic trematodes have a complicated life cycle in two or more hosts, consisting of three (or more) generations. The final stage is usually hermaphroditic, but in blood flukes (schistosomes) it is dioecious. In most Digenea the fertilized egg (Fig. 8–1), after its discharge from the definitive host, hatches in water, with the escape of a ciliated larva *(miracidium)*, which is free-swimming for a relatively short time. To proceed with development, the miracidium must penetrate the tissues of an appropriate mollusc, usually a snail.

In the hemolymph spaces of the mollusc, the miracidium sheds its ciliated epithelium and transforms into a simple elongated sac, a *first-generation sporocyst.* Germ cells developed from the inner wall of the sporocyst give rise either to a number of *second-generation sporocysts* in some species or to *rediae* in other species. The second-generation organisms escape from the first and grow and internally produce larvae called *cercariae;* when mature, the cercariae emerge from the mollusc and temporarily become free-living (Fig. 8–1).

Depending on the particular group, the cercaria (1) becomes attached to the skin of a definitive vertebrate host, discards its tail, penetrates into the tissues aided by enzymes elaborated by penetration glands, and after migration and growth matures in this host (schistosomes or blood flukes); (2) crawls onto an aquatic plant, drops its tail, rounds up and encysts by covering itself with material secreted by cystogenous glands *(Fasciolopsis buski, Fasciola hepatica),* or (3) sheds its tail and penetrates into the tissues of an aquatic animal *(Clonorchis sinensis, Opisthorchis felineus, Paragonimus westermani)* or a terrestrial animal *(Dicrocoelium dendriticum),* in which it becomes encysted. In the latter two types of development the definitive host becomes infected when it ingests the uncooked plant or animal tissues on which or in which the encysted stage occurs.

When the cercaria discards its tail it either becomes encysted to form a *metacercaria,* transforms into a *schistosomulum* (the schistosomes) or forms a *mesocercaria* (the strigeid *Alaria).* Infection with *Alaria* spp. is zoonotic, and in a few cases (one fatal), the mesocercariae were found in the eye or in the lung and other tissues.

The Mature Worm. Trematodes vary in size and shape: some *(Fasciola, Fasciolopsis)* are large and fleshy; others are nearly microscopic (heterophyid species); still others are thin and flabby *(Clonorchis, Opisthorchis, Dicrocoelium),* and the blood-inhabiting schistosomes are more or less delicately cylindrical (Fig. 8–1).

TEGUMENT. The adult trematode is covered with a tegument that may be smooth or bear spines or plaquelike structures. Under the tegument there are successively a circular and a longitudinal muscle

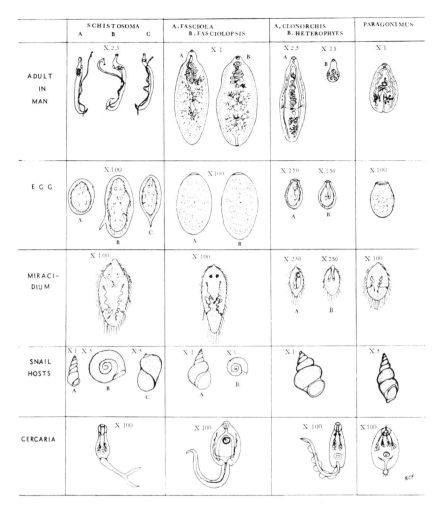

Fig. 8–1. Principal stages and differential characteristics of common digenetic trematode parasites of man. Under *Schistosoma*, *A* represents *Schistosoma japonicum; B, S. mansoni;* and *C, S. haematobium.* (By E.C. Faust)

layer, oblique muscles, and a loose parenchymatous matrix surrounding the internal organs. In addition to a sucker that surrounds the mouth, in most families there is a median ventral sucker or acetabulum.

THE DIGESTIVE SYSTEM. The digestive organs consist of a mouth (buccal cavity), then an esophagus that is provided with a spherical or pyriform, usually muscular pharynx, and finally a pair of ceca, which in most species are simple and end blindly in the subdistal portion of the worm (Figs. 8–6, 8–8, and 8–11).

THE NERVOUS SYSTEM. Relatively large saddle-like nerve commissures are located in the anterior portion of the worm dorsal to the pharynx. Connected with this central nerve mass are three pairs of nerve trunks, one pair each in the lateral, dorsolateral, and ventrolateral positions.

THE EXCRETORY SYSTEM. A median posterior bladder empties through a posterior pore; primary and secondary collecting tubules are bilaterally symmetric, connecting to the capillaries with terminal "flame cells" *(solenocytes).*

THE GENITAL SYSTEM. All digenetic trematodes except the schistosomes are hermaphroditic. Each organism is typically self-fertilizing, so that an isolated worm is able to reproduce its kind.

The usual *male reproductive organs* (Fig. 8–2) are the *testes,* commonly two; for each testis there is a *vas efferens,* a common *vas deferens,* a swollen *seminal vesicle, prostate gland,* and a muscular *cirrus* or penial organ. Usually a *cirrus sac* surrounds these terminal male genital organs. The male system opens into the common *genital atrium,* which is provided with a *genital pore.*

The *female reproductive organs* (Fig. 8–3) con-

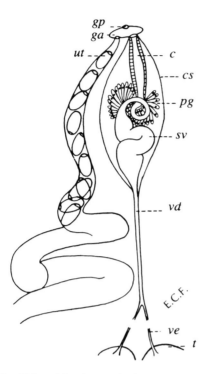

Fig. 8–2. Male and female reproductive organs leading to the genital pore of a digenetic trematode. *c,* Cirrus. *cs,* Cirrus sac. *ga,* Genital atrium. *gp,* Genital pore. *pg,* Prostate gland. *sv,* Seminal vesicle. *t,* Testis. *ut,* Uterus with eggs. *vd,* Vas deferens. *ve,* Vas efferens. (From Faust, E.C. 1949. *Human Helminthology,* 3rd ed. Philadelphia, Lea & Febiger, p. 75.)

sist of a single *ovary,* an *oviduct, seminal receptacle, Laurer's canal,* the *vitellaria* that contain yolk cells and in part shell-gland material, paired and common vitelline collecting ducts, the *ootype,* surrounded by *Mehlis' gland,* and the coiled *uterus,* which originates on the anterior face of the

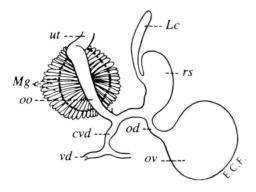

Fig. 8–3. Female reproductive organs of a digenetic trematode. *cvd,* Common vitelline duct. *Lc,* Laurer's canal. *Mg,* Mehlis' gland. *od,* Oviduct. *oo,* Ootype. *ov,* Ovary. *rs,* Seminal receptacle. *ut,* Uterus. *vd,* Vitelline duct. (From Faust, E.C. 1949. *Human Helminthology,* 3rd ed. Philadelphia, Lea & Febiger, p. 75.)

ootype and proceeds in tortuous coils to the genital atrium.

Spermatozoa that reach the genital atrium from the male system proceed through the uterus to the seminal receptacle, where they are stored. The naked *ovum,* the spermatozoa, and the vitelline shell-gland material pass into the ootype. Here the ovum is first surrounded by vitelline cells rich in glycogen, fertilization occurs, and the fused elements form an enveloping shell. The egg is then carried in the uterus to the genital pore.

Eggs of *Fasciola, Fasciolopsis, Paragonimus,* echinostomes, amphistomes (flukes with ventral sucker or acetabulum at the posterior end of the body), and monostomes (flukes having no acetabulum) are unembryonated when deposited in host feces and require a period of development in water before they hatch. Eggs of schistosomes are only partially embryonated when oviposited in the host's tissues but are usually mature when they are discharged in the excreta and soon hatch when they reach fresh water. Although eggs of *Clonorchis, Opisthorchis,* and heterophyid species are mature when they are evacuated in the host's feces, they do not hatch in water but must be ingested by the appropriate snail before the miracidia are released.

The eggs of most digenetic trematodes are operculate; a few, particularly those of schistosomes, are nonoperculate.

INTESTINAL FLUKES

Fasciolopsis buski
(Fasciolopsiasis)

Fasciolopsis buski (Lankester, 1875) Odhner, 1902, the giant intestinal fluke, was first observed by Busk in the duodenum of a Laskar sailor at autopsy in London. Its natural geographic distribution is limited to mainland China, Taiwan, several countries of southeast Asia, and the Indian subcontinent.

Biology and Life Cycle. *Fasciolopsis buski* is a large, fleshy worm that lives attached to the wall of the duodenum or jejunum (Fig. 8–4). It measures 20 to 75 mm long, 8 to 20 mm wide, and 0.5 to 3.0 mm thick. The tegument is spinose. The oral sucker is much smaller than the nearby acetabulum. Conspicuous features of the genital organs are extensive highly branched testes that occupy much of the posterior three fifths of the body, a small branched ovary, and a relatively short, convoluted uterus.

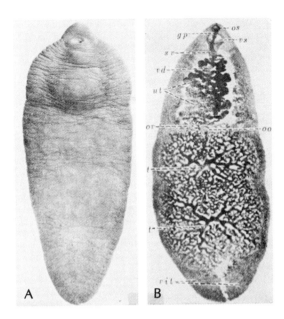

Fig. 8–4. *Fasciolopsis buski. A*, Photograph of living worm, ventral view. (× 3.) (By J.G. Basneuvo.) *B*, Stained specimen, ventral view. (× 3.) *gp*, Genital pore. *oo*, Ootype. *os*, Oral sucker. *ov*, Ovary. *sv*, Seminal vesicle. *t*, Testis. *ut*, Uterus. *vd*, Vas deferens, *vit*, Vitellaria. *vs*, Ventral sucker. (Adapted by E.C. Faust from photo by R. Roudabush, Ward's Natural Science Establishment.)

Eggs of *F. buski* are large, shaped like hen's eggs, measure 130 to 140 μm by 80 to 85 μm, have a thin, transparent shell with a small operculum at one end, and are unembryonated when evacuated in the host's feces. They are difficult to differentiate from the eggs of *Fasciola hepatica* (Fig. 8–9).

To proceed with their development, eggs of *F. buski* must reach quiet fresh water. Here they embryonate in 3 to 7 weeks at a temperature of 26° to 32°C, following which a miracidium emerges through the opened operculum and swims about in the water. On contact with an appropriate small planorbid snail (species of *Segmentina* or *Hippeutis*), the miracidium penetrates the soft tissues and transforms into a sporocyst. In this a generation of rediae is produced, then within each redia a second brood of rediae. The second redial generation produces cercariae, which erupt from the snail and, after swimming about, crawl onto aquatic vegetation and encyst. Man commonly becomes infected while peeling off the hull of the seed pods of the water buffalo nut or the skin of the "water chestnut" with his teeth, so that some of the en-

cysted metacercariae are set free and swallowed. After excysting in the duodenum, the young worms become attached to the mucosa and in about 3 months are mature.

Pathogenesis and Symptomatology. Inflammation and ulceration at the sites of attachment of worms to the mucosa and allergy to products of the worms are the principal mechanisms of disease. The commonest symptoms are diarrhea and abdominal pain. Heavier infections cause edema of the lower extremities and face and ascites, and are sometimes fatal. Peripheral eosinophilia typically is present.

Diagnosis. Infection is demonstrated by finding characteristic eggs in the stools.

Treatment. Praziquantel, given as for other trematode infections, is the drug of choice.

Epidemiology. The natural definitive hosts of *Fasciolopsis buski* are man and the hog. Endemicity is associated with cultivation of buffalo nuts (*Trapa natans* in China, *T. bicornis* in Thailand and Bangladesh), the "water chestnut" (*Eliocharis tuberosa*), the lotus, water bamboo, and other aquatic plants, portions of which are eaten raw by native populations. Use of human excreta containing eggs of *F. buski* to fertilize fields of aquatic plants provides a major source of inoculum for the molluscan stages of the life cycle. In Thailand, however, contamination of the fields where water caltrop and water morning glory are cultivated takes place in areas where there is little or no dry ground and where the people defecate directly into the standing water beneath the houses. Children frequently have heavy infections.

Control. To be effective, control requires that human excreta be treated before use as fertilizer, defecation not be permitted where edible plants are cultivated, and hogs not be allowed to forage in the fields where these plants are grown.

Amphistomate Flukes
(Amphistomiasis)

Two amphistomes have been reported as human parasites. These medium-sized fleshy worms have the following common characteristics: a large acetabulum situated at the posterior end of the worm; large, operculate eggs that are unembryonated when evacuated in the stool; and metacercariae that encyst like those of *Fasciolopsis buski* on vegetation, so that infection results from eating plants bearing the metacercariae. Herbivorous mammals are the usual definitive hosts. *Watsonius watsoni* has been obtained only once from man, a West African who died of severe diarrhea. At necropsy many worms were found attached to the duodenal and jejunal mucosa and free in the colon. Monkeys are considered to be the natural hosts. *Gastrodiscoides hominis* is a relatively common human parasite in

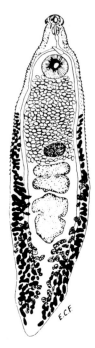

Fig. 8–5. *Echinostoma ilocanum,* ventral view. (× 20.) (Adapted by E.C. Faust from Odhner, T. 1911. *Echinostoma ilocanum* (Garr) ein neurer menschen Parasit aus Ostasien. Zool. Anzeiger, *38*:65–68.)

Bangladesh and adjacent parts of India and has been reported as endemic in parts of southeast Asia. Pigs in India and deer in Malaysia are known reservoirs. The parasite, which is attached to the cecum and ascending colon, produces a mucous diarrhea. The eggs (see Fig. 1–1W) are elongate and spindle-shaped, with bluntly rounded ends, and measure 150 to 152 μm by 60 to 72 μm.

Echinostomate Flukes
(Echinostomiasis)

Echinostomes are characterized by a collar of spines on a circumoral disc, interrupted on the ventral side and also mid-dorsally in the genus *Echinochasmus.* A few echinostomes are natural human parasites in Oriental countries, while several others have been incidentally reported from man.

Echinostoma ilocanum is relatively common among the Ilocano population of Luzon and occurs on other Philippine islands, in Java, and in parts of China. Infection results from eating raw snails containing the encysted metacercarial stage.

The living worms (Fig. 8–5), up to 6.5 mm in length by 1 to 1.35 mm in width, are attached to the wall of the small intestine. The small circumoral disc bears 49 to 51 spines. The large, straw-colored eggs, 83 to 116 μm by 58 to 69 μm, have a small operculum and are unembryonated when discharged in the feces. The molluscan hosts are species of planorbid and lymnaeid snails. After the cercariae escape from the snail, they enter the soft tissues of large edible snails such as *Pila conica* (Philippines) and *Viviparus javanicus* (Java), in which they encyst and are infective when eaten.

The mature worms may produce intestinal colic and diarrhea. Diagnosis is based on recovery of the eggs and their differentiation from those of other echinostomes and from *Fasciolopsis buski* and *Fasciola hepatica.* Treatment is with praziquantel in a single dose of 40 mg/kg body weight.

Other species of echinostomes that have been reported oc-

casionally as human parasites include *Echinostoma malayanum* from Malaysia, Sumatra, and India, *E. melis* from Romania and China, *E. revolutum* from Formosa and Indonesia, *E. cinetorchis* from Japan, Formosa, Korea, and Java, *E. hortense* from Japan, *Paryphostomum sufrartyfex* from Assam, *Himasthla muehlensi* once from New York City, *Echinoparyphium paraulum* from the U.S.S.R., *Echinochasmus perfoliatus* from Japan, and *Hypoderaeum conoideum* from northeastern Thailand.

HETEROPHYID FLUKES

Heterophyids are small, ovoid, pyriform or occasionally tongue-shaped flukes that live attached to the mucosa at the upper levels of the small intestine of birds and mammals. They are found at the base of the mucosal crypts and may be buried in the glands. In routine autopsies they are frequently overlooked but are readily obtained by examining superficial scrapings of the mucosa after shaking for 10 to 15 minutes in a 0.5% solution of sodium sulfate.

The small, ovoid, operculate eggs each contain a fully mature miracidium at the time they are evacuated in the feces, but hatching occurs only after ingestion by an appropriate operculate snail. Within the soft extraintestinal tissues of the mollusc, the miracidium transforms into a sporocyst. There are two generations of rediae that produce cercariae with a pair of pigmented "eye-spots" and a long tail that has a dorsal and a ventral fluted fin (*i.e.,* is lophocercous). The cercaria, after escape from the snail, becomes attached to the underside of the scales of fishes or penetrates into superficial tissues, where it discards its tail, rounds up, and becomes encysted. Infection is acquired when an infected fish is eaten.

Heterophyes heterophyes
(Heterophyiasis)

Heterophyes heterophyes (von Siebold, 1852) Stiles and Hassall, 1900, first found by Bilharz in 1851 at autopsy of a native of Cairo, Egypt, is a common parasite in the lower Nile Valley near the Mediterranean coast. It has been reported from Greece, Turkey, Israel, Morocco, Spain, Senegal and Nigeria. It occurs in the Orient and has been reported from Western India.

Biology and Life Cycle. The mature *H. heterophyes* (Fig. 8–6) is a minute pyriform worm, broadly rounded posteriorly and somewhat narrower anteriorly. It measures 1.0 to 1.7 mm in length by 0.3 to 0.4 mm in breadth. It is covered with minute spines set close together. The oral sucker is very small (90 μm in diameter) and the acetabulum considerably larger (230 μm in diameter). A conspicuous feature is the genital sucker, which lies on the lateral posterior border of the acetabulum. The seminal vesicle lacks an enveloping cirrus sac and there is no cirrus organ.

The eggs (Fig. 8–1) are small (28 to 30 μm by 15 to 17 μm), have a conspicuous conical operculum, and each contains a mature miracidium. When these eggs are ingested by *Pirenella conica* (Egypt) or *Cerithidea cingulata* (Japan), they hatch and proceed with their intramolluscan stages of development. The cercariae that escape from the mollusc encyst superficially in the skin of brackish or freshwater fishes, which constitute the source of infection for man and other mammals.

Pathogenesis and Symptomatology. *Heterophyes* and related species produce superficial irritation of the intestinal mucosa, with excess secretion of mucus. In heavy infections this may be accompanied by colicky pains and a mucous diarrhea. More serious is the occasional deep penetration of the worms so that their minute eggs get into mesenteric venules or lymphatics and are carried to the heart, brain, or spinal cord, where they may stimulate granulomatous reaction with symptoms related to these lesions. Fatalities result from heterophyid myocarditis in the Philippines.

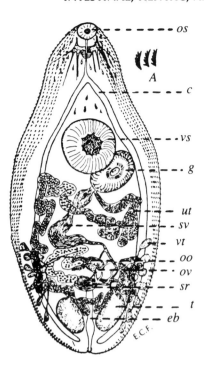

Fig. 8–6. *Heterophyes heterophyes*, ventral view. (× 50.) *c*, Cecum. *eb*, Excretory bladder. *g*, Genital sucker (gonotyl). *oo*, Ootype. *os*, Oral sucker. *ov*, Ovary. *sr*, Seminal receptacle. *sv*, Seminal vesicle. *t*, Testis. *ut*, Uterus. *vt*, Vitellaria. *vs*, Ventral sucker. *A*, Detail of spines of genital sucker. (Adapted by E.C. Faust from Looss, A. 1894. *Ueber den Bau von* Distomum heterophyes *V. Sieb. und* Distomum fraternum *n. sp.* Kassell, Th. G. Fisher & Co., 1894, Plate 1, Fig. 1.)

Diagnosis. Eggs of *H. heterophyes* (Fig. 8–1) and other heterophyid flukes are detected in the feces and must be differentiated from those of *Clonorchis sinensis* and species of *Opisthorchis* that are about the same size and general shape.

Treatment. Praziquantel and niclosamide, in view of their efficacy against other trematodes, probably are effective.

Epidemiology. Infection is acquired from eating brackish or freshwater fish (frequently mullet) in a raw, salted, or dried condition. Brackish water snails become infected when they ingest the eggs of the fluke discharged in the feces of definitive hosts.

Control. Infection can be prevented by not eating uncooked fish.

Metagonimus yokogawai
(Metagonimiasis)

Metagonimus yokogawai Katsurada, 1912 is probably the most common heterophyid fluke in the Orient, Maritime Provinces of U.S.S.R., northern Siberia, the Balkans, and Spain.

Biology and Life Cycle. *M. yokogawai* (Fig. 8–7) resembles *H. heterophyes* in its habitat, shape, size (1.0 to 2.5 mm by 0.4 to 0.75 mm), and life cycle. The distinctive features are in the acetabulum, which is deflected to one side of the midline, and the genital opening, which lacks an independent sucker but has its muscular rim fused with that of the acetabulum.

The eggs of *M. yokogawai*, measuring 26 to 28 μm by 15 to 17 μm, closely resemble those of *H. heterophyes* (Fig. 8–1) and are also easily mistaken for those of *Clonorchis sinensis*. The snail hosts are species of *Thiara, Semisulcospira*, and others

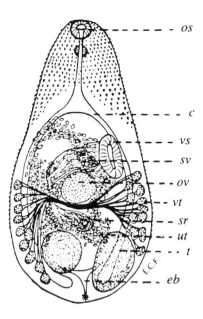

Fig. 8–7. *Metagonimus yokogawai*, ventral view. (× 36.) *c*, Cecum. *eb*, Excretory bladder. *os*, Oral sucker. *ov*, Ovary. *sr*, Seminal receptacle. *sv*, Seminal vesicle. *t*, Testis. *ut*, uterus. *vt*, Vitellaria. *vs*, Ventral sucker. (From Faust, E.C. 1949. *Human Helminthology*, 3rd ed. Philadelphia, Lea & Febiger, p. 226.)

that ingest the eggs. The cercariae that escape from the snail host become attached to freshwater fishes and encyst under the skin. Eating uncooked infected fish provides opportunity for infection.

Pathogenesis and Symptomatology. These minute worms live in mucosal crypts of the upper small intestine, causing excess secretion of mucus, superficial erosion of the mucosa, and granulomatous infiltration around eggs deposited in the tissues.

Diagnosis. Infection is detected by demonstration of eggs in the stool and their differentiation from those of other heterophyid flukes, *Clonorchis sinensis* and species of *Opisthorchis*.

Treatment. Praziquantel is the drug of choice, although niclosamide is also effective and safe.

Epidemiology. Man, fish-eating mammals, and the pelican are the natural hosts, which become infected from freshwater trout *(Plectoglossus altivelis), Odontobutis obscurus*, and *Salmo perryi*. Pollution of water with egg-laden feces of definitive hosts provides the source of infection for the intermediate hosts.

Control. Thorough cooking of freshwater fish will safeguard the human population.

Other Heterophyid Infections

Other heterophyid flukes have been reported from man, most of which occur in the China Sea area. Two species have been diagnosed in Hawaiians and Tokelau islanders who had eaten locally caught mullet. All such heterophyid flukes have the capacity to produce ectopic lesions when their eggs are carried in the lymphatics or bloodstream from the intestinal wall. In some communities of the Philippines, complications involving the heart, brain, spinal cord, liver, lungs, and spleen are not uncommon.

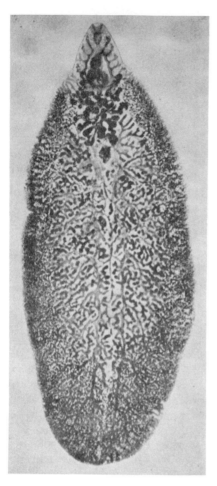

Fig. 8–8. *Fasciola hepatica,* ventral view. (× 4.) (By H.J. Van Cleave.) (From Faust, E.C. 1936. Diseases due to helminths and arthropods. *In* Brennemann's *Practice of Pediatrics,* Vol. II, Ch. 35. Hagerstown, Maryland, W.F. Prior Co., p. 41.)

HEPATIC FLUKES

Fasciola hepatica
(Fascioliasis hepatica)

Fasciola hepatica Linnaeus, 1758 was the first trematode to be described, by de Brie in 1379, and was likewise the first for which the complete life cycle was elucidated, by Leuckart in Germany in 1882 and by Thomas in England in 1883. It is particularly prevalent in sheep-raising areas, following the importation of sheep from Europe. In several countries the incidence of human infection is increasing.

Biology and Life Cycle. The mature *Fasciola hepatica* (Fig. 8–8) is large, measuring up to 30 mm by 13 mm. It is flattened, and at the anterior end there is a distinct, conical projection, while the posterior end is broadly rounded. Conspicuous morphologic features are extensive branching of the intestinal ceca, testes, and vitelline follicles, and a relatively short, convoluted uterus.

F. hepatica adults live in the larger bile ducts and gallbladder. Occasionally they fail to reach the liver and are found ectopically in the peritoneal cavity or other sites.

Eggs pass from the common bile duct into the intestinal tract to be evacuated in the feces. These eggs are large (130 to 150 μm by 63 to 90 μm), relatively thin-shelled, and have a small operculum. Unembryonated when laid, they require 9 to 15 days to mature in fresh water at an optimum temperature of 22° to 25°C (72° to 77°F). Upon hatching, the miracidium invades a lymnaeid snail, shedding its ciliated epithelium as it enters the tissues and transforms into a sporocyst. Within about 30 days, second and third generation rediae and cercariae are produced. Then the cercariae swarm out of the snail, crawl onto moist vegetation, shed their tails, round up, and encyst as metacercariae. These survive for a considerable time in a moist atmosphere but soon succumb to drying.

When metacercariae are ingested by mammals, they excyst and actively burrow through the intestinal wall, migrate to the liver, penetrate Glisson's capsule, and feed upon the tissues as they move through the hepatic parenchyma to the bile ducts, where they develop into adults. The prepatent period is about 2 months in calves, 3 to 4 months in man.

Pathogenesis and Symptomatology. The migrating young flukes passing through the hepatic parenchyma to the bile ducts cause traumatic damage and intense eosinophilic inflammation along their pathways. In the larger bile passages they produce hyperplasia of the biliary epithelium, with leukocytic infiltration and enveloping fibrosis of the ducts.

Early symptoms in human infections consist of right upper quadrant abdominal pain, fever, and hepatomegaly; biliary colic with coughing and vomiting; and marked jaundice. Generalized abdominal rigidity, diarrhea, irregular fever, profuse sweating, urticaria, and a significant eosinophilia may appear. Later there may be macrocytic anemia, empyema of the gallbladder, and cholecystitis or cholelithiasis. Adult worms may cause obstructive jaundice by blocking the common bile duct.

The mature or adolescent worms have been found in abscess pockets in blood vessels, lungs,

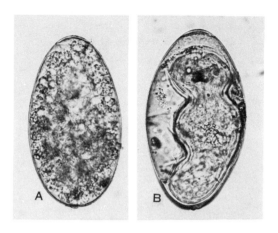

Fig. 8–9. *Fasciola hepatica.* Eggs from patient in Japan. *A*, Recovered from fresh bile. *B*, Containing miracidium after 10 days' incubation in water at 28°C. (× ca. 33.) (From Yoshida, Y., et al. 1974. A case of human infection with *Fasciola* sp. and its treatment with bithionol. Jpn. J. Parasitol., *23*:116–124.)

subcutaneous tissues, ventricles of the brain and the orbit, often associated with the presence of mature worms in the bile passages.

False or *spurious fascioliasis* refers to the appearance of eggs of *Fasciola* in the stool following ingestion of infected livers of sheep, goats, or cattle, raw or cooked.

Diagnosis. Most cases of fascioliasis hepatica are first detected by recovery of the eggs in the feces (Fig. 8–9). In cases of false fascioliasis, eggs will cease to appear in the feces a few days after the patient has been placed on a liver-free diet.

Treatment. The treatment of choice is currently bithionol given orally, but praziquantel is probably as effective as it is for other trematode infections.

Epidemiology. Sheep liver fluke infection is contracted by ingesting vegetation on which the metacercariae of *F. hepatica* have encysted. In the case of sheep and many other herbivorous mammals, exposure results from eating grass that has grown in marshy meadows or around ponds or streams where the infected snail hosts abound. Human infection is usually acquired by eating fresh watercress *(Nasturtium officinale)* to which the metacercarial cysts are attached. Several hundred autochthonous human cases have originated in Latin America, Mediterranean countries, England, Germany, Poland, the U.S.S.R., China, Hawaii, and East and South Africa. In Cuba, Uruguay, Chile and other Latin-American countries, and southern France and Algeria, human infection is relatively frequent and clinically important. Epidemics have been reported from Cuba, Mexico,

France, England, and Italy. High prevalences were reported from some Peruvian villages where the infections may have been acquired from eating raw plants other than watercress. Only one case of human fascioliasis has been demonstrated in the continental United States (Norton and Monroe, 1961), although the disease is prevalent in sheep and cattle in the South and West and has become established in the Middle West.

Control. Control requires measures to eradicate natural infection in sheep and other herbivorous mammals. Since most human infections result from the use of watercress as salad greens, human fascioliasis hepatica usually will be controlled if this food is omitted from the diet in enzootic areas. No satisfactory practical method has been devised for mass treatment of sheep and other reservoir hosts.

Fasciola gigantica
(Fascioliasis gigantica)

Fasciola gigantica Cobbold, 1856, the giant liver fluke, differs from *F. hepatica* in its greater length, more attenuate shape, slightly larger acetabulum, more anterior position of the testes, and larger size of the eggs (160 to 190 μm by 70 to 90 μm). The natural hosts are cattle, water buffalo, sheep, and other herbivorous mammals. The life cycle parallels that of *F. hepatica,* including lymnaeid snails as first intermediate hosts. Human infections have been reported from Senegambia, Cameroon, Zimbabwe, Rwanda, Burundi, Uganda, and Malawi in Africa, and from Vietnam, Uzbekistan (U.S.S.R), Iraq, and Hawaii. Clinical aspects of this infection are essentially the same as those of fascioliasis hepatica. *F. gigantica* has been reported in ectopic locations, especially in subcutaneous nodules and abscesses, more commonly in East Africa than elsewhere (Ongom, 1980).

Dicrocoelium dendriticum
(Dicrocoeliasis)

Dicrocoelium dendriticum (Rudolphi, 1818) Looss 1899 is a common parasite of bile passages of sheep and other herbivorous mammals in Europe, North Africa, northern Asia, and other parts of the Orient and to a lesser extent in North and South America. Numerous diagnoses of human infection have been reported from the U.S.S.R. and elsewhere; most of these are cases of false parasitosis resulting from eating infected livers, with the detection of eggs of *D. dendriticum* in the feces, but genuine human cases have been diagnosed from Europe, Asia, and Africa.

Biology and Life Cycle. The adult worm (Fig. 8–10) lives in the smaller bile ducts. It is lancet-shaped, flat, thin, and transparent. It is relatively small, measuring 5 to 15 mm by 1.5 to 2.5 mm, and has a smooth tegument. The most conspicuous features of its internal anatomy are the position of the testes anterior to the ovary in the anterior half of the body and distribution of the major portion of the long uterine coils in the median field of the posterior half of the body. Eggs are ovoid, thick-shelled, dark brown in color, have a broad convex operculum, measure 38 to 45 μm by 22 to 30 μm, and typically contain a mature miracidium when evacuated in the feces. When eggs are eaten by an appropriate land snail, the miracidium produces two generations of sporocysts, which in turn produce

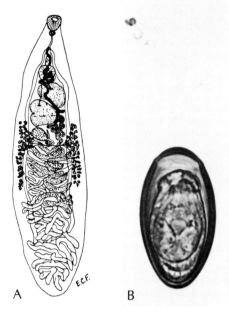

Fig. 8–10. *Dicrocoelium dendriticum, A,* Ventral view. (× 10.) *B,* Egg. (× 900.) (*A,* Adapted by E.C. Faust from original by M. Braun in Faust, E.C. 1949. *Human Helminthology,* 3rd ed. Philadelphia, Lea & Febiger, p. 202; *B,* Courtesy of G.H. Sahba.)

cercariae that have a delicate oral stylet and a long attenuated tail. The cercariae emerge from the molluscan host only when rains succeed a long dry period, and become massed in slime balls. A second intermediate host, a foraging ant *(Formica fusca),* eats the slime balls and the metacercariae become encysted. If the metacercaria is encysted in the brain of the ant, contraction of the mandibles causes the ant to remain fixed to vegetation. This enhances the fortuitous ingestion of the ant by the grazing animal or by man.

Pathogenesis and Symptomatology. The pathogenic effects of dicrocoeliasis are similar to those of fascioliasis but relatively less marked. The common symptoms are biliary colic, hepatitis, abdominal distress, flatulence, diarrhea, vomiting, and chronic constipation. Diagnosis is based on the continued recovery of the characteristic eggs in the stool or from biliary drainage (Fig. 8–10B). No dependable chemotherapy for human infection has been discovered. Praziquantel, which is effective against other trematodes, should be tried.

Dicrocoelium hospes occurs in West Africa and is responsible for some human infections. It is more slender and smaller than *D. dendriticum* and also differs from the latter species in some details of the genital organs (Malek, 1980).

Clonorchis sinensis
(Clonorchiasis)

Clonorchis sinensis (Cobbold, 1875) Looss, 1907, the Chinese liver fluke, was first reported by McConnell in 1875 from the bile passages of a Chinese carpenter at autopsy in Calcutta. The endemic-enzootic areas of *C. sinensis* extends from Japan to Vietnam.

Biology and Life Cycle. The mature *C. sinensis* lives typically in bile passages, most frequently in

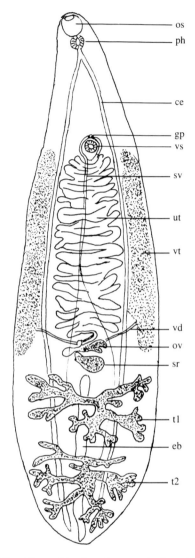

Fig. 8–11. *Clonorchis sinensis,* ventral view. (× 7.) *ce,* Cecum. *eb,* Excretory bladder. *gp,* Genital pore. *os,* Oral sucker. *ov,* Ovary. *ph,* Pharynx. *sr,* Seminal receptacle. *sv,* Seminal vesicle. *t1, t2,* Testes. *ut,* Uterus. *vs,* Ventral sucker (acetabulum). *vt,* Vitellaria. *vd,* Vitelline duct. (By E.A. Malek.)

the more distal tributaries. The worms (Fig. 8–11) are lanceolate, flat, transparent, pinkish in the living condition, and measure 10 to 25 mm long by 3 to 5 mm broad. The tegument is smooth. Internal structures are visible in the unstained living worm. At the anterior tip there is a globose oral sucker, and at about one fifth body length posteriorly there is a smaller acetabulum. Life cycle stages are shown in Fig. 8–1.

The eggs (Fig. 8–12) are broadly ovoid, have a moderately thick, light yellowish-brown shell with a distinct convex operculum that fits into a circular rim of the shell, and usually a small knob at the

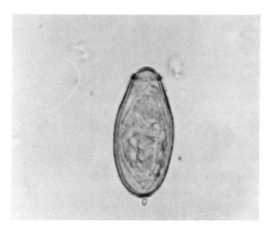

Fig. 8–12. *Clonorchis sinensis.* Egg with mature miracidium. (× 1000.) (From Beaver, P.C., Jung, R.C., and Cupp, E.W. 1984. *Clinical Parasitology,* 9th ed. Philadelphia, Lea & Febiger, p. 475.)

opposite end. They measure 27 to 35 μm in length by 12 to 20 μm in greatest diameter and are fully embryonated when discharged in the feces. They hatch only when ingested by a suitable species of operculate snail *(Parafossarulus, Bithynia, Alocinma);* the miracidia transform into sporocysts, one or two generations of rediae are produced, and these generate cercariae (Fig. 8–13). The cercariae escape from the rediae and continue their development in the snail's tissues; then they leave the snail and swim about for a short time in the water. On contact with freshwater fishes, the cercariae penetrate into the flesh and become encysted. On being eaten in uncooked fish, the metacercariae are digested out of the flesh and excyst in the duodenum, thereupon the larvae migrate through the ampulla of Vater to the smaller bile radicles, become attached, and develop into adult worms.

Pathogenesis and Symptomatology. Mature *C. sinensis* in the bile passages provoke hyperplasia of the biliary epithelium with subsequent dense fibrous envelopment of the duct. The number of worms may reach several thousand, and practically all the terminal bile ducts may have fibrous thickening of the walls with pressure necrosis of adjacent hepatic parenchyma.

In an epidemic of clonorchiasis described by Koenigstein in 1949, prodromal symptoms were observed less than a month after exposure, before eggs were detected in the stools. The clinical onset was gradual or sudden, with chills and fever up to 40°C. The liver was large and tender, and the sclerae were icteric. In some cases there was congestive splenomegaly. Eosinophil counts

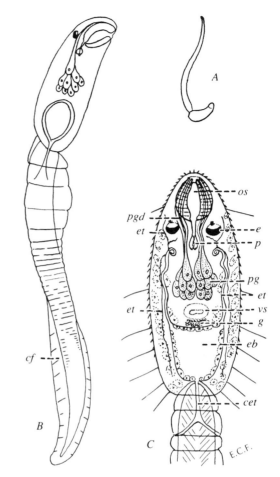

Fig. 8–13. *Clonorchis sinensis. A,* Cercaria as seen at rest in water. (× ca. 30.) *B,* Entire cercaria. (× 125.) *C,* Details of cercaria. (× 260.) *cet,* Caudal excretory tubule. *cf,* Caudal fin. *e,* Eyespot. *eb,* Excretory bladder. *et,* Excretory tubule. *g,* Genital primordium. *os,* Oral sucker. *pgd,* Penetration gland ducts. *pg,* Penetration glands. *p,* Pharynx. *vs,* Ventral sucker. (Adapted by E.C. Faust from Yamaguti, S. 1935. Ueber der Cercarie von *Clonorchis sinensis* (Cobbold). Z. Parasitenk., 8:183–187.)

ranged from 10 to 40%. Some weeks later the picture was one of cholecystitis and hepatitis. On the other hand, in light infections clonorchiasis may be essentially asymptomatic.

Diagnosis. The characteristic eggs may be demonstrated in direct fecal films, by a concentration technique, or by duodenal or biliary drainage.

Treatment. Praziquantel is the most effective and safest drug currently available (Rim *et al.,* 1981). Heavy infections complicated by the development of obstructive jaundice may require surgical relief of the obstruction.

Epidemiology. Infection is acquired by eating freshwater fish that is raw, pickled in brine or rice

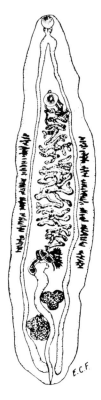

Fig. 8–14. *Opisthorchis felineus.* (× 10.) (Adapted by E.C. Faust from Stiles, C.W. 1904. *Illustrated Key to the Trematode Parasites of Man.* Washington, D.C., Hygienic Laboratory Bull. 17., U.S. Public Health and Marine Hospital Service, p. 32.)

wine, smoked or dried containing the encysted metacercariae.

Control. Cooking all fish that is intended to be eaten will safeguard the human population.

Opisthorchis felineus
(Opisthorchiasis felineus)

Opisthorchis felineus (Rivolta, 1884) Blanchard, 1895 was originally described from a cat in Italy and a few years later from man in Siberia. It has wide distribution in eastern and southeastern Europe and the Asiatic U.S.S.R. It has been recovered from man in India.

The adult worm (Fig. 8–14) closely resembles *Clonorchis sinensis* in size and general appearance. One notable difference is the smaller size and lesser notching of the testes. Eggs of *O. felineus* are narrower (30 by 11 μm) than those of *Clonorchis* but otherwise bear a close resemblance. The snail hosts are species of *Bithynia.* Freshwater fishes serve as second intermediate hosts. In addition to man, the dog, cat, fox, wolverine, and seal have been found to be naturally infected.

Clinical aspects and treatment of *O. felineus* infection are similar to those of clonorchiasis.

Opisthorchis viverrini
(Opisthorchiasis viverrini)

Opisthorchis viverrini (Poirier, 1886) Stiles and Hassall, 1896 is closely akin to *O. felineus.* It is endemic in northeastern

Thailand, where up to 25% of the population is infected. It also occurs in Laos, Malaysia, and probably other countries in southeast Asia. The infection commonly causes diarrhea, hepatic enlargement and tenderness, jaundice, and moderate fever. Symptoms increase progressively. Praziquantel is the drug of choice for treatment (Bunnag and Harinasuta, 1981).

PULMONARY FLUKES

Paragonimus westermani
(Paragonimiasis)

Paragonimus westermani (Kerbert, 1878) Braun, 1899, the Oriental lung fluke, was discovered in the lungs of two Bengal tigers that died in Hamburg and Amsterdam. The next year a Portuguese resident of Formosa was found by Ringer to have a pulmonary worm. In 1880 Manson found eggs of this fluke in the rusty-brown sputum of a Chinese patient. Baelz found similar eggs in the bloody sputum of a native Japanese, and 3 years later he discovered the flukes in the lungs of Japanese subjects. The life cycle was elucidated by Kobayashi in 1918 in Korea and by Yokogawa in 1919 in Formosa (Taiwan).

The most heavily endemic regions of Oriental paragonimiasis are in central China, Korea, Japan, the Philippines, and Taiwan. It occasionally has been reported from Manchuria, Nepal, and Thailand. It is known to be present in animals in Eastern USSR, Sri Lanka, India, Indonesia, Malaysia, and elsewhere in southeast Asia.

Biology and Life Cycle. The adult fluke normally lives in a fibrous capsule in the lungs, but it may also develop in other soft tissues of the body. This worm (Fig. 8–15) is stout and reddish-brown in the living state. It measures 7.5 to 12 mm in length, 4 to 6 mm in breadth, and 3.5 to 5 mm in thickness. The tegument bears scalelike spines. The oral sucker and acetabulum are subequal (0.75 to 0.8 mm) in diameter.

Eggs of *P. westermani* (Fig. 8–16A) are ovoid, relatively thick-shelled, golden-brown in color, have a somewhat flattened operculum, and measure 80 to 118 μm by 48 to 60 μm. They are unembryonated when laid.

When deposited the eggs reach the respiratory passages and are coughed up, imparting a rusty tinge to the sputum. Many are swallowed and evacuated in the feces. Eggs reaching clear, cool, running water embryonate and hatch in 16 or more days. The free-swimming miracidia (Fig. 8–16B) enter suitable operculate snails (species of *Semisulcospira, Thiara,* and *Brotia*). Development in the snail through sporocyst and redia stages pro-

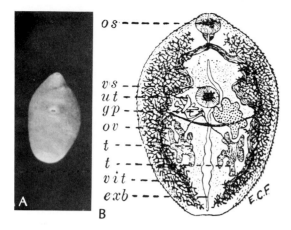

Fig. 8–15. *Paragonimus westermani. A,* Ventral view. (× 2.) *B,* Compressed, stained specimen, ventral view (× 5.) *exb,* Excretory bladder. *gp,* Genital pore. *os,* Oral sucker. *ov,* Ovary. *t,* Testis. *ut,* Uterus. *vit,* Vitellaria. *vs,* Ventral sucker. (Adapted by E.C. Faust from Leuckart, P. 1889. *Parasiten des Menschen,* Band 1, Lief. 4. Leipzig u. Heidelberg, C.F. Winter'sche Verlagshaundlung, p. 405.)

duces a brood of cercariae, which escape from the snail and are temporarily free in the water.

The cercaria is minute, about 200 μm long, with a large oral sucker beset with a dorsal stylet and a delicate knoblike tail. These nonswimming cercariae are transported by water currents and invade the viscera and muscles of freshwater crabs or, in Korea, a species of crayfish *(Procambarus clarkii),* and become encysted in their soft tissues.

When cysts are ingested by the definitive host, the young worms excyst and migrate through the intestinal wall to the peritoneal cavity, burrow

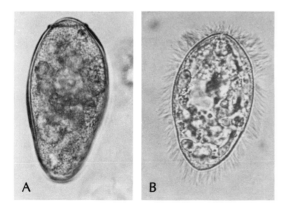

Fig. 8–16. *Paragonimus. A,* Egg of *P. westermani* from human feces. (× 450.) In either feces or sputum the eggs contain a clear ovum or immature embryo surrounded by yolk cells. *B,* Miracidium of *Paragonimus* species hatched from the egg after 3 weeks of incubation in a Harada-Mori test tube–filter paper culture of feces from an infected animal. (× ca. 450.) *(A,* By P.C. Beaver. *B,* By M.D. Little.)

through the diaphragm, enter the lungs, and finally settle down, usually in pairs, near a bronchiole, where they develop into adult worms within a fibrous capsule laid down by the host.

Pathogenesis and Symptomatology. In the pulmonary parenchyma, the host-tissue reaction consists of an eosinophilic and neutrophilic infiltration around the growing worm, followed by development of a thick fibrous capsule about 1 cm in diameter. Leakage from the cystic cavity into a bronchiole causes paroxysmal coughing frequently resulting in hemorrhage, with blood in the sputum.

The young worms often migrate into ectopic locations, including the liver, intestinal wall, mesenteric lymph nodes, peritoneum, muscles, myocardium, testes, pleura, brain, and subcutaneous tissues. In these abnormal sites there is a tendency for development of abscesses and pseudotubercules, or the lesion may be ulcerative.

Paragonimiasis of the lungs is usually insidious in its onset and mildly chronic in its course. There may be no symptoms other than occasional cough with rusty sputum. However, dyspnea, fever, malaise, and anorexia have been observed in cases of extensive pulmonary involvement.

Paragonimiasis in ectopic locations usually causes significant symptoms. In the pleura there may be a thick purulent effusion containing an abundance of the fluke's eggs. Glandular involvement characteristically provokes leukocytosis with fever. In the brain the worms reside in granulomatous tissues, characteristically producing a Jacksonian type of epilepsy and often intracranial calcification, which is revealed in skull radiographs. Impaired vision is common in cerebral paragonimiasis.

Diagnosis. Specific diagnosis can readily be made by recovery of the eggs of *P. westermani* (Fig. 8–16) in sputum, feces, pleural aspirate, or from abscesses. Intradermal and serodiagnostic tests provide evidence of infection. A roentgenogram may be helpful in making a tentative diagnosis of pulmonary paragonimiasis, although the chest shadows strongly parallel those of pulmonary tuberculosis. Cerebral paragonimiasis can be determined only after exploratory operation and recovery of the worm or its eggs.

Treatment. Since 1962 the drug of choice for treatment has been bithionol in 10 to 15 doses on alternate days. Niclofolan is effective in a single oral dose but produces side-effects, which make it less desirable than a 3-day course of praziquantel.

Epidemiology. The crustacean hosts typically live in clear, fresh water, usually in mountain streams that are contaminated with the egg-laden excreta of human and reservoir hosts. These provide the inoculum for the molluscan hosts and subsequently the crustaceans. Belief in the medicinal value of raw crustaceans is a factor in the prevalence of infection. Similarly, raw crabs are eaten by women in West Africa to increase fertility.

Control. For the individual in endemic areas, the disease can be prevented by taking care not to eat crabs or crayfish unless they have been thoroughly heated and not to contaminate the fingers while preparing raw crustaceans for the table. No public health program has been developed to control the infection. With effective mass treatment, the disease should eventually die out.

Other *Paragonimus* Species

Species of *Paragonimus* other than *P. westermani* cause infection in people in various parts of the world. Species causing human infections are *P. skrjabini*, *P. heterotremus*, and *P. heuitungensis* in China, *P. miyazakii* in Japan, *P. philippinensis* in the Philippines, *P. mexicanus* and probably other species in Mexico and Central and South America, *P. kellicotti* in the United States, and two species in West Africa, *P. africanus* and *P. uterobilateralis*. As the natural hosts of these species are wild crab- or crayfish-eating mammals, the infections are largely or entirely zoonotic. In their life cycles and the infections they cause in man, all *Paragonimus* species closely resemble *P. westermani*.

SUMMARY

1. Trematode parasites of man are digenetic, i.e., their life cycle involves alternating sexual and asexual generations. Adult worms, hermaphroditic except in schistosomes, by sexual reproduction generate eggs that develop into miracidia, and on entering a snail host the miracidia initiate a series of asexual generations of sporocysts or redia or both, and these produce cercariae, which generally encyst to become metacercariae on or in second intermediate hosts (plants or animals) to be eaten by man or other final host, in which they develop directly into the adult worms.

2. The principal intestinal flukes of man are *Fasciolopsis buski*, a large species common in the hog in the Orient, and various heterophyids, minute species found in fish-eating birds and mammals in the Near and Far East. *F. buski* infection is acquired when aquatic plants bearing metacercariae are eaten. Infective metacercariae of heterophyids are in freshwater fish. When numerous, intestinal flukes cause symptoms of enteritis. Diagnosis is based on identification of eggs in the feces. The drug of choice for treatment is praziquantel. Prevention consists in cooking the suspected sources of infective metacercariae.

3. The principal liver flukes of man are *Fasciola hepatica*, *Clonorchis sinensis*, and species of *Opisthorchis*. *Fasciola* infection, found mainly in sheep-raising areas of Europe and Latin America, is acquired by eating watercress or other aquatic plants bearing encysted metacercariae; clonorchiasis and opisthorchiasis are acquired from eating raw freshwater fish; the former is prevalent in the Orient, notably China, the latter in eastern Europe, the U.S.S.R., and parts of Southeast Asia. *Fasciola* enters the liver through Glisson's capsule and slowly migrates through the liver parenchyma to reach the larger bile ducts and causes massive eosinophilic infiltration of the damaged tissues, whereas *Clonorchis* and *Opisthorchis* species reach the biliary passages via the common bile duct. All liver flukes live in the biliary passages and cause hyperplasia of the epithelium and fibrosis of the walls. Diagnosis is based on detecting eggs in the feces or biliary drainage. The drug of choice for treatment is praziquantel. Prevention consists in avoiding raw salads containing watercress and cooking all freshwater fish in endemic areas.

4. The lung fluke *Paragonimus westermani* is distributed extensively in the Orient. Other *Paragonimus* species are found in the same areas and in small foci in West Africa and in central and northern South America. Infection is acquired by eating raw freshwater crabs (or crayfish in Korea) containing metacercariae. The ingested metacercariae (young flukes) migrate from intestine to lungs directly through tissues and body cavities and occasionally are found developing in abscesses in the brain, peritoneal cavity, and other ectopic locations. Usually found in pairs in the lung parenchyma, they induce host-tissue encapsulation with a channel to a bronchiole for discharge of eggs, which cause cough with blood-tinged sputum. Diagnosis is made by demonstrating eggs in sputum or feces. The drug of choice for treatment is praziquantel. Prevention consists of not eating freshwater crabs and crayfish, except when well cooked.

REFERENCES

Bunnag, D., and Harinasuta, T. 1981. Studies on the chemotherapy of human opisthorchiasis. III. Minimum effective dose of praziquantel. S. E. Asian J. Trop. Med. Publ. Hlth., *12*:413–417.

Koenigstein, R.P. 1949. Observations on the epidemiology of infections with *Clonorchis sinensis*. Trans. R. Soc. Trop. Med. Hyg., *42*:503–506.

Malek, E.A. 1980. *Snail-Transmitted Parasitic Diseases*, Vol. II. Boca Raton, Fla., CRC Press, 324 pp.

Norton, R.A., and Monroe, L. 1961. Infection by *Fasciola hepatica* acquired in California. Gastroenterology, *41*:46–48.

Ongom, V.L. 1980. Episternal abscess due to fascioliasis in an Etesot in Uganda. Trans. R. Soc. Trop. Med. Hyg., *74*:417.

Rim, H-J., Lyu, S-S., and Joo, K-J. 1981. Clinical evaluation of the therapeutic efficacy of praziquantel (Embay 8440) against *Clonorchis sinensis* infection in man. Ann. Trop. Med. Parasitol., *75*:27–33.

Chapter 9

Blood Flukes or Schistosomes

E. A. Malek

The digenetic trematodes that inhabit the bloodstream of vertebrate hosts are commonly referred to as blood flukes, and those of birds and mammals are known as schistosomes, so-called because of the "split body" on the ventral side of the male, in which the female is held during insemination and egg laying. All blood flukes of man are dioecious.

SCHISTOSOMES AS A GROUP

Human infection with blood flukes is often referred to as bilharziasis in honor of Theodor Bilharz, who in 1851 discovered the parasite *(Schistosoma haematobium)* at the post mortem of a man who died in Cairo, Egypt. The disease caused by blood flukes is often insidious. On the other hand, there are notable instances of the course of world history's being influenced by this disease's dramatic effects on military operations.

Adult Blood Flukes. The male and female worms in continuous copula live in portal venous blood vessels or in the vesical venules of the caval system. At times, however, they are carried or migrate into the intrahepatic portal vessels, pelvic veins, pulmonary arterioles, or to distant ectopic sites.

The mature schistosomes are delicate and cylindroidal, accommodated to the smaller veins by usually lying with the anterior end directed toward the capillaries. The somewhat larger, more muscular male is attached by its suckers to the wall of the vessel, holding the threadlike female in its sex canal and thus enabling the female to extend its anterior extremity into the smaller venules in which it deposits its eggs. The worms may live for 30 years in the human host. However, the average life span of schistosomes is possibly less than 5 years.

Life Cycle. Eggs of schistosomes are relatively thin-shelled and nonoperculate. They are laid in the smaller venules, where they obstruct the normal flow of blood. Obstruction of the venules, pressure exerted by the worm, increase in size of the egg, and hypermotility of the parasitized organ cause the blood vessel to rupture and discharge the eggs into surrounding tissues. Maturation of the miracidium inside the egg while in the tissues takes place within about 1 week *(S. mansoni* and *S. haematobium)* or 12 days *(S. japonicum)*, after which the egg is sloughed into the lumen of the organ and evacuated in the feces (intestinal types) or urine (vesical type).

When the eggs in feces or urine reach fresh water, hatching occurs and the miracidia become free-swimming. The miracidium eventually penetrates any of several species of snails, but only in an appropriate snail can it develop into a sporocyst. Within the first-generation sporocyst several second-generation sporocysts are developed, and these escape from the parent sporocyst and migrate further into the snail's tissues. Here fork-tailed cercariae are produced over a period of several weeks. When mature, the cercariae emerge from the snail and swim about in the water (Fig. 9–1).

On contact with the skin, the cercariae penetrate the outer layers, shedding the tail as they enter. After entry they are called *schistosomula*. On reaching the dermis they enter a venule or lymph vessel and soon reach the right side of the heart and then the lungs. After growth and development in the lungs, they migrate to the liver, where they develop to maturity. The route by which the schistosomula reach the liver is unknown. They may return to the heart by crawling against the bloodstream along the walls of the pulmonary arteries

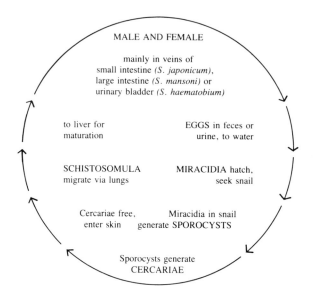

Fig. 9–1. *Schistosoma* species. Diagram of the life cycle.

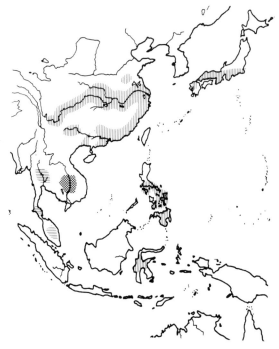

Fig. 9–2. Map showing the distribution of *Schistosoma japonicum (vertical shading), Schistosoma mekongi (diagonal shading),* and *Schistosoma japonicum*-like *(horizontal shading)* schistosomes in the Orient. (By E.A. Malek and R.C. Jung.)

and continue to move against the current through the atrium, posterior vena cava, and hepatic vein into the liver (Kruger *et al.,* 1969). An alternative theory is that the schistosomula force their way through the pulmonary capillaries into the veins, where they are passively carried to the liver through the left side of the heart and arterial channels to the hepatic artery or through the intestinal arteries and intestinal capillaries to the portal vein and liver (Miller and Wilson, 1980). This route was described by Faust and Meleney in 1924. On reaching sexual maturity, each male embraces a female and migrates against the incoming portal bloodstream to the location where egg-laying occurs—primarily in the venules of the small intestine for *S. japonicum,* the colon for *S. mansoni,* and the urinary bladder for *S. haematobium.*

Pathogenesis. Pathologic changes resulting from blood fluke infection in a susceptible host are divided into three consecutive periods: (1) *prepatent period,* from skin penetration to the appearance of eggs in the excreta, (2) *acute stage,* which is one of active egg deposition and extrusion, and (3) *chronic stage,* which consists of stable egg output, tissue proliferation, and repair.

Symptomatology, Diagnosis, and Treatment. These topics are considered separately for each species.

Epidemiology. The usual means of human exposure consist of wading, swimming, bathing, or washing clothes in shallow fresh water near the infected snail hosts. Excreta of man and reservoir hosts containing viable schistosome eggs provide the inoculum that initiates the extrinsic phase of the parasite's life cycle. *Schistosoma japonicum* has numerous mammalian reservoirs, yet the use of human feces as fertilizer for crops in endemic areas probably constitutes the most important source of infection. In contrast, *S. mansoni* and *S. haematobium* are perpetuated almost exclusively by the promiscuous discharge of human waste into nearby water.

The geographic distribution of these three blood flukes is shown in Figs. 9–2 and 9–3.

Control. The possibilities for control are through effective mass treatment to eliminate the sources of infection in snails, sanitation to eliminate contamination of water where the vector snails live, and destruction of the snails or their habitats to eliminate an essential part of the parasite's life cycle (Ansari, 1973). Thus far the most successful approach has been through snail control (Hunter *et al.,* 1982).

Schistosoma japonicum
(Schistosomiasis japonica)

The Oriental blood fluke, *Schistosoma japonicum,* was first described and named by Katsurada

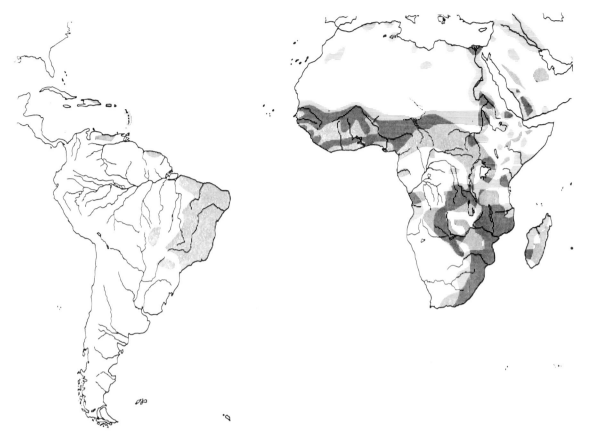

Fig. 9–3. Map showing distribution of *Schistosoma haematobium (horizontal shading)* and *Schistosoma mansoni (vertical shading)*. (By E.A. Malek and R.C. Jung.)

in 1904. In 1909 Fujinami and Nakamura demonstrated that the portal of entry into the definitive host was through the skin, and in 1913 and 1914 Miyairi and Suzuki elucidated the extrinsic stages of the life cycle.

Schistosomiasis japonica is confined to the Far East and occurs mainly in China, Japan, and the Philippines (Fig. 9–2). In Taiwan, *S. japonicum* is enzootic and, except in one endemic focus, produces patent infection only in nonhuman hosts. It has been discovered in an isolated community at Lake Lindu on the island of Sulawesi in Indonesia. *S. japonicum*-like eggs have been found at autopsy or on rectal biopsy of aborigines in Malaysia.

Biology and Life Cycle. Adult males of *S. japonicum* (Fig. 9–4) measure 12 to 20 mm by about 0.5 mm. The tegument is smooth. Conspicuous features of the body are the subequal oral sucker and acetabulum, the long ventral sex canal, and the relatively large testes (there are usually 7) behind the acetabulum.

Females are much more delicate, with a length

of 15 to 30 mm and a breadth of 0.1 to 0.3 mm. Eggs discharged in the feces are usually rotund, measure 70 to 100 μm, and each contains a ciliated miracidium (Fig. 9–5). A minute blunt projection may be seen on the outer surface halfway between the equator and one pole. This is often obscured by adherent cellular debris.

The earliest habitat of the young adult *S. japonicum* is the tributaries of the superior mesenteric vein of the small intestine. Later, some worms migrate into the inferior mesenteric vein. In these locations, females continue to lay eggs daily over a period of years.

Fully embryonated viable eggs in feces (Fig. 9–5) soon hatch on contact with fresh water and the miracidia attack and enter the tissues of various snails. In an appropriate snail (species of the genus *Oncomelania*), the intramolluscan phase is completed and cercariae begin to emerge into the water in 6 to 7 weeks at summer temperatures (Fig. 9–6). On contact with skin the cercariae become attached, penetrate into cutaneous capillaries, and

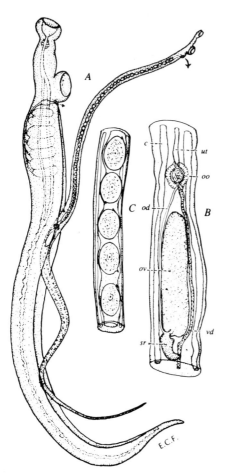

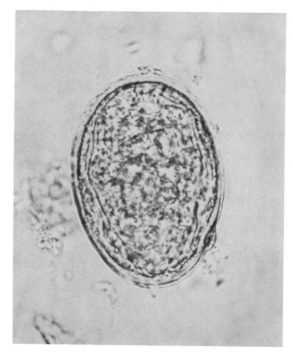

Fig. 9–5. *Schistosoma japonicum.* Egg containing fully developed miracidium in freshly passed feces. (× 650.) (By M.D. Little.)

Fig. 9–4. *Schistosoma japonicum,* adult male and female. *A,* Female in gynecophoral canal of male, in position for laying eggs. *Arrows* indicate genital pores. *B,* Detail of female at level of ootype and ovary. *C,* Portion of uterus. *c,* Cecum. *od,* Oviduct. *oo,* Ootype. *sr,* Seminal receptacle. *ut,* Uterus. *vd,* Vitelline duct. (From Faust, E.C. 1949. *Human Helminthology,* 3rd ed. Philadelphia, Lea & Febiger, p. 141.)

begin their blood migration. Approximately 4 to 5 weeks later they have matured in the smaller branches of the superior mesenteric vein, and egg-laying begins.

Pathogenesis and Symptomatology. The tissue and humoral changes produced by *S. japonicum* conform in general to what is described for other schistosome species, but the following points require special emphasis: the prepatent period is relatively short, *i.e.,* 4 to 5 weeks; the number of eggs produced by each female *S. japonicum* is greater than that produced by the other common species; and the brunt of the damage is borne by the small intestine and the liver.

Damage is produced as each egg escapes from a venule, filters through the tissues, and is extruded into the lumen of the intestine through the ruptured mucosa, with accompanying hemorrhage. The eggs pass down the intestinal canal and are evacuated in the feces, sometimes mixed with bloody mucus. Meanwhile, the worms' metabolites continue to produce systemic sensitization, resulting in eosinophilic leukocytosis that occasionally reaches 90% of the total leukocyte count. Over a period of 5 years in heavy infections the picture may assume grave proportions, with the development of fibrosis, papillomas, and stenosis of the intestinal tract, hepatic fibrosis with ascites, splenomegaly, and at times pulmonary fibrosis.

Toward the end of the prepatent period the patient begins to have late afternoon fever, night sweats, and diarrhea, usually with an enlarged tender liver, epigastric distress, and pain in the back, groin, or legs. In some cases giant urticaria develops about this time or somewhat later.

The acute stage is characteristically ushered in with diarrhea and the appearance of eggs in the feces, daily fever, epigastric pain, and continued enlargement of the liver. The patient loses appetite and weight and takes to his bed, but after a few weeks he may feel better and return to work, only to have a recurrence of symptoms on physical ex-

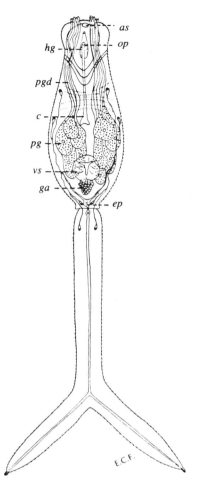

Fig. 9–6. *Schistosoma japonicum,* cercaria. *as,* Opening of anterior sucker. *c,* Cecum. *ep,* Excretory pore. *ga,* Genital anlage. *hg,* Head gland. *op,* Oral pore. *pg,* Penetration glands. *pgd,* Penetration gland ducts. *vs,* Ventral sucker. (× 340.) (From Faust, E.C. 1949. *Human Helminthology,* 3rd ed. Philadelphia, Lea & Febiger, p. 146.)

ertion. The blood picture is one of anemia and an increase in serum globulin levels, with continued high eosinophilia.

As the chronic stage develops, the liver becomes increasingly fibrosed, with multiple minute granulomas in the parenchyma and on the surface (Figs. 9–7 and 9–8). The mesentery and omentum may be thickened so as to bind down the colon and separate the abdomen into an upper and a lower portion. Somewhat later, increasing ascites and emaciation develop along with hepatic facies, dyspnea on slight exertion, dilatation of the superficial abdominal veins, and in some patients a myocarditis due to infiltration of eggs into the cardiac wall. The patient gradually goes into a decline

and may die of exhaustion or a supervening infection.

Diagnosis. During the prepatent period, specific diagnosis is not possible. With development of the acute stage eggs can usually be recovered in the feces, although sedimentation, acid-ether concentration, or Kato thick-smear techniques may be required to discover the eggs. Intradermal and other serologic tests with schistosome antigen (see Technical Aids) will provide additional evidence of the infection.

Treatment. See page 107.

Epidemiology. Most mammals are susceptible to *S. japonicum* infection. Exposure occurs when cercariae in infected water come in contact with the skin, most frequently during wading, bathing, or washing clothes in infested canals. The principal source of infection in the snail is fecal contamination by man, although eggs are shed by cattle, buffalo, and other mammals.

Control. Schistosomiasis japonica is most difficult to control because of the numerous reservoir hosts. Moreover, it may be impractical for natives in endemic enzootic areas to avoid contact with infested water.

A method of control that may become practical in the extensive endemic territories in the Far East is the application of chemicals to kill the snail host. Niclosamide (Bayluscide) was found to be very effective in the Philippines and sodium pentachlorophenate worked well in Japan. A Japanese product, Yurimin, is also effective against the amphibious snail hosts in the Orient. Where the terrain is not suitable for application of molluscicides, naturalistic methods such as draining, filling, ponding, or pumping of flood plains and low-lying marshy and swampy ground may be effective. In Japan, cement lining of irrigation ditches has been successful in reducing the snail population (Hunter *et al.,* 1982).

Schistosoma mekongi
(Mekong schistosomiasis)

S. mekongi Voge, Bruckner and Bruce, 1978 is a schistosome related to *S. japonicum* and is found in Laos and Cambodia. It differs from *S. japonicum* in that it has smaller eggs, a longer prepatent period in the mammalian host, its intermediate host is an aquatic hydrobiid snail, *Tricula aperta,* and thus far it has not been found capable of infecting *Oncomelania* spp., the amphibious snail hosts of *S. japonicum* (Voge *et al.,* 1978). In Laos, *S. mekongi* was reported on Khong Island, in the Mekong River, and in Cambodia it is found near Kratie, a floating village on the lower Mekong River. The identity of the schistosome producing *S. japonicum*-like eggs in Thailand has not been determined with certainty.

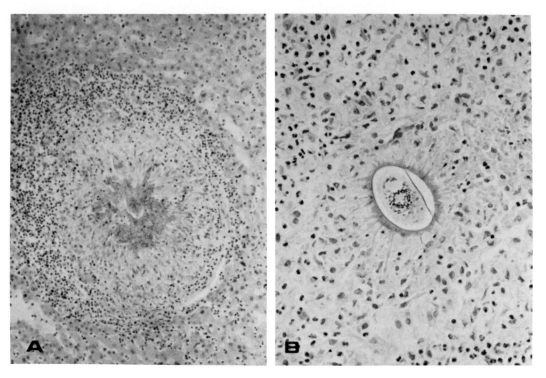

Fig. 9–7. *Schistosoma japonicum.* Eggs in liver of man in the Philippines. *A,* In a granuloma with chronic inflammatory cells at the periphery (× 100). *B,* Egg at center of granuloma with eosinophilic material radiating from the eggshell, known as the Hoeppli reaction (× 250). (From Beaver, P.C., Jung, R.C., and Cupp, E.W. 1984. *Clinical Parasitology,* 9th ed. Philadelphia, Lea & Febiger, p. 422.)

Schistosoma mansoni
(Schistosomiasis mansoni)

While studying human blood fluke infection in Egypt, Bilharz in 1852 found that some female worms contained lateral-spined eggs. In 1907 Sambon proposed the name *mansoni* for this type of schistosome. In 1918 Leiper described morphologic and life-cycle differences between *Schistosoma mansoni* and *S. haematobium.*

Manson's blood fluke is fundamentally a parasite of man on the continent of Africa (Fig. 9–3). It is hyperendemic in the Nile Delta and is present immediately south of Cairo but absent elsewhere in Egypt. It is common throughout practically all of tropical Africa, where it sometimes coexists with *S. haematobium.* It is present in several foci of the Arabian peninsula. Importation of infected African slaves to tropical America provided opportunity for establishing the disease in Brazil, Surinam, Venezuela, and several of the West Indies.

Biology and Life Cycle. Males of *S. mansoni* (Fig. 9–9) have a length of 6.4 to 9.9 mm, females, 7.2 to 14 mm. The tegument of the male is provided with numerous warty excrescences. The testes,

numbering 6 to 9, form a grapelike cluster a short distance behind the acetabulum. The most striking internal feature of the female is a short uterus, containing very few eggs. The worms usually reside in tributaries of the inferior mesenteric vein adjacent to the lower colon, although they may be found at higher levels of the intestine, in intrahepatic portal veins, in vesical venules, in pulmonary arterioles, and rarely in other ectopic foci.

Fully developed eggs of *S. mansoni* as recovered from feces (Fig. 9–10) are large, rounded at both ends, and provided with a conspicuous lateral spine near one pole, extending at an obtuse angle from the shell's long axis. The eggs range in size from around 120 × 45 μm when laid to 170 × 65 when ready to hatch.

On dilution of the host's feces with fresh water, the fully embryonated eggs hatch and the miracidia are attached to and penetrate and develop in freshwater snails of the genus *Biomphalaria.* The cercariae that later emerge from the snail become attached to and enter human skin, and after development in the lungs and liver, they migrate to the mesenteric-portal vessels. The time required

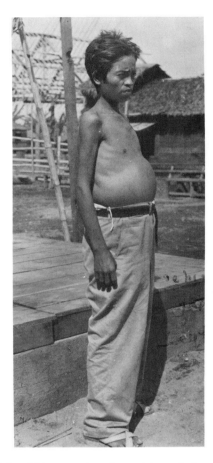

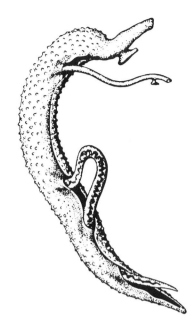

Fig. 9–9. *Schistosoma mansoni,* adult male and female in copula. Note the tegumental tuberculations on the male. (× 10.) (From Gönnert, R. 1948. Die Struktur der Korperoberfläche von *Bilharzia mansoni* (Sambon, 1907). Ztschr. Tropenmed. u. Parasitol., *1*:105–112.)

Fig. 9–8. *Schistosoma japonicum.* Advanced disease in a Philippino boy from an endemic area on the Island of Leyte. (Courtesy of U.S. Public Health Service, 1945.)

for their maturation to the egg-laying stage is about 6 to 7 weeks. Infections are known to persist for more than 32 years (Harris *et al.,* 1984).

Pathogenesis and Symptomatology. Humoral and tissue changes caused by *S. mansoni* closely resemble those of infection with *S. japonicum* but (1) the incubation period is about 2 weeks longer; (2) the early intestinal lesions typically develop in the colon rather than the small intestine, and (3) the number of eggs produced by each *S. mansoni* female is less, and therefore for each worm there are fewer eggs extruded from the intestinal wall and fewer that later become trapped in the perivascular tissues of the intestine and liver. Thus intestinal and hepatic fibrosis develop more slowly in Manson's schistosomiasis (Fig. 9–11).

There is no notable difference in the prepatent symptoms between infection with *S. mansoni* and *S. japonicum.* There may be evidence suggestive of peptic ulcer, malabsorption syndrome, gastroin-

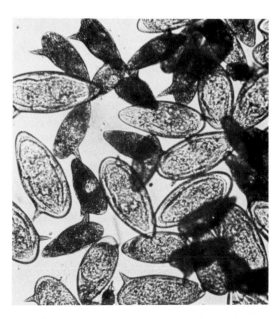

Fig. 9–10. *Schistosoma mansoni.* Eggs obtained from worms *in vitro* and incubated for 12 days. Eggs failing to develop remained as small as when laid, whereas the dimension of eggs that developed a mature miracidium increased markedly in all parts except the spine. (× 180.) (Courtesy of T.H Weller.) (From Beaver, P.C., Jung, R.C., and Cupp, E.W. 1984. *Clinical Parasitology,* 9th ed. Philadelphia, Lea & Febiger, p. 429.)

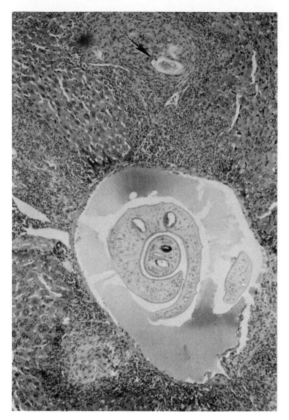

Fig. 9–11. *Schistosoma mansoni.* Egg in granuloma in parenchyma *(arrow)* and male and female worms in intrahepatic blood vessel in section of liver of experimental animal. (× 100.) (Adapted from Malek, E.A. 1980. *Snail-Transmitted Parasitic Diseases.* Vol. I, Boca Raton, Florida, CRC Press, p. 265.)

testinal bleeding, rectal polyps, thrombophlebitis, and hepatic fibrosis. Hepatic fibrosis develops much more gradually than in schistosomiasis japonica, frank ascites is less frequent, and fibrosis of the mesentery and omentum is rarely demonstrated. Nevertheless, very heavy infections with *S. mansoni* produce severe toxic symptoms and may be fatal. Pulmonary lesions and symptoms are relatively common in Manson's schistosomiasis. The severity of the disease depends largely on the number of worms causing it.

Diagnosis. A diagnosis usually is made on demonstration of characteristic eggs of *S. mansoni* in the feces (Fig. 9–10). As eggs rarely are abundant, a concentration technique must be used routinely. Rectal biopsy can be a particularly fruitful procedure, the specimen being cut into small portions and examined fresh under pressure of a coverglass. The large eggs are readily seen under low magnification of the microscope. Several immunodi-

agnostic tests are available, but they are more useful for epidemiologic than for clinical studies. These include the circumoval precipitin test, Cercarien-Hüllen Reaktion, immunodiffusion, immunoelectrophoresis, and varieties of fluorescent antibody tests. The circumoval precipitin test is both highly sensitive and specific for infections with *S. mansoni.*

Treatment. See page 107.

Epidemiology. Although several species of mammals have been found to be infected with *S. mansoni,* both in Africa and Brazil, the only important definitive host is man. Human exposure results from contact with cercaria-infested water.

Control. Because there are no important reservoir hosts for Manson's schistosomiasis, unsanitary disposal of human excreta constitutes the main obstacle to control. Rice fields and sugar cane plantations under irrigation and other cultivated areas provide a challenge for the sanitary engineer. Chemotherapy combined with snail control can be effective in stable communities. Niclosamide (Bayluscide) is an effective available molluscicide. Frescon, though effective, is not readily available. Because of their relatively low cost in some areas, molluscicides derived from plants may become useful. Biologic control with predators can be effective against medically important snails in restricted habitats such as ponds. The large, operculate ampullarid snail, *Marisa cornuarietis,* was found to be an effective competitor of *B. glabrata* in irrigation ponds in Puerto Rico. In some habitats of Puerto Rico and the Dominican Republic, the Oriental snail *Thiara granifera,* which was accidentally introduced, has displaced *B. glabrata.* Field trials with *T. granifera* in St. Lucia extended these observations (Prentice, 1983).

Schistosoma haematobium
(Schistosomiasis haematobia)

Vesical blood fluke disease caused by *Schistosoma haematobium* (Bilharz, 1852) Weinland, 1858 was prevalent in Egypt in ancient times, as demonstrated by examination of mummies. Adult worms were first recovered at autopsy by Theodor Bilharz, in 1851, from the mesenteric veins of a native in a Cairo hospital. In 1918, Leiper provided conclusive evidence that *S. haematobium* and *S. mansoni* were separate species.

In spite of evidence of the antiquity of human schistosomiasis in Egypt, it is now believed that this was not the geographic area where the parasites

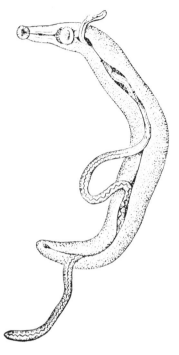

Fig. 9–12. *Schistosoma haematobium,* adult male and female. Note fine tegumental spinosities on male (× 12.) (Adapted by E.C. Faust from Looss, A. 1896. Recherche sur la faune parasitaire de l'Egypte. Premier partie. Mem. Inst. Egypt., 3:1–252.)

originated. The central East African Lake Plateau harbors a complexity of snail hosts and schistosomes, and it is probable that the simpler varieties in Egypt were carried down the Nile from this region. The migration of the Bantu southward probably also carried the parasites from the same central East African region to the southern part of Africa. The present day distribution of urinary schistosomiasis (Fig. 9–3) includes practically the entire African Continent (with the exception of desert regions), Malagasy, areas in the Arabian peninsula and Lebanon, several centers in Syria near the Turkish border, the lower Tigris-Euphrates valley, and western Iran. Endemic centers formerly in southern Portugal and Cyprus are now extinct. Controversy exists as to the specific identity of a schistosome causing urinary infection in two villages in Bombay State, India.

Biology and Life Cycle. The male, measuring 10 to 15 mm in length by about 1 mm in greatest girth (Fig. 9–12), has 4 to 5 small subglobose testes immediately behind the acetabulum. The female is delicately formed, with a length of about 20 mm and a diameter of 0.25 mm. The genital organs, exclusive of the vitellaria, occupy the median longitudinal field and the uterus is long. On oviposition the eggs are immature, but when shed from the tissues and excreted, they usually have become fully embryonated (Fig. 9–13A).

The mature egg of *S. haematobium* (Fig. 9–14) is rounded at one pole and has a terminal spine at the other. It measures up to 170 μm in length by 70 μm in breadth and is straw-colored and relatively transparent. When these eggs reach fresh water they soon hatch, and escaping miracidia are attracted to and penetrate the soft tissues of appropriate snails, species of *Bulinus,* in which they undergo development and multiplication, with emergence of large numbers of fork-tailed cercariae beginning 4 to 8 weeks later.

On contact with human skin the cercariae penetrate and migrate in blood vessels through the lungs into portal blood, where they feed and grow; about 3 weeks after skin exposure they begin to migrate against the venous current into the inferior mesenteric vein and rectal vessels. In this location some worms mature and oviposit, but a majority migrate through the hemorrhoidal anastomoses and pudendal vein to the vesical plexus, the optimum location for this species. Usually eggs first appear in the urine 10 to 12 weeks after skin penetration.

Like *S. japonicum* and *S. mansoni,* in exceptional cases *S. haematobium* may live for 20 to 30 years.

Pathogenesis and Symptomatology. The symptoms during the prepatent period in schistosomiasis haematobia parallel those of the two intestinal types of the disease, but there is usually less evidence of acute hepatitis.

Egg deposition and extrusion cause local damage to the tissues of the rectum or urinary bladder. Ulceration and irritation of the epithelium of the bladder lead to formation of polyps, which may undergo malignant change. Numerous eggs become calcified, giving the inner surface a "sandy" appearance, and calculi may form in the lumen (Fig. 9–13B). Extensive fibrosis of the bladder wall leads to marked contraction of the organ, whereas fibrosis of the bladder neck obstructs the flow of urine and leads to the development of hydroureter and hydronephrosis. The latter may be associated with bacteriuria, most often involving *Salmonella* species. In women the vulva frequently is hyperplastic and indurated. Advanced cases of vesical schistosomiasis often have septic involvement.

During the prepatent period, the patient may be essentially symptomless or may have increasing

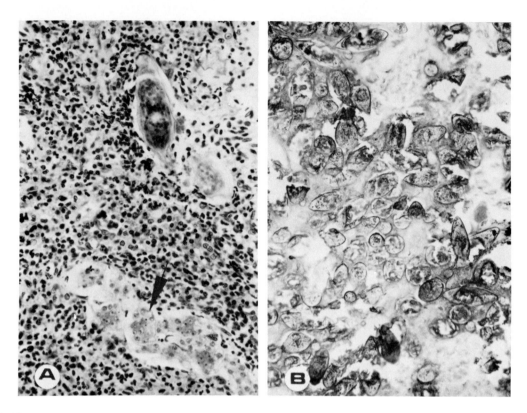

Fig. 9–13. *Schistosoma haematobium.* Eggs in histological section of bladder wall. *A,* From early infection showing an egg with well-developed shell and miracidium, and several freshly deposited eggs with shell only vaguely evident and miracidium immature *(arrow).* (× 250.) *B,* From late heavy infection showing numerous calcified eggs in a matrix of fibrous tissue. (× 100.) (From Beaver, P.C., Jung, R.C., and Cupp, E.W. 1984. *Clinical Parasitology,* 9th ed. Philadelphia, Lea & Febiger, p. 439.)

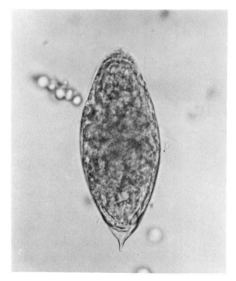

Fig. 9–14. *Schistosoma haematobium.* Egg from urine containing fully developed miracidium with its anterior end at the egg's spine. Miracidia may face either pole of the egg. (× 400.) (From Beaver, P.C., Jung, R.C., and Cupp, E.W. 1984. *Clinical Parasitology,* 9th ed. Philadelphia, Lea & Febiger, p. 440.)

malaise with late afternoon fever, moderate hepatic pain or epigastric distress, and an elevated eosinophil count. If worms mature in the rectal veins, there may be severe tenesmus with dysentery. More often the first evidence of the infection is the painless passage of blood at the end of micturition, but more and more there is also discharge of pus cells and necrotic tissue debris, decrease in the intervals between urination, and eventually incontinence or anuria due to urethral stricture. Bladder colic is a cardinal symptom.

Diagnosis. Infection is diagnosed by identifying characteristic eggs (Fig. 9–14) in urine sediment. Immunologic tests may be valuable, especially in epidemiologic surveys. Bladder biopsy may be useful in demonstrating the eggs. Because of the common involvement of the rectum in this infection, rectal examination may be diagnostically helpful.

Treatment. See page 107.

Epidemiology. Man is the only important definitive host of *S. haematobium.* Since the eggs of this worm are extruded from the wall of the bladder and excreted in the urine, urination into bodies of fresh water such as ponds, irrigation canals, and primitive latrines situated over small rivers or ponds, and the emptying of excreta from night pails into streams all provide sources of infection for the snail hosts, which are species of *Bulinus (Bulinus),* and *Bulinus (Physopsis).*

The prevalence of schistosomiasis haematobia varies from small percentages to near the total of a native population. The infection is particularly prevalent among young boys who wade or swim in polluted water.

Extension of irrigation projects throughout Africa and the Middle East is responsible for the spread of vesical schistosomiasis into previously uninfected contiguous areas as a result of transport of the snail hosts into the new canals.

Control. Theoretically, vesical schistosomiasis is amenable to practical control, since there are essentially no mammalian reservoir hosts. As is the case in schistosomiasis japonica and mansoni, the most effective measures are snail control combined with chemotherapy. Useful molluscicides have been mentioned under *S. japonicum* and *S. mansoni.*

Schistosoma intercalatum

Schistosoma intercalatum adults are similar morphologically to those of *S. haematobium,* and the eggs also have a terminal spine, though they differ in size. However, *S. intercalatum* causes human intestinal schistosomiasis instead of the urinary form. It has been reported from Zaire, Cameroon, Gabon, Guinea, and the Central African Republic.

Other Schistosomes Reported As Human Parasites

Several species of schistosomes that are natural parasites of wild or domestic mammals occur in man (Malek, 1980). *Schistosoma mattheei* of cattle, sheep, baboons, and antelopes causes a significant number of human infections in Zimbabwe and South Africa, especially the latter. Human infections occasionally have been reported as resulting from the following animal schistosomes: *S. margrebowiei* of equines, cattle, sheep, and antelopes in South Africa, Chad, and Zaire; *S. leiperi* of antelopes, cattle, and sheep in Zambia and South Africa; *S. rodhaini* of rodents and dogs in Zaire, Uganda, and Kenya; *S. incognitum* of pigs and dogs in India, Indonesia, and Thailand, and *S. bovis* of cattle, sheep, camels, and equines in Sudan, Egypt, and elsewhere in the Middle East.

TREATMENT OF SCHISTOSOMIASIS

The following basic principles may be helpful in the consideration of various chemotherapeutic agents:

1. Treatment cannot be expected to undo the chronic inflammatory lesions (fibrous) that occur in the stages of healing and repair.

2. Of the human blood fluke infections, schistosomiasis japonica, the most pathogenic, is the least responsive to treatment; schistosomiasis haematobia, the least pathogenic, is the most responsive.

3. Only when eggs are demonstrated either in excreta or in a biopsy specimen should treatment be given.

Praziquantel, administered orally in a single day, is effective and relatively well tolerated. It is therefore generally preferred for the treatment of human schistosomiasis caused by any species. Side-effects of abdominal discomfort, drowsiness, headache, backache, fever, sweating, and giddiness do occur.

Oxamniquine and metrifonate, which are highly effective against schistosomiasis mansoni and schistosomiasis haematobia, respectively, are ineffective against schistosomiasis japonica. Oxamniquine has been observed to cause seizures, and metrifonate, although relatively free of side-effects, is related to dangerously toxic congeners.

Niridazole, formerly a drug of choice, causes side-effects involving the heart, liver, and brain, the latter including psychosis and convulsions. Its efficacy with regard to cure is also less than that of the previously mentioned drugs.

SCHISTOSOME DERMATITIS

In 1928 Cort demonstrated that cercariae of certain nonhuman schistosomes were the causal agents of a form of dermatitis in Michigan, where it was called *swimmer's itch.* Investigations in many other regions have demonstrated that this infection usually occurs during the warm months and is caused by skin penetration of the schistosome cercariae. Nonoperculate snails in bodies of fresh water serve as intermediate hosts for these schistosomes, the adults of which are usually parasites of aquatic migratory birds. The birds pollute the water with their excreta, which contain eggs of the parasite, and the miracidia hatched from the eggs initiate infection in the snails.

General Aspects. Schistosome dermatitis resulting from contact with cercaria-infested fresh water has been reported from many regions of the United States, Europe, Latin America, India, Thailand, Australia, and New Zealand. Species of *Lymnaea, Stagnicola, Physa, Planorbis, Gyraulus, Polypylis, Segmentina, Chilina,* and other genera serve as snail hosts and the definitive hosts are commonly ducks and geese, but some passerine birds are naturally infected with avian schistosomes. Schistosomes that are principally responsible for cercarial dermatitis belong to the genera *Trichobilharzia, Ornithobilharzia,* and *Gigantobilharzia.*

Other areas of schistosome dermatitis are found along salt-

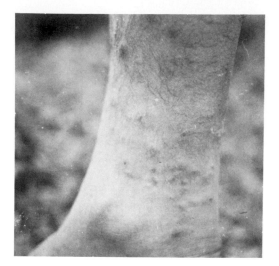

Fig. 9–15. Schistosome dermatitis of 7 days' duration on the ankle of a rice-field worker in the Caspian Sea region of Iran, caused by *Orientobilharzia turkestanicum,* a cattle schistosome. (Courtesy of E.A. Malek.) (From Beaver, P.C., Jung, R.C., and Cupp, E.W. 1984. *Clinical Parasitology,* 9th ed. Philadelphia, Lea & Febiger, p. 443.)

water beaches in Hawaii, southern California, Florida, Rhode Island, and Connecticut. In these areas marine snails are intermediate molluscan hosts of the blood flukes, and terns, as well as other water and migratory birds, are the natural definitive hosts. The adult worm of a common marine cercaria is a species of *Microbilharzia.* Cercariae of certain species of *Austrobilharzia, Ornithobilharzia,* and *Gigantobilharzia* also are responsible for dermatitis along saltwater beaches.

A third epidemiologic type of schistosome dermatitis is caused by invasion of the human skin with schistosomes of mammals, including the cattle schistosomes *Schistosoma bovis* and *S. spindale* in Thailand, and *Orientobilharzia turkestanicum* in northern Iran and southern Russia, the schistosome of rodents, *Schistosomatium douthitti,* and of the raccoon and dog, *Herterobilharzia americana. Orientobilharzia harinasutai,* a blood fluke of the water buffalo in Thailand, has not been associated with naturally occurring dermatitis but is of special interest because its lateral-spined egg resembles that of *S. mansoni.* It is probable that the cercariae of essentially all mammalian and avian schistosomes are capable of penetrating the skin of man.

Clinical Aspects of Schistosome Dermatitis. The lesions produced in schistosome dermatitis (Fig. 9–15) consist of an initial prickling or nettling sensation, which may be accompanied by erythema of the invaded area and by local or generalized urticaria. Soon the initial irritation subsides, leaving only a macule at each site of penetration, but in a few hours there is intense itching of the involved area and the macules transform into papules. The reaction reaches its maximum between the second and third day, then gradually decreases.

Treatment consists of trimeprazine orally, or application of palliatives such as calamine lotion topically to relieve the itching, and, if required, sedation.

Control. If the schistosome cercariae causing dermatitis are coming from freshwater snails, copper salts or other molluscicidal chemicals such as those used against the snail hosts of human schistosomes may be dissolved in the water along the shore of lakes or in canals and ditches where the snails are found. Along saltwater beaches the control of schistosome der-

matitis poses a more difficult problem, the solution to which has not been explored.

SUMMARY

1. Blood flukes or schistosomes are typically dioecious; mated pairs normally live in the smaller vessels of the mesenteric-portal and caval blood systems, where they lay nonoperculate, partially embryonated eggs. These escape into the lumen of the intestine or urinary bladder and are evacuated in the excreta, meanwhile completing embryonation. They hatch in fresh water and active ciliated larvae (miracidia) enter susceptible species of snails, in which they metamorphose into sporocysts, with production internally of a brood of second-generation sporocysts; these, in turn, produce fork-tailed larvae (cercariae). These larvae swarm out of the snails and, on contact with the skin of man or mammalian reservoirs, enter the cutaneous blood vessels and initiate infection.
2. Three species, *Schistosoma japonicum* in the Far East, *S. mansoni* in Africa and tropical America, and *S. haematobium* in Africa and the Middle East, are important parasites of man.
3. The cercariae of blood flukes migrate in or along blood vessels from the skin, through the lungs, and into the intrahepatic portal blood. When mature, they migrate into veins of the intestine *(S. japonicum* and *S. mansoni)* or the urinary bladder *(S. haematobium).*
4. Pathologic changes produced by schistosomes consist of (1) intoxication and sensitization during the prepatent period and intermittently thereafter, (2) tissue damage due to egg extrusion, and (3) reaction to eggs remaining in the tissues.
5. *S. japonicum* and *S. mansoni* cause toxic and allergic symptoms; fever and acute hepatitis develop early, followed by epigastric distress, dysentery, enlargement of liver and spleen, and later profound intestinal and hepatic dysfunction. *S. haematobium* causes hematuria, followed by increasing dysfunction of the urinary organs.
6. Diagnosis is made by recovery of characteristic eggs in the feces or urine, or by rectal or bladder biopsy. Praziquantel is the drug of choice for treatment.
7. Pollution of fresh water by excreta of man or reservoir hosts containing viable eggs of the blood flukes initiates the extrinsic phases of the life cycle, allowing eggs to hatch, emerging miracidia to infect susceptible snails, and, after two generations of multiplication in the snails, the emergence of cercariae that leave the snail and on contact with skin initiate infection in man or reservoirs. Eggs of *S. japonicum* and *S. mansoni* are evacuated in the feces, those of *S. haematobium* in the urine. Only *S. japonicum* has important reservoir hosts.
8. Control of blood fluke infection is by sterilization of human excreta, avoidance of contact with infested water, destruction of the snail hosts and modification of snail habitats, and anthelmintic treatment of infected people.
9. Schistosome dermatitis results from human exposure to schistosome cercariae of birds or mammals in fresh or brackish water.

REFERENCES

Ansari, N., ed. 1973. *Epidemiology and Control of Schistosomiasis (Bilharziasis).* Basel, Switzerland, S. Karger.
Harris, A.R.C., Russell, R.J., and Charters, A.D. 1984. A review of schistosomiasis in immigrants in Western Aus-

tralia, demonstrating the unusual longevity of *Schistosoma mansoni*. Trans. R. Soc. Trop. Med. Hyg., *78*:385–388.

Hunter, G.W., Yokogawa, M., Akusawa, M., Sano, M., Araki, K., and Kobayashi, M. 1982. Control of schistosomiasis japonica in the Nagatoishi area of Kurume, Japan. Am. J. Trop. Med. Hyg., *31*:760–770.

Kruger, S.P., Heitman, L.P., Van Wyk, J.A., and McCully, R.M. 1969. The route of migration of *Schistosoma mattheei* from the lungs to the liver in sheep. J.S. Afr. Vet. Med. Assoc., *40*:39–43.

Malek, E.A., 1980. *Snail-Transmitted Parasitic Diseases,* Vol. I. Boca Raton, Florida, CRC Press.

Miller, P., and Wilson, R.A. 1980. Migration of the schistosomula of *Schistosoma mansoni* from the lungs to the hepatic portal system. Parasitology, *80*:267–288.

Prentice, M.A. 1983. Displacement of *Biomphalaria glabrata* by the snail *Thiara granifera* in field habitats in St. Lucia, West Indies, Ann. Trop. Med. Parasitol., *77*:51–59.

Voge, M., Bruckner, D. and Bruce J.I. 1978. *Schistosoma mekongi* sp. n. from man and animals compared with four geographic strains of *Schistosoma japonicum*. J. Parasitol., *64*:577–584.

Chapter 10

Cestodes (Tapeworms)

M. D. Little

TAPEWORMS AS A GROUP

The cestodes or tapeworms, class Cestoidea, along with the mostly free-living Turbellaria and the exclusively parasitic Trematoda, constitute the phylum Platyhelminthes. Cestodes are parasitic in all, or nearly all, stages of the life cycle. Typically the adults are intestinal parasites of vertebrates and the larval stages generally are parasitic in the tissues or body cavities of vertebrate or invertebrate hosts. Parasites of man include both adult and larval cestodes.

Adult Tapeworms

The mature tapeworms live attached to the mucosa of the small intestine. All adult tapeworms of man consist of the following parts: (1) a *scolex* or "head," which is the organ of attachment and serves to orient rather than to support the rest of the worm; (2) a "neck" immediately behind the scolex, the region of growth and proliferation from which the more distal portion of the worm is derived; and (3) a strand of *proglottids* or segments, beginning with *immature* ones, followed in turn by those that are *mature* with fully developed reproductive organs, and last by the distalmost *gravid* ones that contain mature eggs. The entire series of proglottids and neck is a *strobila*. The number of proglottids varies from 3 or 4 in the *Echinococcus* species to 1,000 or more in the beef tapeworm *(Taenia saginata)* and 3,000 or 4,000 in the fish tapeworm *(Diphyllobothrium latum)*. All parts are mobile, and the strobila may form several loops in the intestine.

The worm is typically flattened dorsoventrally, creamy to chalky white in color, and covered with a relatively transparent layer, the tegument, which is a syncytium with an outer covering of microvilli (microtrichs). Internal to the tegument are 2 thin layers of muscle fibers, the outer one being circular, the inner longitudinal. Immediately under the muscles are the nuclei of the tegumental syncytium. These layers encircle a loose meshwork of undifferentiated parenchyma, within which are the nervous, excretory, and genital organs. A digestive tract is lacking.

The *scolex* in most species of human tapeworms (Fig. 10–1) is more or less knoblike and is provided with four cupped suckers symmetrically arranged, with two being situated ventrolaterally and two dorsolaterally. In species of *Diphyllobothrium*, the scolex is spatulate and is provided with a long median ventral and a similar dorsal sucking groove.

The *excretory system* consists of paired ventrolateral and dorsolateral longitudinal canals joined by anastomoses in the scolex and by a transverse anastomosis near the posterior margin of each proglottid. Opening into the longitudinal canals at frequent intervals are numerous tubules that originate from *flame cells* in the tissues.

The *genital organs* begin to develop in the more distal immature proglottids and reach full growth and function in the mature proglottids. In most species, there is one complete set of male and female organs for each proglottid. In *Taenia saginata* and other Cyclophyllidea, the genital openings are midlateral in position (Fig. 10–2). In the Pseudophyllidea, the group to which species of *Diphyllobothrium* belong, these openings are midventral in the anterior half of the proglottid (Fig. 10–1).

In egg production, the naked ovum is passed through the oviduct, is fertilized on its way into the *ootype* or soon thereafter and then is provided

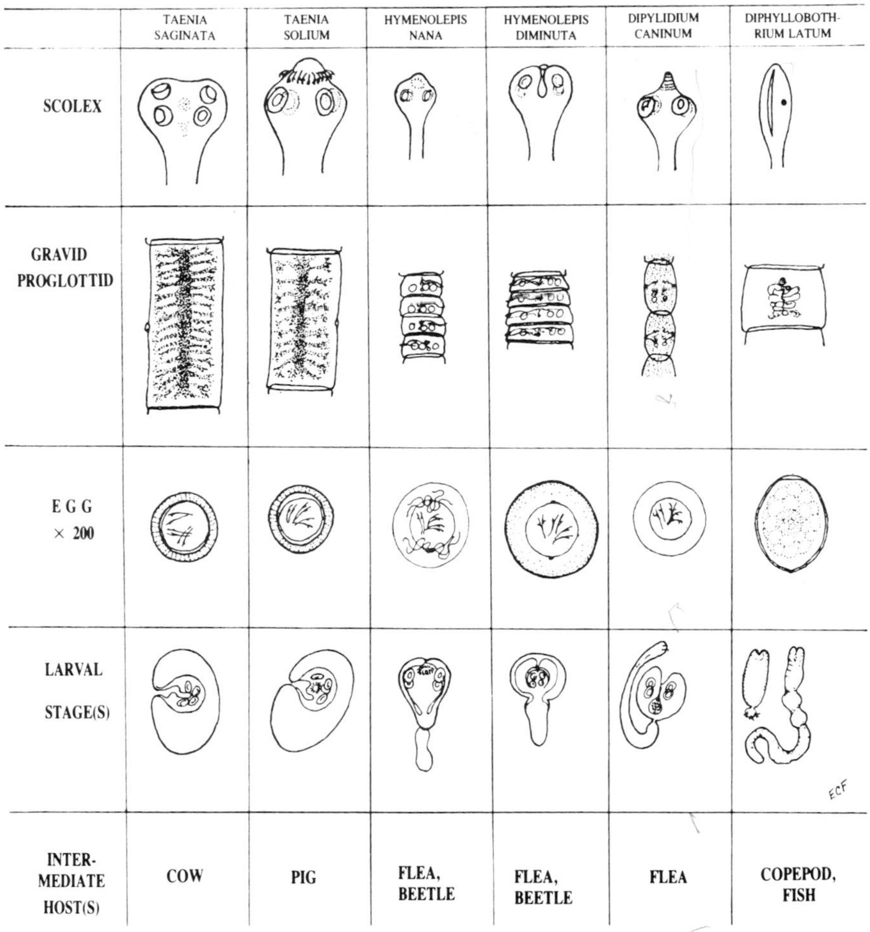

	TAENIA SAGINATA	TAENIA SOLIUM	HYMENOLEPIS NANA	HYMENOLEPIS DIMINUTA	DIPYLIDIUM CANINUM	DIPHYLLOBOTH-RIUM LATUM
SCOLEX						
GRAVID PROGLOTTID						
E G G × 200						
LARVAL STAGE(S)						
INTER-MEDIATE HOST(S)	COW	PIG	FLEA, BEETLE	FLEA, BEETLE	FLEA	COPEPOD, FISH

Fig. 10–1. Cestodes of man. Principal life-cycle stages and diagnostic features. (By E.C. Faust.)

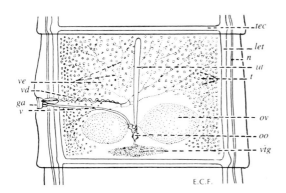

Fig. 10–2. *Taenia saginata.* Mature proglottid. *ga,* Male and female genital atrium. *let,* Lateral excretory trunk. *n,* Lateral nerve trunk. *oo,* Ootype. *ov,* Ovary. *t,* Testes. *tec,* Transverse excretory canal. *ut,* Uterus. *v,* Vagina. *vd,* Vas deferens. *ve,* Vas efferens. *vtg,* Vitelline gland. (By E.C. Faust.)

with yolk material. A thick shell is then formed and the egg is carried into the uterus, where it matures.

The essential difference between the genital system of *Taenia saginata* and that of species of *Diphyllobothrium* lies in the fact that the uterus of the latter group is provided with a pore, through which unembryonated eggs are discharged.

Although attached by its scolex to the intestinal mucosa, the worm is a lumen parasite. During periods of hypermotility of the small bowel, the main portion frequently breaks away from the scolex and is evacuated in the stool. However, as long as the scolex remains attached, a new strobila will be formed from it.

Lacking a digestive system, the worms absorb nutrients selectively through the highly absorptive tegument. Tapeworms have a high ratio of gly-cogen, lipids, and phospholipids to protein, stored in the parenchymal cells. There is a large amount of calcium carbonate throughout the parenchyma in the form of numerous rounded granules, the *calcareous corpuscles*.

Developmental Stages of Tapeworms

In species of *Hymenolepis*, the fully developed eggs are passed in the feces; in species of *Taenia* and in *Dipylidium caninum*, gravid proglottids be-come detached and pass out of the bowel, usually liberating only a small portion of their eggs. The mature egg contains the *hexacanth embryo* or *on-cosphere*, provided with three pairs of hooklets (Fig. 10–1).

Oncospheres developing in the eggs of species of *Diphyllobothrium* and their relatives have a cil-iated epithelium and are referred to as *coracidia*. All other human tapeworms produce eggs that de-velop oncospheres lacking a ciliated epithelium. Developing from the oncosphere in intermediate hosts are several morphologic types of larvae that are characteristic of different species of tapeworms (Fig. 10–1). *Diphyllobothrium* has two distinct lar-val stages, *procercoid* and *plerocercoid*, both solid organisms lacking a bladder. In *Hymenolepis nana*, *H. diminuta*, and *Dipylidium caninum*, the larval stage, or *metacestode* infective for the final host is a *cysticercoid*, a small solid larva with the scolex enveloped by tissues of its body. In species of *Taenia* the infective stage is a *cysticercus*, which has a conspicuous bladder surrounding the inva-ginated scolex. In *Taenia multiceps* there is a some-what larger bladder, the *coenurus*, which forms a number of invaginated scolices. In *Echinococcus* the larva is a large bladder, or *hydatid*, which in-ternally produces multiple scolices (protoscolices) and numerous daughter bladders or brood capsules.

When the mature larva surrounded by the tissues of the intermediate host is ingested by the definitive host and reaches the small intestine, it is digested out of the tissues and the scolex evaginates and becomes attached to the intestinal mucosa; in a few weeks or months, it develops into a complete stro-bilate worm.

ADULT TAPEWORM INFECTIONS

Taenia saginata

(Taeniasis saginata, beef tapeworm infection)

The beef tapeworm, *Taenia saginata* Goeze, 1782 was widely known in ancient Egypt and

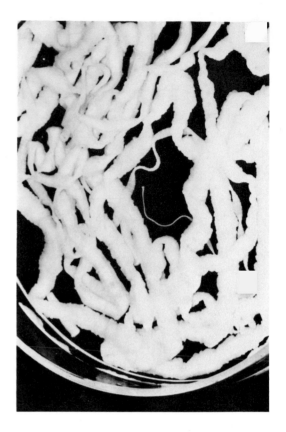

Fig. 10–3. *Taenia saginata*. Showing characteristic delicate scolex and neck at center, and relatively massive remaining parts of the strobila. (Ca. one half natural size.) (From Naka-bayashi, T., *et al.* 1984. A new therapy for *Taenia saginata* and *Diphyllobothrium latum* infections by duodenal adminis-tration of gastrografin. Jpn. J. Parasitol., *33*:215–220.)

Greece and was prevalent in Europe during the Middle Ages. The larva was reported from the mus-cles of cattle by Wepfer in 1675. Leuckart in 1862 first demonstrated that human infection resulted from eating infected raw beef. Beef tapeworm in-fection is widely distributed in Australia, New Zea-land, Africa, Europe, Latin America, and to a lesser extent the United States.

Morphology, Biology, and Life Cycle. The adult worm typically develops in the middle third of the small intestine. The average length of the relaxed worm is approximately 5 meters, although there are records of specimens of far greater length. It has 1000 to 2000 proglottids, of which from one third to one half are nearly gravid. Usually only a single specimen occurs in an infection, but there may be more.

The fully developed worm is delicate anteriorly and more robust posteriorly (Fig. 10–3). The scolex (Fig. 10–1) bears four suckers and a slight

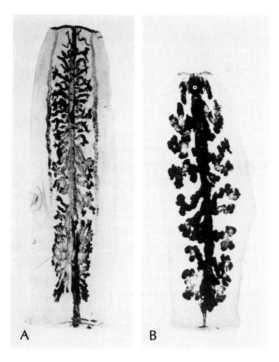

Fig. 10–4. *Taenia* proglottids with uterus filled with India ink to show lateral branches. *A, T. saginata. B, T. solium.* (× ca. 4) (By M.D. Little.)

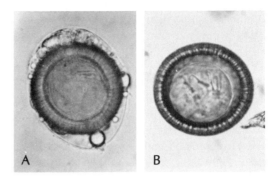

Fig. 10–5. *Taenia saginata. A,* Egg with outer membrane intact, freshly shed from motile proglottid. One of three pairs of hooklets is evident. *B,* Egg recovered from feces. (× ca. 700.) (By M.D. Little.)

apical depression. Immediately behind the delicate unsegmented "neck" is a region of immature proglottids in which the genital organs are not yet developed. Gradually the more distal of these proglottids increase in breadth and width until they reach a maximum width of 12 mm. These are the mature proglottids, each of which contains a full set of functioning male and female reproductive organs (Fig. 10–2). Still more distally, the mature units have transformed into more elongated, narrower, gravid ones as a result of the development of the large number of branched lateral arms of the uterus (15 to 20) characteristic of *T. saginata* (Fig. 10–4A). The terminal proglottids become separated from the strobila and actively migrate out of the bowel or are evacuated in the stool with only partial loss of eggs. The eggs are essentially spherical, measure 31 to 43 μm in diameter, and have a thin, transparent outer embryonal envelope and a thick brown shell composed of many slender rods cemented together. Within this shell is a hexacanth embryo, which has three pairs of delicate lancet-shaped hooklets (Fig. 10–5).

The evacuated gravid segments extrude the eggs while crawling in a measuring-worm fashion on the ground, vegetation, or other surface. Cattle grazing on infested ground pick up the eggs, which hatch in the duodenum. The emerging embryos penetrate into the mesenteric venules or lymphatics and reach skeletal muscles or the heart, where in about 2 months they transform into the typical cysticercus stage *(Cysticercus bovis),* which measures roughly 5 by 10 mm and has a head like that of the adult worm, invaginated into the fluid-filled bladder (Fig. 10–6). Thereafter, for a period of more than a year, a person who eats the raw infected beef is subject to infection. The prepatent period usually is 10 to 12 weeks.

Pathogenesis and Symptomatology. Infection with *T. saginata* is ordinarily asymptomatic except for the discomfort, inconvenience, or embarrassment resulting from the gravid proglottids crawling out of the anus. In this respect the infection resembles that of *Enterobius vermicularis.* However, toward the end of the prepatent period diarrhea and

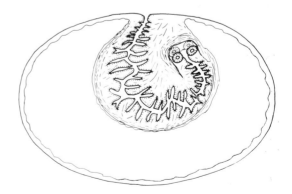

Fig. 10–6. *Taenia saginata.* Optical section view of cysticercus from beef muscle, showing scolex with four suckers at end of scolex canal. (× 7.) (Adapted by M.D. Little from photo by H. Thornton in Soulsby, E.J.L. 1982. *Helminths, Arthropods and Protozoa of Domesticated Animals,* 7th ed. Philadelphia, Lea & Febiger, p. 110.)

abdominal cramps may occur. Rarely, a mass of tangled worms may cause acute intestinal obstruction.

Diagnosis. Eggs of *T. saginata* are often found in the feces. They are indistinguishable from those of *T. solium*. In mature infections gravid proglottids are evacuated or migrate from the rectum onto the skin or clothing. When the fresh proglottids are compressed between glass slides and held over a bright light, it is usually possible to count the number of main lateral arms of the uterus (15 to 20) on each side of the main uterine stem (Fig. 10–4*A*). The gravid proglottids deposit eggs in the perianal area as they crawl from the rectum. For this reason the diagnosis may be made by use of an adhesive cellophane tape technique, as for enterobiasis. Diagnosis is more likely to be made by identifying proglottids or eggs from the anus than by examination of feces.

Treatment. By virtue of its efficacy and low toxicity, the treatment of choice has been niclosamide (Yomesan) (see Table 21–1, p. 265). A newer, equally effective drug is praziquantel. If these drugs are not available, quinacrine hydrochloride is preferable to other older preparations.

Epidemiology. Cattle acquire the larval stage of *T. saginata* by grazing on moist pasture polluted with feces or raw sewage containing the eggs; under optimal conditions of moisture and temperature the eggs may remain viable for 6 months, but under natural conditions they usually are nonviable after about 2 months. The eggs can withstand temperatures of 24°F (−4.5°C) for 2 weeks or longer. Approximately 2 months after the cattle are exposed, the larvae have matured and the meat is infective. After a year or more, however, the cysticerci often become calcified. Infection of young calves provides relatively solid immunity to subsequent exposure. In some human communities infection results from eating raw beef. In most endemic areas it is due to eating undercooked steaks or hamburgers. While a majority of infections in the United States are contracted from heavily infected uninspected beef, about 0.3% of inspected beef in large slaughterhouses contains a minimal infection. Man is the only natural definitive host of *T. saginata*.

Control. Basically, control of taeniasis consists of sanitary disposal of human feces, so that eggs of *T. saginata* in the excreta or community sewage do not reach pastures where cattle graze. Workers at cattle feedlots should be examined periodically

for signs of infection. Cysticerci are killed in beef that has been kept 24 hours or longer in a deep freezer (−20°C). Likewise, heating the meat to 65°C is a safeguard.

Taenia solium
(Taeniasis solium, pork tapeworm infection)

The larval stage of the pork tapeworm *(Cysticercus cellulosae)* was described from swine by Greek naturalists. Gessner in 1558 and Rumler in 1588 first reported human infection with the cysticercus. Linnaeus in 1758 gave this worm its specific name and placed it in the genus *Taenia*. Goeze in 1782 first differentiated the adult *T. solium* from *T. saginata*, and Kuchenmeister in 1855 and Leuckart in 1856 first conducted life cycle studies.

Pork tapeworm infection occurs wherever raw or lightly cooked pork is eaten. It is relatively common in the Balkan states, all Slavic countries, North China and Manchuria, India, and widespread in Latin America, from Mexico to Chile. Autochthonous *T. solium* infection in the United States apparently has ceased to exist.

Morphology, Biology, and Life Cycle. In most respects *Taenia solium* resembles *T. saginata*, but it is shorter, usually having a length of less than 3 meters due to a smaller number of proglottids (fewer than 1000) and smaller gravid proglottids. Anterior to the 4 suckers on the scolex is a rostellum with a double circle of alternating large and small hooks, numbering from 22 to 36 and measuring 140 to 200 μm and 100 to 150 μm, respectively (Fig. 10–1).

The mature proglottid of *T. solium* closely resembles that of *T. saginata* but is usually readily differentiated because it contains approximately one half the number (usually 9 or 10) of main lateral uterine arms on each side of the longitudinal uterine stem (Fig. 10–4*B*). Eggs of *T. solium* are indistinguishable from those of *T. saginata*.

Gravid proglottids actively migrate from the anus or are passed in the feces. Eggs are discharged by migrating proglottids or are freed when they disintegrate on the ground. To develop, the eggs must be ingested by a pig or by man himself. The hexacanth embryos hatch in the duodenum, migrate through the intestinal wall, and reach the blood and lymphatic channels, which carry them to skeletal muscle and myocardium. Here the embryos transform in 2 to 3 months into cysticerci *(Cysticercus cellulosae)*, glistening pearly white and measuring about 5 mm by 8 to 10 mm (Fig. 10–7). The scolex

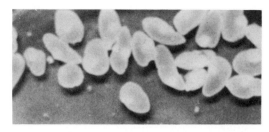

Fig. 10–7. *Cysticercus cellulosae.* Viable cysts digested from muscle of pig. (× ca. 1.5.) (From Tellez-Giron, E., Ramos, M.C., and Montante, M. 1981. Effect of flubendazole on *Cysticercus cellulosae* in pigs. Am. J. Trop. Med. Hyg., *30*:135–138.)

is deeply invaginated into the fluid-filled bladder and is provided with 4 suckers and a rostellum, as in the adult scolex. When people eat pork containing viable cysticerci, the larvae are digested out of the meat and the heads evaginate from the bladder, become attached to the wall of the small intestine, and mature in 5 to 12 weeks.

Pathogenesis and Symptomatology. Infection with the adult *T. solium* produces the same clinical manifestations as infection with *T. saginata* (see page 113). However, because of its shorter length, there is less likelihood that intestinal obstruction will develop. The extraintestinal development of cysticerci of *T. solium* and the serious clinical consequences of human cysticercosis are considered on page 119.

Diagnosis. Although eggs of *T. solium* may be found in the feces or on anal swabs, specific diagnosis is based on demonstration of the relatively small number of main lateral arms of the uterus (7 to 13, usually about 9) in the gravid proglottids (Fig. 10–4B).

Treatment. Niclosamide and praziquantel are the drugs of choice. However, although niclosamide is as effective against *T. solium* infection as against *T. saginata,* it is not recommended by several authorities because it causes the proglottids to disintegrate and release the eggs into the bowel lumen, possibly increasing the hazard of cysticercosis. Praziquantel or quinacrine is recommended instead. There is, however, no evidence that eggs released from proglottids into the bowel lumen are infective or that quinacrine, which causes vomiting, is less prone to cause cysticercosis.

Epidemiology. Human infection with *Taenia solium* results from eating essentially raw pork containing viable *Cysticercus cellulosae.* The pork may be fresh or smoked ham or sausage. Man is the only natural host of the adult worm. However,

man is also a suitable host for the cysticercus (page 119).

Control. The serious, frequently disabling, and at times fatal consequences of human cysticercosis resulting from larval *T. solium* infection indicate the need for control. In endemic areas human feces should not be deposited in locations where hogs have access to them. Pork should be adequately cooked before it is eaten or held in a deep-freezer for at least 24 hours. Persons harboring this worm should be freed of the infection by anthelmintic treatment.

Hymenolepis nana
(Dwarf tapeworm infection)

Hymenolepis nana (von Siebold, 1852) Blanchard, 1891, the dwarf tapeworm, was discovered by Bilharz in 1851, in the small intestine of a boy at autopsy in Cairo, Egypt. Its life cycle was elucidated by Grassi in 1887 and by Grassi and Rovelli, who in 1892 demonstrated that no intermediate host is required.

Dwarf tapeworm infection in humans is primarily limited to children in warm climates. It is prevalent throughout India, parts of the U.S.S.R., countries bordering on the Mediterranean, all of the countries of Latin America, Hawaii, and some of the islands of the South and Southwest Pacific. It is the most frequently detected tapeworm in the United States.

Morphology, Biology, and Life Cycle. *H. nana* is the smallest of the tapeworms of man. The entire worm has a length of only 25 to 40 mm and a maximum breadth usually not exceeding 1 mm. The scolex is provided with 4 suckers and a rostellar crown of 20 to 30 minute hooklets (Fig. 10–1). The neck is long and slender, all of the approximately 200 proglottids are broader than they are long, and the terminal gravid proglottids usually disintegrate before separating from the strobila, so that the eggs are randomly mixed with the feces. The average infection consists of a few to several worms, but thousands have been reported from some patients. The eggs of *H. nana* (Fig. 10–8) are nearly spherical, 30 to 47 μm in diameter. There are two thin membranous shells, the inner one of which has polar thickenings, each provided with 4 to 8 long threadlike filaments extending into the space between the inner and outer shells.

When eggs are swallowed, they hatch in the duodenum, and the liberated embryos penetrate

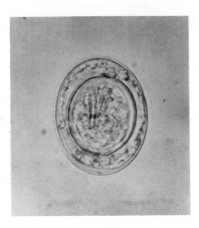

Fig. 10–8. *Hymenolepis nana.* Egg from human feces. (× ca. 800.) (By M.D. Little.)

into the stroma of villi, where in 5 to 6 days they transform into cysticercoid larvae (Fig. 10–1). These then attach to the mucosa, and in about 2 weeks they develop into complete worms. Thus, both the larval and adult stages develop in the same individual. Moreover, in heavy infections it seems entirely probable that internal autoinfection may have occurred as a result of hatching of eggs in the upper levels of the small intestine following regurgitation into the stomach. *H. nana* also can utilize fleas and beetles for development of the cysticercoid stage (Fig. 10–9).

Pathogenesis and Symptomatology. Infection with *Hymenolepis nana* may produce no detectable

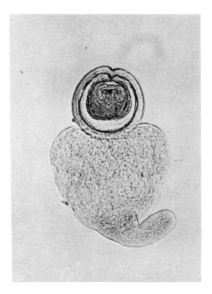

Fig. 10–9. *Hymenolepis nana.* Cysticercoid from body cavity of experimentally infected grain beetle *(Tenebrio molitor).* (× 100.) (By M.D. Little.)

symptoms or it may be responsible for diarrhea, anorexia, vomiting, insomnia, loss of appetite and weight, irritability, pruritus of the nose and anus, urticaria, and, rarely, choreiform symptoms. Heavy infection invariably is pathogenic, causing diarrhea, abdominal pain, anorexia, and nervous disorders.

Diagnosis and Treatment. Diagnosis is based on demonstration of the characteristic eggs (Fig. 10–8) in the stools. Niclosamide in a course of 5 to 7 days is the treatment of choice. (See Table 21–1, page 265.)

Epidemiology. *H. nana* (human strain) requires no extrinsic development and has only a single host; infection commonly is acquired by anus-to-mouth transmission of eggs. For this reason infection is particularly prevalent among groups of younger children. Although infection can be acquired from *H. nana* eggs in feces of rodents, this type of infection probably is uncommon. The generally high prevalence of the infection in arid regions has not been explained.

Control. Good personal hygiene and sanitation are important in preventing transmission.

Hymenolepis diminuta
(Rat tapeworm infection)

Hymenolepis diminuta (Rudolphi, 1819) Blanchard, 1891 is a cosmopolitan parasite of rats, mice, and other rodents. It has been reported from human hosts, usually children, from India, Indonesia, the U.S.S.R., Japan, the Philippines, southern Europe, Latin America from Argentina to Mexico and Cuba, and from several parts of the United States. The *H. diminuta* recovered from man is identical to that found in rodents.

H. diminuta measures 20 to 60 cm in length by 3.5 to 4.0 mm in maximum width at its distal end and may consist of 1,000 or more proglottids. The scolex is provided with 4 relatively small suckers and a rudimentary unarmed rostellum (Fig. 10–1). The neck is short and stout. The gravid proglottids disintegrate while still attached to the strobila, liberating fully embryonated ovoid to subspherical eggs measuring 72 to 86 by 60 to 79 μm (Fig. 10–10). There is considerable space between the tanned outer egg membrane and the hyaline inner membrane. The latter is provided with a pair of polar thickenings but lacks the polar filaments characteristic of *H. nana* eggs.

For larval development, the eggs voided in the feces of the definitive host must be ingested by an arthropod, usually the larval stage of rodent fleas which breed in rats' nests, but many species of beetles and also meal moths, earwigs, and diplopods have been found naturally or experimentally to be suitable intermediate hosts. When the infected arthropod is ingested by the definitive hosts, the cysticercoid is digested out of its vector-host and the scolex attaches to the duodenal or jejunal mucosa and develops into the adult worm.

H. diminuta infection usually produces no symptoms. Diagnosis is made on the recovery of typical eggs (Fig. 10–10) in the stool and their differentiation from those of *H. nana* (Fig. 10–8). Treatment is similar to that employed in *H. nana* infection. Control consists fundamentally of measures to eradicate rats around the home.

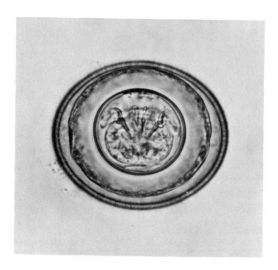

Fig. 10–10. *Hymenolepis diminuta*. Egg from feces of wild rat. (× 600.) (By M.D. Little.)

Dipylidium caninum
(Dipylidiasis or dog tapeworm infection)

Dipylidium caninum (Linnaeus, 1758) Railliet, 1892, a cosmopolitan tapeworm of dogs and cats, has been found in humans, mostly in children, including infants, in Europe, the Orient, Africa, Latin America, and the United States.

The adult worms are medium-sized, measuring from 10 to 70 cm in length, and consist of several hundred proglottids. Mature proglottids contain paired reproductive organs and have a genital pore at each lateral margin. The distalmost gravid proglottids resemble a cucumber seed in size, shape, and color. The scolex is roughly rhomboidal in shape, measures about 0.3 to 0.5 mm in diameter, and has 4 conspicuous suckers and an introversible apical club-shaped proboscis provided with 6 rows of minute hooklets. In dogs and cats the infection typically consists of several to many worms; in children it is frequently solitary. The intact gravid proglottids, containing polygonal-shaped masses of egg capsules, separate from the strobila and pass down the intestinal canal and migrate out of the anus or are passed in the feces.

Each proglottid contains numerous egg capsules filled with 1 to about 20 fully embryonated eggs (Fig. 10–1). When the larva of the dog flea or the cat flea, the dog louse, or possibly another arthropod, ingests the egg capsule, hatching occurs and the liberated embryos migrate into the arthropod's hemocoel and transform into cysticercoid larvae (Fig. 10–1). The definitive host becomes infected by ingesting the infected insect.

This infection in a child may produce diarrhea and unrest. Occasionally there may be severe sensitization reactions, such as urticaria, fever, significant eosinophilia and, rarely, convulsions. Diagnosis is made on recovery of the characteristic gravid proglottids evacuated in the stool or migrating from the anus and by observing the egg capsules in the uterus and double genital pores. Treatment is the same as that recommended for *Taenia saginata*.

Control of dog tapeworm infection consists of periodic administration of taeniafuges to dogs and cats to remove their tapeworms and of applying insecticides to get rid of their ectoparasites.

Uncommon Cyclophyllidean Tapeworms of Man

The following species have been reported:

Bertiella studeri and *B. mucronata* are common in monkeys of the Eastern and Western Hemispheres, respectively. They are relatively short (up to 30 cm), thick, and about 1 cm wide, with extremely short proglottids that usually are shed in strands of several to many. Intermediate hosts are mites.

Inermicapsifer madagascariensis is a parasite of rodents in Africa. It is slender, up to about 40 cm long, and its rice grainlike proglottids are shed singly in the feces. The mode of infection is unknown.

Mesocestoides species are found in carnivorous mammals in Europe, the Middle East, and North America. In man, the strobila of most species is slender, up to about 40 cm long, and its proglottids are shed singly or in strands of various lengths in the feces. The mode of infection is unknown.

Raillietina celebensis and other *Raillietina* species are found in rats in the Orient, Indonesia, and Australia, and one species is found in Cuba and South America. As in *Inermicapsifer* infection, rice grainlike proglottids are shed in the feces. Intermediate hosts of *R. celebensis* are ants.

Diphyllobothrium latum
(Fish tapeworm infection, diphyllobothriasis)

Diphyllobothrium latum (Linnaeus, 1758) Lühe, 1910 was undoubtedly prevalent in the Baltic Sea area at an early period and became widely disseminated as the people of that area migrated to other parts of Europe and elsewhere. Today *D. latum* is indigenous throughout many parts of the U.S.S.R., in the Baltic Sea countries, Central and Southeastern Europe, Lake Ngami (Botswana), northern Manchuria and Japan, and New South Wales, Australia. In the Americas it is found in northern Minnesota, extensive areas of Canada and Alaska, and the lakes of southern Chile and Argentina.

Morphology, Biology, and Life Cycle. The fully developed strobila of *D. latum* (Fig. 10–11) is up to 10 meters or more in length and has up to 4000 proglottids. The elliptical or spatulate scolex measures about 2.5 mm in length by 1 mm in breadth and is provided with a median ventral and a median dorsal grooved sucker. Organs of a mature proglottid are shown in Fig. 10–12.

The eggs within the fully developed proglottid are continuously discharged through the uterine pore. Terminal proglottids gradually become exhausted and disintegrate. The broadly ovoid, light golden-yellow eggs (Fig. 10–13) have an operculum at one end and a small inconspicuous thickening of the shell at the opposite end. They are unembryonated when passed in the host's feces and measure 58 to 76 μm by 40 to 51 μm.

Embryonation of eggs that reach cool fresh water (15 to 25°C) requires 11 to 15 days. Then the cil-

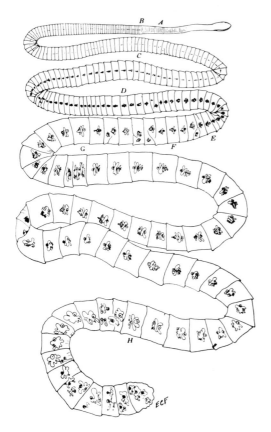

Fig. 10–11. *Diphyllobothrium latum.* Complete strobila with terminal proglottid still attached, obtained from a dog 24 days after experimental infection by feeding sparganum larvae in a fish *(Salmo irideus)*. *A* to *F,* Progression in differentiation and maturation of reproductive organs. *G,* Proglottids with organs fully developed but not producing eggs. *H,* Proglottids producing eggs. (× ca. 5.) (From Faust, E.C. 1952. Some morphologic characters of *Diphyllobothrium latum.* An. Inst. Trop. Med. Lisboa, 9:1277–1300.)

iated oncosphere, *coracidium*, escapes through the opened operculum and swims about in the water. In order to proceed with development, it must be eaten within 12 hours by an appropriate species of copepod (*Diaptomus* or *Cyclops* in Europe, *Diaptomus* in North America). Once ingested by a copepod, the embryo burrows into the hemocoel and transforms into the *procercoid* larva (Fig. 10–1). If the infected copepod is then eaten by a freshwater fish, the larva migrates into the flesh or connective tissue of this host and transforms into a *plerocercoid* larva (sparganum) (Fig. 10–1). The plerocercoid larva is usually passed by predation through one or more small paratenic fish hosts before reaching one that is, or grows to be, of edible size. When the infected fish is eaten raw by the definitive host, the worm develops to maturity and begins laying eggs in about 4 weeks.

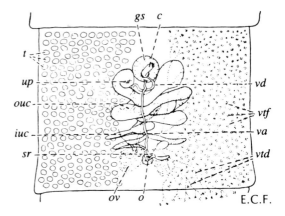

Fig. 10–12. *Diphyllobothrium latum.* Mature proglottid, ventral view. *c,* Cirrus. *gs,* Genital sucker. *iuc,* Inner uterine coils. *o,* Ootype. *ouc,* Outer uterine coils. *ov,* Ovary. *sr,* Seminal receptacle. *t,* Testes (shown only in left field but symmetrically present also in right field). *up,* Uterine pore. *va,* Vagina. *vd,* Vas deferens. *vtd,* Vitelline ducts. *vtf,* Vitelline follicles (shown only in right field but symmetrically present in left field). (× 15.) (Adapted from Faust, E.C. 1952. Some morphologic characters of *Diphyllobothrium latum.* An. Inst. Trop. Med. Lisboa, 9:1277–1300.)

Pathogenesis and Symptomatology. *D. latum* may produce no symptoms, but infections often cause digestive disturbances, including diarrhea, heartburn, a sense of fullness in the epigastrium, hunger pains or loss of appetite, anorexia, nausea, and vomiting. Sudden vomiting of a portion of the worm may occur, accompanied by symptoms suggesting peptic ulcer, cholelithiasis, ileus, or appendicitis. The infection may be multiple.

In certain instances, notably in Finland, carriers develop pernicious anemia, the so-called "bothriocephalus anemia." In 1956 Von Bonsdorff found that severe symptoms are associated with jejunal attachment, causing impairment of the interaction of the extrinsic and intrinsic factors of

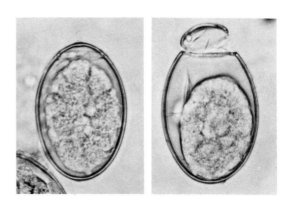

Fig. 10–13. *Diphyllobothrium latum.* Eggs, one with operculum intact, the other with operculum forced open by coverglass pressure. (× 500.) (By P.C. Beaver.)

Castle (*i.e.*, failure to assimilate vitamin B_{12}). Usually the only change in the blood picture is moderate eosinophilia and slight leukocytosis.

Diagnosis and Treatment. Diagnosis depends on finding the characteristic egg (Fig. 10–13), or strands of proglottids in the stool, or the occasionally vomited proglottids. A single worm at the height of productivity may produce up to 15,000 eggs per gram of feces, amounting to 15 or more eggs per average fecal smear.

Treatment is similar to that recommended for *Taenia saginata* infection (see Table 21–1, p. 265).

Epidemiology. Several epidemiologic conditions must exist before the life cycle of *Diphyllobothrium latum* can be completed: (1) eggs must be discharged into cool fresh water, where they embryonate and hatch; (2) the emerging ciliated embryo must be eaten by a copepod *(Diaptomus* or *Cyclops)*, in which the embryo transforms into a procercoid; (3) the infected copepod must then be eaten by a plankton-feeding fish, in the flesh of which the procercoid transforms into the plerocercoid (sparganum), and (4) the infected fish must be eaten raw by the definitive host, in whose intestine the larva develops into the adult worm. In a recent outbreak of diphyllobothriasis in the western United States, fresh salmon (*Oncorhynchus* spp.) was implicated as the source of infection (Ruttenber *et al.*, 1984). Because of the increasing popularity of raw or slightly cooked fish, such outbreaks are likely to continue to occur.

Although dogs and in some areas probably bears are reservoirs of *D. latum*, man is primarily responsible for establishing and maintaining the life cycle in which he is involved.

Control. Control of fish tapeworm infection in endemic areas requires (1) sanitary disposal of human feces so that viable eggs of *D. latum* do not reach bodies of fresh water in which the intermediate hosts breed, and (2) thorough cooking of all fish obtained from the area. Freezing at a temperature of $-18°C$ for 48 hours also will kill the infective larva.

Pseudophyllidea Rarely Found in Man

Diphyllobothrium cordatum, a common intestinal parasite of the seal, the walrus, and the dog in Greenland and Iceland, of the dog in Japan, and of the bear in Yellowstone National Park, Wyoming (U.S.A.), has been reported as a human parasite in Greenland and, doubtfully, in Japan. The distinguishing external character of this species is the inverted heart-shaped scolex. The eggs are indistinguishable from those of *D. latum*. *Diphyllobothrium dalliae* is reported to be a common parasite of man, dog, Arctic fox, and gulls in western Alaska. The pler-

ocercoid is found in blackfish. *Diphyllobothrium dentriticum*, a parasite of gulls and terrestrial mammals, has been found twice in man in Alaska. The plerocercoid is found in salmon. *Diphyllobothrium pacificum*, a parasite of seals, has been reported numerous times from man in Peru, twice in Chile, and once in Japan. *Diphyllobothrium ursi*, a parasite of bears that has its plerocercoid stage in salmon, has been found in man three times in North America, twice in Alaska, and once in Canada.

Diplogonoporus grandis, a common intestinal parasite of whales, has been reported 55 or more times in Japanese patients. The proglottids are very broad compared with their length, and each one has two sets of genital organs.

Spirometra erinacei, a parasite of dogs and cats, has been found in man five times in Japan. *Spirometra houghtoni*, an intestinal parasite of the dog and cat in China, has been recovered twice from man in that country.

LARVAL TAPEWORM INFECTIONS

While the majority of tapeworms parasitize man in their adult stage in the small intestine, a few produce human infection in their larval stage, always in extraintestinal foci, *viz.*, the cysticercus of *Taenia solium*, the coenurus of *Taenia multiceps* and related species, the hydatid cyst of *Echinococcus granulosus* and related species, and the sparganum (plerocercoid) of species of *Spirometra*. Except for the coenurus, all these larval forms are relatively common in the human host in certain geographic areas.

Cysticercus of *Taenia solium*
(Cysticercosis)

The larval stage of *Taenia solium*, the pork tapeworm, is often referred to as *Cysticercus cellulosae*. Although other species may be involved, it is generally presumed that any cysticercus found in man is *Cysticercus cellulosae*. Man is the only proven host of the definitive stage of *T. solium*, and the pig is the usual intermediate host in which the hexacanth embryo hatched from the egg develops into the cysticercus, or bladder worm (Fig. 10–1). However, man is also a satisfactory host for development of this larva.

Pathogenesis and Symptomatology. The lesions produced and the symptoms evoked by cysticercosis depend primarily on the tissues in which the embryos become established but also on the number of cysticerci that develop. In most endemic areas, it is reported that the central nervous system is the most frequent location for cysticerci to develop, followed by the muscle and subcutaneous tissues, the eye, lungs, heart, liver, and other visceral locations. Infection is more frequently multiple than solitary (Fig. 10–14). If there are many visible or palpable cysticerci in the subcutaneous

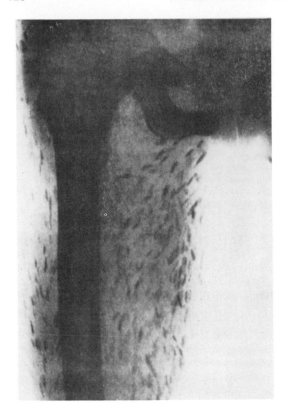

Fig. 10–14. *Taenia solium.* Numerous calcified cysticerci in the thigh tissues of man. (From Evans, R.R. 1939. Cysticercosis in an athlete. Trans. R. Soc. Trop. Med. Hyg., 32:549–550, Plate 1.)

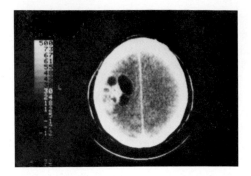

Fig. 10–15. *Cysticercus racemosus.* Computed tomogram of proliferating cysticercus in human brain, demonstrating both solid and cystic components. (From Jung, R.C., Rodriguez, M.A., Beaver, P.C., Schenthal, J.E., and Levy, R.W. 1981. Racemose cysticercus in human brain. A case report. Am. J. Trop. Med. Hyg., 30:620–624.)

tissues or superficial muscles, one or more are likely to have matured in the brain or other internal organs.

The cysticerci may remain viable in man up to 4 or 5 years. Except in the *racemosus type,* or when present in the vitreous, pia mater, or ventricles of the brain, cysticerci in human tissues are surrounded by a tough adventitious capsule. The racemosus type is an unencapsulated larva that develops in the subarachnoid spaces at the base of the brain and occasionally in the choroid plexus (Fig. 10–15). It may reach an overall length of 15 cm, and it produces numerous branches; hence the designation "racemosus."

Cysticerci that develop in the subcutaneous and muscle tissues cause essentially no pain. In the brain, cysticerci are commonly found in meningeal and ventricular locations as well as in the parenchyma. They often occur in multiple locations. Epileptic seizures, hydrocephalus, and stroke are the most common serious effects (McCormick *et al.,* 1982). In addition, patients may experience severe headaches, nausea, vomiting, dizziness, di-

plopia, and other ocular manifestations and undergo psychic changes. Racemose cysticerci develop primarily in the ventricles and subarachnoid spaces and usually produce the more serious forms of the disease. When in the eye, the living unencapsulated cysticerci are constantly changing shape. Usually the subjective symptoms are minimal except for discomfort caused by the shadows cast in front of the retina. However, the parasite may cause damage to any tissue of the eyeball resulting in uveitis, iritis, detachment of the retina, or atrophy of the choroid membrane. The larva may also invade the palpebral conjunctiva, the subconjunctiva, or become encapsulated in the eyelid.

Diagnosis. A diagnosis may be made from a nodule excised from subcutaneous tissue or superficial muscles compressed between glass slides and examined under low power of the microscope. The presence of a scolex having four suckers and a crown of rostellar hooks is specifically diagnostic. The first suggestion of cysticercosis may consist of a patient presenting with defective vision or a series of epileptiform seizures without a history of epilepsy in early childhood. The ophthalmoscope frequently will reveal the motile organism in the eye. In patients with neurologic symptoms, computed tomography (CT) of the brain (Fig. 10–15) along with serologic tests (IHA or HA) may permit a preoperative diagnosis of neurocysticercosis (Botero and Castano, 1982; Grisolia and Wierderholt, 1982). Specific diagnosis of the causative agent can be made only after exploratory removal of the specimen or at necropsy.

Treatment. Although surgery was formerly the sole therapeutic procedure in cysticercosis, chemotherapy with praziquantel following or accompanying administration of corticosteroids has recently been shown to be effective, even in neurocysticercosis (Botero and Castano, 1982; deGhetaldi *et al.*, 1983). Surgical intervention may be required in some ocular or cerebral cases. Removal of superficial nodules is useful only for diagnostic purposes.

Epidemiology. Human exposure to cysticercosis results when the eggs of *T. solium* are ingested. This may occur when eggs that have been liberated from disintegrating gravid proglottids passed by one individual are ingested by another in contaminated food or water (heteroinfection), or when eggs are transferred from anus to mouth of an individual who has an intestinal infection with *T. solium* (external autoinfection). Internal autoinfection may occur if gravid proglottids in an individual harboring the adult *T. solium* become detached from the main strobila, are regurgitated into the stomach and then returned to the duodenum, where they liberate ripened eggs, but conclusive evidence for this occurrence is lacking. Heteroinfection is the usual mode of transfer. Some cases are attributable to the custom of fertilizing vegetable gardens with human feces.

Control. Prevention of cysticercosis involves (1) prompt treatment of humans infected with the adult worm, (2) good personal hygiene, (3) sanitary measures to prevent pigs from becoming infected, and (4) adequate cooking or prior freezing of pork to prevent human infection with the adult worm.

Cysticercus of *Taenia crassiceps*

Taenia crassiceps, a parasite of foxes in Europe and northern North America, utilizes various rodents as intermediate hosts. The cysticercus in these hosts may reproduce asexually by exogenous budding. A large budding cysticercus of *T. crassiceps* was found in the eye of a young woman in Canada.

Coenurus of *Taenia* Species
(Coenurosis)

The *coenurus* resembles the cysticercus except that its bladder generally is much larger and bears numerous protoscolices rather than one (Fig. 10–16). Final hosts are dogs and their wild relatives, and the coenurus stage occurs in animals preyed upon by them. The coenurus is the larval stage of several species of *Taenia*, all very similar. *T. multiceps* is found in sheep-raising areas, not including the United States; its coenurus characteristically develops in the brain and spinal cord of the sheep and causes symptoms characteristic of central nervous system lesions. *T. serialis* is a North American species and its coenurus characteristically develops in the subcutaneous tissues of rabbits and hares. *T. brauni* occurs in Africa, especially East Africa, and is common in small rodents. *T. glomerata,* also an African species whose coenurus is found in small rodents, is known mainly in West Africa. Each of these four species has been

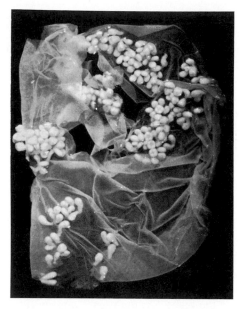

Fig. 10–16. *Taenia multiceps*. *Coenurus* from base of brain of a 2-year-old boy in California. ($\times$ 3.) (Courtesy of H.D. Johnstone.)

identified in man—in the brain in cases reported from California and South Dakota in the United States and in France, England and Africa; in the subcutaneous or intramuscular tissue in cases reported from the United States (Texas), Canada, and Africa; and in the eye in numerous cases in both West and East Africa, especially the latter. In *T. multiceps*, the protoscolices tend to be distributed in clusters. In the other species, notably in *T. serialis,* the protoscolices characteristically have a linear distribution.

HYDATID CYSTS OF *ECHINOCOCCUS* SPECIES
(Echinococcosis, hydatid disease)

A hydatid (or hydatid cyst) is the larval stage of species of *Echinococcus,* the adults of which are parasites attached to the intestinal mucosa of dogs, wolves, foxes, and related carnivorous mammals. Usually there are several adult worms in an infection, and at times there may be hundreds or thousands. The adults of all species of *Echinococcus* are small, rarely over a centimeter in length. The strobila consists of scolex, neck, and one immature, one mature, and one or two gravid proglottids. In addition to 4 minute suckers, the scolex is provided with a double row of alternating rostellar hooks. Gravid proglottids disintegrate in the intestine and eggs are evacuated in the feces. These eggs cannot be distinguished from those species of *Taenia* that are parasites of dogs.

In a suitable intermediate host, eggs hatch in the duodenum and the hexacanth embryos work their way through the wall of the intestine, reach a mesenteric venule (or lymphatic vessel), and become lodged in hepatic, pulmonary, or other tissues. The embryo then transforms into a hydatid, having a mother cyst wall and many protoscolices, that are derived from a germinal membrane. The hydatids of three species, *Echinococcus granulosus, E. multilocularis,* and *E. vogeli* develop in the human host. That of a fourth species, *E. oligarthrus,* is not known to occur in man (D'Alessandro *et al.,* 1979).

Hydatid of *Echinococcus granulosus*
(Unilocular hydatid disease)

Although hydatid cyst was known to ancient physicians and historians, Goeze in 1782 first demonstrated that the causative organism was a cestode. The adult worm in the dog's intestine was discovered by Hartmann in 1695. In 1786 Batsch gave it the name "granulosus," and in 1805 Rudolphi placed it in the genus *Echinococcus.* In 1852 von Siebold first fed cysts from cattle to dogs and in 3 weeks recovered the minute adult worms from the intestine.

E. granulosus is widely distributed throughout temperate and subtropical regions where sheep are extensively raised. Human infection is common in southern South America, much of Africa, eastern and southern Europe, the Middle East, southern Australia, New Zealand, and extensive areas of Asia. A few autochthonous cases are diagnosed each year in the United States and southern Canada. In northern Canada and Alaska the disease is highly enzootic. In the Central Valley of California the infection occurs in sheep and in dogs, coyotes, and deer, as well as in man. Human infections have been acquired in Utah (Crellin *et al.,* 1982).

Morphology, Biology, and Life Cycle. The adult *E. granulosus* lives in the small intestine of the canine host, with its scolex embedded between the villi. The worm (Fig. 10–17*A*) measures up to 6 mm long. It has a pyriform scolex provided with 4 suckers and a rostellar crown of 28 to 50 hooks. When eggs are swallowed by sheep, cattle, hogs, other herbivores, or man, they hatch in the intestine and the hexacanth embryos migrate through blood and lymphatic channels to the liver and less frequently to other viscera. Here they develop, rather slowly, into *unilocular hydatids,* characterized by an external, milky white laminated membrane and an internal germinal layer typically producing multiple protoscolices and daughter cysts within the parent cyst. Usually the primary cyst has a dense

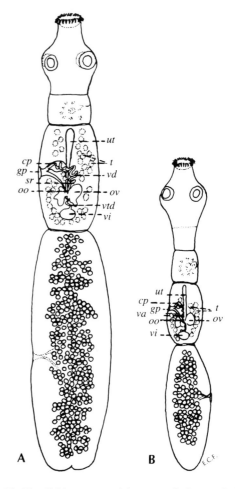

Fig. 10–17. *Echinococcus,* adult worms, the larvae of which produce two of the three known types of hydatid cysts in man. *A, E. granulosa* from small intestine of dog, Yugoslavia. *B. E. multilocularis* from fox, South Germany. *cp,* Cirrus pouch. *gp,* Genital pore. *oo,* Ootype. *ov,* Ovary. *sr,* Seminal receptacle. *t,* Testes. *ut,* Uterus. *va,* Vagina. *vd,* Vas deferens. *vi,* Vitellaria. *vtd,* Vitelline duct. (× 25.) (Adapted from original of E.C. Faust.)

layer of host connective tissues over the laminated membrane. A majority of human hydatids develop in the liver; infection of the lungs is next in prevalence; if they pass the pulmonary filter, the embryos may settle down in any organ or tissue, including bone, and proceed to develop into hydatids. In some areas of South America and Canada, the pulmonary location is more frequent than the hepatic one.

Pathogenesis and Symptomatology. There are two morphologic types in human tissues, unilocular and osseous. The *unilocular cyst* has a fluid-filled cavity lined with a germinal membrane, surrounded by a friable laminated membrane that is covered with a host-tissue capsule (Figs. 10–18 and

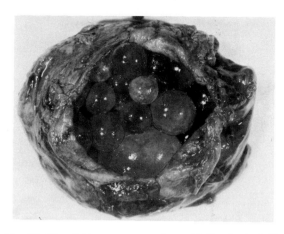

Fig. 10–18. *Echinococcus granulosus.* Unilocular hydatid cyst, 12 cm in diameter and containing numerous daughter cysts ranging up to 7 cm in diameter, removed from the liver of a Greek seaman from whom two similar cysts had been removed 6 years earlier. (Courtesy of U.S. Marine Hospital, New Orleans, Louisiana.)

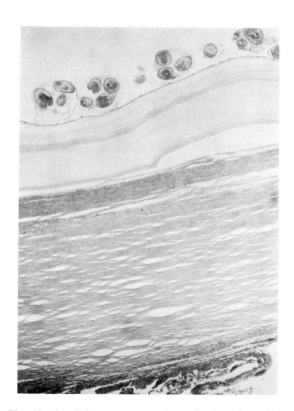

Fig. 10–19. *Echinococcus granulosus.* Section of a unilocular hydatid cyst from lung, showing brood capsules with protoscolices, a thin cellular germinal membrane, thick, noncellular laminated membrane, and much thicker, fibrous host-tissue capsule. (× 40.) (By P.C. Beaver.)

10–19). A majority of human hydatids are unilocular, but if the hexacanth embryo reaches bony tissues, outer membranes are not produced and the organism proceeds to grow as a protoplasmic stream that erodes the cancellous tissues, particularly of the long bones and the pelvic arch, forming an *osseous hydatid.*

The size of the unilocular hydatid depends on the site of implantation and on its age. After 12 to 20 years, it may be 15 cm or more in diameter, containing a liter or more of clear, sterile hydatid fluid, typically with numerous protoscolices and daughter hydatids (Fig. 10–19). If a large abdominal cyst bursts, either spontaneously or following a blow on the abdomen, anaphylaxis may be precipitated by the sudden liberation of hydatid fluid into the peritoneal cavity. Moreover, protoscolices spilled out of the cyst cavity will become implanted in the peritoneum and produce multiple secondary growths. Rupture of a pulmonary cyst into a bronchus results in the patient's coughing up the contents, with possible spontaneous clearance of the infection. Hydatid of the brain produces increasing symptomatic evidence of an intracranial tumor. Osseous hydatid is insidious, gradually eroding the bone to a stage at which fracture or crumbling suddenly occurs.

Diagnosis and Treatment. In endemic areas, experienced clinicians may obtain strong suspicion of hydatid disease from the patient's history, presenting symptoms, and x-ray films. More specific diagnosis can be obtained by the intradermal test employing a known amount of hydatid antigen. A positive reaction of the immediate type, *i.e.,* within 15 minutes, indicates that the patient has or has had hydatid disease. Immunologic tests may be useful, but their interpretation requires experience and judgment (Schantz *et al.,* 1983). Final diagnosis consists of demonstration of free protoscolices or daughter cysts from aspirated hydatid fluid or of the histologic structure of the cyst wall, with its laminated membrane.

Chemotherapy of hydatid disease has been studied extensively in animals and in humans. Although a standard treatment has not evolved (Schantz *et al.,* 1982), chemotherapy with mebendazole provides some benefit. The standard procedure is surgical removal of the cyst. If surgical removal is not possible, oral therapy with mebendazole may be tried. Dosage has not yet been established. In many people infected with unilocular hydatid, the parasite eventually dies and becomes calcified if it is located in an anatomic site where it does not produce important pressure effects.

Epidemiology. Human infection with the hydatid cyst of *E. granulosus* is apt to occur where dogs harbor the adult worms and sheep or hogs serve as common reservoirs of the larval stage. The hydatid in cattle is characteristically sterile. Exposure commonly occurs in childhood, particularly among boys who play with infected dogs. Herders of infected sheep and swine are likewise frequently exposed. The hydatid may grow for 5 to 20 years before it causes serious concern. Hence, exposure usually occurs several to many years before diagnosis is made. In different parts of the world there are distinct populations of *Echinococcus* parasites insofar as their normal host ranges are concerned. In England the horse is a significant reservoir. In Switzerland, cattle are important intermediate hosts.

Control. Control must be directed against the dog, the carrier of the adult *Echinococcus granulosus,* and sheep, the common reservoirs of the viable hydatid. All infected carcasses should be deeply buried or incinerated. Stray dogs should be destroyed. Domestic dogs should be periodically dewormed. Personal hygiene in endemic areas includes care to avoid contamination of food and drink with the feces of dogs.

Hydatid of *Echinococcus multilocularis*
(Alveolar hydatid disease)

In 1855 Virchow recognized a morphologic form of human hydatid that differed from the usual unilocular type. In 1863 Leuckart named it *multilocularis*. Yet until 1951 there was no accepted proof that there existed more than one species of hydatids that infect man and herbivorous mammals. Soon thereafter it was shown that in the Arctic region of Alaska and in South Germany foxes and other wild canines are the definitive hosts of *E. multilocularis* and that the natural hosts of the hydatids are wild mice.

Alveolar hydatid in man occurs in Central and Eastern Europe, the Balkans, the U.S.S.R., Siberia, among Eskimos in Alaska, in Minnesota, and on Rebun Island, Japan.

Morphology, Biology, and Life Cycle. The adult *E. multilocularis* (Fig. 10–17*B*) is smaller than *E. granulosus*—1.2 to 3.7 mm long—and the disposition of the genital pore with respect to the reproductive organs as well as the number of testes is consistently different in the two species. The eggs are indistinguishable. In nature and in experimental tests, when eggs are ingested by field mice, tundra voles, ground squirrels and shrews (Alaska),

and mice (South Germany), the hatched hexacanth embryos migrate from the intestine to the viscera, mostly the liver, where they lodge and proceed to grow by exogenous budding, in this way developing into alveolar hydatids. When the infected viscera are eaten by a canine host, each hydatid scolex transforms into an adult *E. multilocularis*.

Pathogenesis and Symptomatology. The site of the alveolar hydatid in man, a relatively poor intermediate host, is commonly the liver and rarely the lungs. Here the hydatid develops minute irregular cavities, each within a hyaline membrane, frequently without fibrous encapsulation, so that the organism grows without capsular confinement, producing destruction of the surrounding host tissues. Often scolices in the alveolar hydatid in man are few or none. Normal fertile cysts can be grown from portions of the sterile cyst by inoculation into the peritoneal cavity of rodents.

The hepatic alveolar hydatid produces neither fever nor hepatomegaly, but jaundice, ascites, and splenomegaly may appear in the later stages, resulting from intrahepatic portal hypertension. This infection is usually fatal.

Diagnosis and Treatment. Specific diagnosis is likely to be missed in the living patient and may be missed at autopsy because of the general unfamiliarity of pathologists with this type of hydatid infection. Alveolar hydatid is not amenable to surgical removal. Successful treatment with mebendazole has been reported, but a standard treatment has not evolved.

Epidemiology. In agricultural and woodland areas in Central Europe, man probably acquires alveolar hydatid from eating raw fruits and vegetables picked off the ground and contaminated with the feces of infected foxes and other Canidae; in boreal regions, sledge dogs and foxes are the sources of eggs that cause human infection.

Control. No effective control measures have been devised.

Hydatid of *Echinococcus vogeli*
(Polycystic hydatid disease)

Echinococcus vogeli was described by Rausch and Bernstein in 1972. The adult differs from *E. granulosus* in its greater length and more slender proglottids. The natural cycle of infection involves the bush dog as final host and the paca as intermediate host. The hydatid, referred to as *polycystic,* is alveolar in character but less so than that of *E. multilocularis*. Human infections have been reported in Colombia, Costa Rica, Panama, Ecuador, and Venezuela.

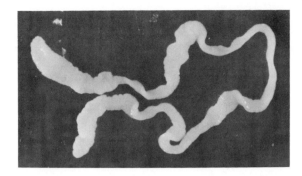

Fig. 10–20. *Sparganum,* probably *S. mansoni.* Live specimen in saline after removal from the abdominal cavity of a man in Thailand. (× 2.) (From Khamboonruang, C., Premasathian, D., and Little, M.D. 1974. A case of intra-abdominal sparganosis in Chiang Mai, Thailand. Am. J. Trop. Med. Hyg., 23:538–539.)

Sparganum of *Spirometra* Species
(Sparganosis)

In 1882 at Amoy, China, Patrick Manson discovered at autopsy a dozen glistening, ribbonlike worms, which Cobbold designated *Ligula mansoni* and which were later found to be the sparganum (plerocercoid stage) of *Spirometra mansoni,* a common parasite of dogs and cats in the Orient and in other parts of the world.

Several species of *Spirometra* are intestinal parasites of canine and feline hosts. For these pseudophyllidean tapeworms, *Cyclops* is the first intermediate host. Second intermediate hosts are various species of vertebrates such as fishes, frogs, snakes, birds, and mammals. The life cycle of *Spirometra* species follows the same pattern as that of *Diphyllobothrium* species. Human infection can be acquired by swallowing a procercoid in a copepod or a plerocercoid in a second intermediate or paratenic host.

A large majority of human infections with unbranched spargana (Fig. 10–20) occur in the China Sea area (Japan and Korea, southern China, Vietnam, Thailand) and in Indonesia. Cases have also been reported from Africa, India, Holland, Australia, and the Western Hemisphere, including the southern United States, Uruguay, Colombia, Ecuador, British Guiana, Puerto Rico, and Belize.

Pathogenesis and Symptomatology. Early in the infection there is relatively little host tissue reaction, but eventually the parasite provokes an infiltration of eosinophils and other inflammatory cells and a tender, puffy area develops around the parasite. Later the parasite may die, causing an intense inflammatory reaction, with a preponderance of eosinophils and Charcot-Leyden crystals.

Ocular sparganosis is characterized by intense pain, irritation, and palpebral edema, with excessive lacrymation. If the worm lodges under the conjunctiva it is likely to provoke nodule formation; if its position is retrobulbar, it causes lagophthalmea and corneal ulceration.

Diagnosis. Unless physicians live in endemic areas and have had experience with cases of sparganosis, the living, contracting, and elongating larva removed from a superficial furuncle or nodule will be a distinct novelty. It can be diagnosed only as the sparganum of a species of *Spirometra* unless recovered intact in the living condition, fed to a young cat or dog, and grown to the adult stage.

Treatment. A single sparganum in superficial tissues is easily removed after incision of the skin under local anesthesia and withdrawal of the worm by gentle traction. Ocular sparganosis is a more serious matter and requires skill to remove the parasite without additional damage to the tissues of the eye.

Epidemiology. Human infection with the sparganum stage of species of *Spirometra* results from (1) drinking pond, lake, or stream water containing procercoid-infected *Cyclops;* (2) eating a raw infected frog, snake, or small mammal, or (3) applying plerocercoid-infected flesh of frogs, snakes, or possibly warm-blooded animals as a poultice on an inflamed eye or finger. As spargana are known to develop in pigs, human infection may occasionally be acquired by eating raw pork. In the United States 65 or more cases of sparganosis have been reported, mostly in Florida and the central Gulf States.

Control. Sparganosis can be avoided by drinking only safe water, eating only well-cooked flesh of animals, and using no flesh poultices.

Sparganum proliferum
(Malignant sparganosis)

Sparganum proliferum, a branching type, has been reported in man in Japan, Taiwan, Paraguay, Venezuela, and the U.S.A. (Florida). The adult form of this type of sparganum is unknown. By malignant asexual proliferation and metastasis, the parasite spreads through the cutaneous and subcutaneous tissues or expands to form massive tumors in the body cavities. The infection usually is fatal (Beaver and Rolon, 1981; Moulinier *et al.,* 1982).

SUMMARY

1. The principal tapeworms of man are *Taenia saginata, Taenia solium, Hymenolepis nana,* and *Diphylloboth-*

rium latum. All of these parasites inhabit the small intestine, with the minute scolex (head) attached to the mucosa and the body of the worm (strobila) absorbing nutrients from the intestinal contents and maintaining its position against the intestinal current by its own motility. The delicate neck region proliferates hermaphroditic proglottids (segments), which in turn generate eggs. Eggs pass from the host's body in motile gravid proglottids *(Taenia* species) or are distributed randomly in the feces *(Hymenolepis, Diphyllobothrium).* Eggs of *Taenia* and *Hymenolepis* are infective when passed, but those of *Diphyllobothrium* require development in cool, clear fresh water.

2. Infection is acquired by ingestion of larvae in the flesh of intermediate hosts (the cysticercus of *T. saginata* in beef, that of *T. solium* in pork, and the plerocercoid of *D. latum* in fish) or in the egg directly by fecal contamination of food or water *(H. nana).*

3. Tapeworms in the intestine generally are well tolerated. Gravid proglottids of *T. saginata* crawling from the anus during the day are an annoyance and those of *T. solium* distribute eggs where they may be ingested and cause cysticercosis in the infected person or others. In some individuals *D. latum* causes anemia, and all tapeworms, including *H. nana,* may cause intestinal symptoms.

4. Diagnosis is made by detecting and identifying free proglottids *(T. saginata)* or the eggs or proglottids in the feces. Drugs of choice for treatment, both of which are usually effective, are niclosamide and praziquantel.

5. The principal larval cestodes causing disease in man are the cysticercus of *Taenia solium (Cysticercus cellulosae),* the coenurus of *Taenia multiceps* and related species, and the hydatid of *Echinococcus* species. Infections with cysticercus are acquired by ingesting eggs passed in the feces of human *(T. solium)* or canine (coenurus and hydatid) hosts. The cysticercus and at least one species of coenurus frequently develop in the central nervous system and eye; the most frequent locations of hydatid cysts are the liver and lungs, but all may develop in other sites. A fourth type of larval cestode causing disease in man is the sparganum (plerocercoid) of *Spirometra* species, which is acquired by ingesting a procercoid in a copepod in water from lakes or streams, or a plerocercoid in the raw flesh of a frog, snake, or mammal that had eaten an infected copepod.

6. The pathologic effects and symptoms caused by larval cestodes depend largely on their size and location. The preferred treatment is surgical removal. When surgery is not feasible, treatment with mebendazole or other benzimidazole or with praziquantel may be beneficial.

REFERENCES

Beaver, P.C., and Rolon, F.A. 1981. Proliferating larval cestode in a man in Paraguay. A case report and review. Am. J. Trop. Med. Hyg., *30*:625–637.

Botero, D., and Castano, S. 1982. Treatment of cysticercosis with praziquantel in Colombia. Am. J. Trop. Med. Hyg., *31*:810–821.

Crellin, J.R., Andersen, F.L., Schantz, P.M., and Condie, S.J. 1982. Possible factors influencing distribution and prevalence of *Echinococcus granulosus* in Utah. Am. J. Epidemiol., *116*:463–474.

D'Alessandro, A., Rausch, R.L., Cuello, C., and Aristizabal, N. 1979. *Echinococcus vogeli* in man, with a review of polycystic hydatid disease in Colombia and neighboring countries. Am. J. Trop. Med. Hyg., *28*:303–317.

DeGhetaldi, L.D., Norman, R.M., and Douville, A.W., Jr. 1983. Cerebral cysticercosis treated biphasically with dexamethasone and praziquantel. Ann. Intern. Med., *99*:179–181.

Grisolia, J.S., and Wiederholt, W.C. 1982. CNS cysticercosis. Arch. Neurol., *39*:540–544.

McCormick, G.F., Zee, C.S., and Heiden, J. 1982. Cysticercosis cerebri. Review of 127 cases. Arch. Neurol., *39*:534–539.

Moulinier, R., Martinez, E., Torres, J., Noya, O., de Noya, B.A., and Reyes, O. 1982. Human proliferative sparganosis in Venezuela: Report of a case. Am. J. Trop. Med. Hyg., *31*:358–363.

Ruttenber, A.J., Weniger, B.G., Sorvillo, F., Murray, R.A., and Ford, S.L. 1984. Diphyllobothriasis associated with salmon consumption in Pacific Coast states. Am. J. Trop. Med. Hyg., *33*:455–459.

Schantz, P.M., Van den Bossche, H., and Eckert, J. 1982. Chemotherapy for larval echinococcosis in animals and humans: Report of a workshop. Z. Parasitenkd., *67*:5–26.

———, Wilson, J.F., Wahlquist, S.P., Boss, L.P., and Rausch, R.L. 1983. Serologic tests for diagnosis and post-treatment evaluation of patients with alveolar hydatid disease *(Echinococcus multilocularis).* Am. J. Trop. Med. Hyg., *32*:1381–1386.

Chapter 11

Nematodes of the Digestive Tract and Related Species

M. D. Little

NEMATODES AS A GROUP

Nematodes are unsegmented, typically elongate and cylindrical, with a fundamentally bilateral symmetry. They have a complete digestive tract and a body cavity (pseudocele) not lined with mesothelium. With few exceptions they are *dioecious*. They range in size from minute, too small to be readily seen by the unaided eye, to many centimeters in length and several millimeters in diameter.

The *body wall* consists of an outer cuticula, an inner muscular layer, and an intermediate thin syncytial hypodermis that secretes the cuticula and binds it to the outer surface of the muscle fibers. Arising from the hypodermis, cords project toward the body cavity at the dorsal, ventral, and lateral lines, dividing the muscles into distinct quadrants (Fig. 11–1). The muscle fibers, several in each quadrant, are oriented parallel to the long axis of the body; thus locomotion is essentially like that of eels and snakes.

Specialized structures at the anterior end of the body serve for attachment, penetration, and sensory purposes. The cuticula may also bear scales or spines, especially over the anterior portion, but the body surface of nematodes generally is finely ridged transversely or smooth.

The *alimentary tract* (Fig. 11–2) is divided into three main portions: (1) an anterior part consisting of buccal cavity and esophagus, both lined with cuticula; (2) a midgut with a single layer of epithelial cells, without cuticular lining, and (3) a hindgut or rectum, which is lined with cuticula.

The *excretory system* consists fundamentally of two longitudinal tubules embedded in the lateral cords. These tubules end blindly at the posterior

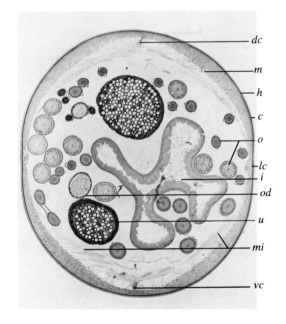

Fig. 11–1. *Ascaris lumbricoides.* Transverse section at midbody level. *c,* Cuticle. *dc,* Dorsal cord. *h,* Hypodermis (between cuticle and muscles). *i,* Intestine. *lc,* Lateral cord, bearing minute excretory canal. *m,* Muscles. *mi,* Muscle innervation processes. *o,* Ovary. *od,* Oviduct. *u,* Uterus. *vc,* Ventral cord. (× 13.) (By P.C. Beaver.)

end; anteriorly they have a transverse ventral connection with a single midventral excretory pore, usually near the nerve ring or the mouth.

The *nervous system* is composed of a circumesophageal nerve ring and short anterior and posterior trunks that run along the ventral, dorsal, and lateral cords and unite near the caudal extremity.

Sense organs of importance in the nematodes are the amphids and the phasmids. The *amphids* consist of a pair of minute, lateral bodies at the anterior end of the body, each with an external chamber

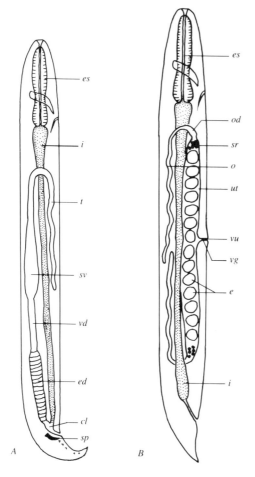

Fig. 11–2. Nematode, male and female. Diagram of principal organs. *cl*, Cloaca. *e*, Eggs. *ed*, Ejaculatory duct. *es*, Esophagus. *i*, Intestine. *o*, Ovary. *od*, Oviduct. *sp*, Spicule. *sr*, Seminal receptacle. *sv*, Seminal vesicle. *t*, Testis. *ut*, Uterus. *vd*, Vas deferens. *vg*, Vagina. *vu*, Vulva. (By M.D. Little.)

that may be a simple pore or a circular, spiral, helical, or elongate tubule. Most nematodes have a pair of minute organs called *phasmids* that are postanal in position.

Nematodes usually are bisexual. However, in a few instances the female may be *parthenogenetic*. Males generally are somewhat smaller than females and may be much smaller, as in *Dracunculus*.

The *male* reproductive system consists typically of a single tubule, beginning as a testis, then a seminal vesicle, a vas deferens, and an ejaculatory duct, opening into the cloaca (Fig. 11–2*A*). Accessory copulatory structures consist of one or two copulatory spicules, which may be of equal length and bristlelike or unequal and variously shaped, and usually a supporting structure, the gubernaculum. In hookworms and their relatives the pos-

terior end of the male is extended into an umbrellalike structure of cuticula supported by fleshy rays *(bursa copulatrix)*, which is applied around the female at the vulva for copulation.

The *female* reproductive system (Fig. 11–2*B*) may be composed of a single reproductive set, as in *Trichinella* and *Trichuris*, but in most nematodes the inner organs are paired. The following regions can usually be recognized: ovary, oviduct, seminal receptacle, uterus, vagina, ovejector, and vulva, which is ventral in position.

The *ovum* characteristically contains yolk material. After passing down the oviduct and being fertilized, it secretes around itself a thin vitelline membrane, a somewhat thicker chitinous layer, and an inner very resistant lipid membrane. In some roundworms such as *Ascaris*, an additional outer shell layer is laid on as a secretion of the wall of the uterus.

The daily production of eggs per female varies greatly in different species. The stage of development at the time of oviposition also varies. Eggs of *Ascaris* and *Trichuris* are unembryonated; those of hookworms are in early stages of cleavage, and those of *Strongyloides* frequently are in the morula or a more advanced stage. In *Trichinella, Dracunculus*, and the filariae, the eggs develop completely and the larvae hatch *in utero* to be discharged as larvae or microfilariae, *i.e.*, these nematodes are *larviparous*.

The fundamental stages in the nematode life cycle are the egg, four larval stages, and the adult. At the end of each larval stage a new cuticula is secreted and the old one is molted.

Several groups of parasitic nematodes require two hosts. In *Trichinella spiralis* all stages in the life cycle are in one host, but transmission of infection to a new host is dependent on ingestion of the larvae encapsulated in the striated muscles of the first host. *Dracunculus* infection in the definitive host results from ingesting copepods *(Cyclops)*, which as intermediate hosts harbor the larval stage. Blood-sucking arthropods are essential intermediate hosts of the filarial worms.

When intermediate hosts are not involved, as in the majority of intestinal roundworms of man, there is a necessary period of development outside the body, frequently in soil, after which the larva in the egg, or free, is infective. Eggs freshly passed in the feces are not infective.

The nematode parasites of man, including numerous zoonotic species, mainly belong to 11 major groups (superfamilies): Trichinelloidea *(Trichinella, Trichuris, Capillaria)*, Dioctophymatoidea *(Dioctophyma)*, Oxyuroidea *(Enterobius)*, Ascaridoidea *(Ascaris, Toxocara)*, Ancyclostomatoidea *(Necator, Ancylostoma)*, Trichostrongyloidea *(Trichostrongylus)*, Metastrongyloidea *(Angiostrongylus)*, Rhabditoidea *(Strongyloides)*, Dracunculoidea *(Dracunculus)*, Gnathostomatoidea *(Gnathostoma)*, and Filarioidea *(Wuchereria, Brugia, Mansonella, Loa, Onchocerca)*.

TRICHINELLA AND RELATED SPECIES
(Trichinelloidea)

In the *Trichinella* group, which in addition to *Trichinella spiralis* includes species of *Trichuris* and *Capillaria*, the forebody is filiform and filled with linearly arranged, relatively large cells *(stichocytes)*, referred to collectively as the *stichosome*. The esophagus, proportionately slender and mostly nonmuscular, is embedded in the stichosome through most of its length. The hindbody, relatively stout, contains the reproductive organs, which in both sexes are single.

Trichinella spiralis
(Trichinosis)

Trichinella spiralis (Owen, 1835) Railliet, 1895 was first observed in human striated muscle at necropsies in London in 1828. In 1835 Paget found the same stage of the parasite in a cadaver. In the same year Richard Owen described the organism and gave it the specific name *spiralis*. Von Siebold (1844) and Dujardin (1845) suggested that the form was the underdeveloped larval stage of a roundworm; Leuckart (1861) and Virchow (1861) proved that this hypothesis was correct. Meanwhile pathologists in other European countries found trichina cysts in human muscle, while Joseph Leidy (1846), in Philadelphia, first demonstrated their presence in domestic swine. In 1860, Zenker provided evidence that the infection in man was responsible for serious and at times fatal disease (Campbell, 1983).

Until recent decades, trichinosis was an important clinical and public health problem in Europe; today it is still prevalent in Poland, Hungary, and the lower Danube countries. In the United States and parts of Latin America, outbreaks occur in small groups of the population.

Morphology, Biology, and Life Cycle. The adult is minute, barely visible to the unaided eye

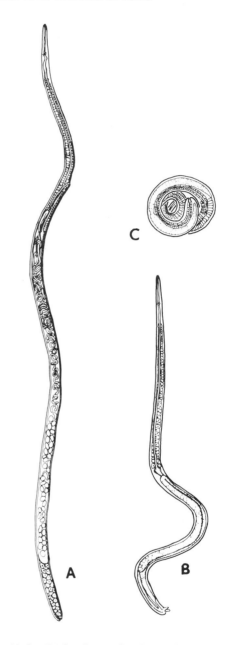

Fig. 11–3. *Trichinella spiralis.* Camera lucida drawings of stained specimens in permanent preparations. *A*, Adult female. *B*, Adult male. *C*, Coiled larva from cyst in muscle. (*A* and *B*, × 75; *C*, × 100.) (From Beaver, P.C. 1952. The detection and identification of some common nematode parasites of man. Am. J. Clin. Pathol., 22:481–494.)

(Fig. 11–3). The male usually measures 1.4 to 1.6 mm in length by 30 to 40 μm in diameter. The cloacal opening is terminal and is guarded by a pair of conical papillae. The female usually is 2.2 to 3.5 mm long by 50 to 60 μm in diameter. The vulva lies midventrally approximately one fifth the body length from the anterior end.

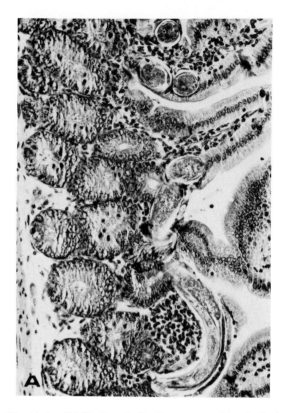

Fig. 11–4. *Trichinella spiralis.* Transverse and longitudinal sections of an adult male in mucosal epithelium at base of villi in small intestine of mouse at 30 hours of infection. (× 180.) (From Gardiner, C.H. 1976. Habitat and reproductive behavior of *Trichinella spiralis.* J. Parasitol., 62:865–870.)

When raw or undercooked meat containing infective *Trichinella* larvae is eaten, digestion in the stomach frees the larvae from their capsules. Upon reaching the intestine, the larvae immediately invade the mucosal epithelium of the glandular crypts (Fig. 11–4), typically at the level of the duodenum and adjacent segment of the jejunum (Gardiner, 1976). Here they develop through four molting stages to maturity and copulate as early as 30 hours postinfection (Kozek, 1971). By the 6th day, the females begin depositing motile larvae measuring about 100 by 6 μm. It is during the 2nd week that the rate of larva production is highest, but larviposition continues for 4 to 16 weeks, with a total output of several hundred per female. In light infections in mice, each female produces about 500 larvae.

After leaving the female, the larvae migrate into the lamina propria, enter lymphatic vessels or venules, and eventually reach the general circulation, which carries them to all parts of the body. Only the larvae that reach striated skeletal muscle are

able to undergo further development. The larva penetrates a muscle fiber and begins rapid growth and development within the cell. As the larva grows, it coils upon itself and induces the host cell to redifferentiate and form a capsule around it (Fig. 11–5). The larva assumes some of the features of the adult and reaches full size, 1 mm long by 30 μm in diameter, about 20 days after entering the fiber and is by then infective for another host. The encapsulation process continues until the 4th or 5th week of infection. Most heavily parasitized are the muscles of the diaphragm, larynx, tongue, and abdomen and the intercostal, masseter, biceps, psoas, pectoral, deltoid, and gastrocnemius muscles. In man, encapsulated larvae may remain viable for many years, but calcification of some may occur within 6 to 9 months (Fig. 11–6).

Pathogenesis. Entry of the young excysted worms into the epithelium of the intestinal mucosa causes an acute eosinophilic cellular reaction. Once larviposition has begun and larvae are distributed among the tissues, their temporary lodgment provokes the same type of cellular response. This is particularly notable in the myocardium, through which larvae migrate but in which they do not encyst, with necrosis and fragmentation of the muscle fibers followed by fibrocytic repair. Similarly, if they lodge in capillaries of the brain, eyes, lungs, or other organs, an acute inflammatory reaction occurs around the invaders (Fig. 11–7).

Invasion of a skeletal muscle fiber by the minute larva causes a redifferentiation of the cell. The contractile filaments are disrupted and within 2 to 4 days the myofibrillar striations disappear. The cell then becomes granular and basophilic, and the sarcolemma nuclei become larger, more numerous, and move to the interior of the fiber. An inner membrane is formed around the larva within an adventitious capsule (Fig. 11–5). In addition to the intense focal infiltration of eosinophils around the adults and larvae in the tissues, there is a characteristic hypereosinophilia of the circulating blood.

Symptomatology. Light infections generally are asymptomatic, although a history of gastrointestinal upset after eating infected meat, followed by muscular pains, can at times be elicited in such cases.

In heavier infections, with invasion of the duodenal and jejunal mucosa by a large number of excysted larvae, the symptoms mimic those of acute food poisoning. This syndrome lasts through the 7th day. Later, larval migration to the muscles

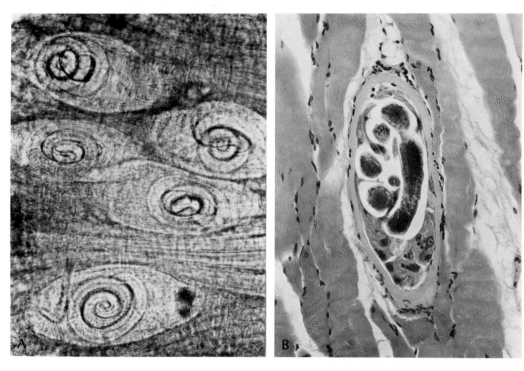

Fig. 11–5. *Trichinella spiralis.* Encapsulated larvae in muscle. *A*, In a press preparation. (× ca 120.) *B*, In longitudinal section. (× ca 200.) (By M.D. Little.)

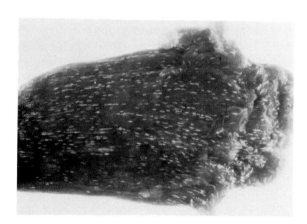

Fig. 11–6. *Trichinella spiralis.* Calcified cysts of unknown age in muscle of a woman who died of leukemia. (Unstained, about natural size.) (From Jacobson, E.S., and Jacobson, H.G. 1977. Trichinosis in an immunosuppressed human host. Am. J. Clin. Pathol., *68*:791–794.)

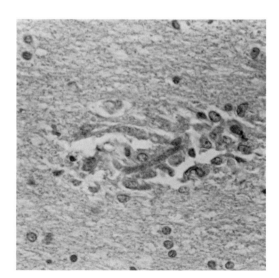

Fig. 11–7. *Trichinella spiralis.* Larva in brain from human autopsy 20 days after onset of illness. The larva, showing no growth or development, is surrounded by scattered glial cells in a small area of necrosis. (× 400.) (By P.C. Beaver; tissue courtesy of F.F. Katz.)

is responsible for severe and at times completely incapacitating myositis, producing difficulty in breathing, mastication, speech, and use of the extremities. Dyspnea may be intense, and edema, particularly of the face, is characteristic, as is fever of 39 to 40°C, occasionally 41°C, remittent in type. Petechial hemorrhages of the skin and mucous membranes, conjunctivae, and retinal vessels commonly occur. These signs and symptoms are most prominent during the 2nd week but may continue throughout the period of larviposition (1 to 3 months). An eosinophilic leukocytosis of up to 50% or higher develops during this period.

The third clinical stage is a culmination of the traumatic and toxic effects of the infection. Edema persists, especially around the eyes. There may be profound cachexia. Migration of the larvae through the cerebral capillaries may cause motor and psychic disturbances, while the lesions in the myocardium may be responsible for congestive heart failure. Fatal outcome or chronic invalidism is not infrequent in heavy infections.

Diagnosis. Without a clear picture of the typical symptoms, a diagnosis of trichinosis must depend on laboratory evidence. This usually cannot be obtained until the larvae produced by the female worms have migrated into striated muscles 14 to 21 days after exposure. Meanwhile severe illness and irreversible pathologic changes may have occurred.

There are two available methods of laboratory diagnosis: (1) biopsy and microscopic examination of a small piece of muscle to demonstrate larvae, either under compression or after digestion in artificial gastric juice, and (2) immunologic tests. The immunologic tests commonly used are flocculation and precipitin reactions (see Chapter 20).

Treatment. There is no established specific therapy for the tissue phase of trichinosis. In patients who are critically ill because of allergic reactions to or intoxication with substances derived from the worms, administration of ACTH or adrenocorticosteroids ameliorates the crisis (see Chapter 21). Mebendazole and related benzimidazoles are effective against the enteric stages in experimental animals and have been reported to be effective in humans. In severe acute infections, mebendazole therapy along with corticosteroids is used until symptoms subside or toxic effects occur (Pawlowski, 1983). Treatment may be accompanied by marked toxic or allergic reactions.

Prognosis. In heavy infections the prognosis is poor to grave, in lighter infections it is fair to good. In severe epidemics the mortality is highly variable; the average probably is about 1%.

Epidemiology. In nature trichinosis is an enzootic disease, for the most part propagated among black and brown rats which are cannibalistic. Although all stages in the life cycle of *T. spiralis* are developed in a single host, in order that enzooticity may continue, it is necessary that the infected muscle of one host be eaten by another. In East Africa the infection is maintained largely by hyenas, which feed on other carnivores and on each other.

Human trichinosis usually is acquired from eating inadequately cooked pork, but at times it may be acquired from eating bear meat (northwestern United States, Alaska) or walrus meat (Greenland). In the United States, pigs fed on grain or forage have fewer infections than those fattened on uncooked municipal garbage. Striking reductions in prevalence, mortality, and severity of infection with *T. spiralis* in man and pigs in the United States during the past 25 years have been brought about by legislation requiring heat treatment of garbage fed to swine and by extensive use of lowtemperature storage of pork, increased use of prepared pork products, and education of the public as to proper methods of cooking pork. The sporadic cases and outbreaks of the disease that still occur are the result of carelessness in feeding, processing, and cooking pigs raised for personal use. The high frequency with which people eat rare or undercooked pork is illustrated by an outbreak in Spain in which at least 452 cases of trichinosis in 5 neighboring provinces were traced to the same small abattoir (World Health Organization, 1983). In Latin America, human trichinosis occurs with high frequency only in Chile. Outbreaks have occurred in recent years in the United States, Canada, Czechoslovakia, Lebanon, Spain, Poland, and the U.S.S.R. Outbreaks from eating bear meat are becoming more frequent; in recent years approximately 10% of recorded cases in the northern states, Canada, and Alaska have been traced to bear meat. Outbreaks traced to horsemeat have occurred in France and Italy.

Control. As the main source of infection is domestic pork, condemning infected carcasses based on microscopic examination of muscles of each slaughtered hog would be desirable but is impracticable. Serologic detection of infected pigs is at present an inadequate safeguard (Seawright *et al.*, 1983). Larvae in pork can be killed by two practical methods: freezing and cooking. In a home freezer (about −15°C), storage for 20 days is required to provide safe pork. Storage of pork in deep-freeze units is simple, effective, and particularly applicable to rural areas. Thorough cooking of pork is always a safeguard, but the danger lies in failure to heat the inside of the meat sufficiently to kill the larvae, even though the outside may be golden brown (Kotula *et al.*, 1983). When the meat temperature reaches 60°C, larvae are killed immediately. Significantly, larvae of Alaskan strains of *T. spiralis* in the meat of bears and other animals remain infective after storage at −15 to −18°C for several months (Dick, 1983).

Trichuris trichiura
(Trichuriasis)

The human whipworm, *Trichuris trichiura* (Linnaeus, 1771) Stiles, 1901, is cosmopolitan in distribution but it is prevalent only in warm or temperate moist climates.

Morphology, Biology, and Life Cycle. Adult whipworms are thread-like in the anterior three fifths of the body and wider in the posterior portion. The anterior end is threaded into the mucosal epithelium of the cecum or appendix, but when large numbers are present the worms are distributed posteriorly throughout the colon, even in the rectum. Whipworms live for several years.

The male measures 30 to 45 mm in length. Its posterior end is curved ventrally into a coil of 360 degrees or more (Fig. 11–8*B*). The female measures 35 to 50 mm in length. Its posterior portion is club-shaped (Fig. 11–8*A*). The egg output of the mature female is not definitely known, but the average probably lies between 3,000 and 6,000 daily. Reduced production can be expected in heavy infections when the worms are crowded. The narrow, barrel-shaped eggs, about 25 by 55 μm, are laid in the one-celled stage (Fig. 11–9). They have a thin, transparent inner shell, a brownish outer shell, and a transparent blisterlike prominence at each pole. Under favorable conditions of soil, moisture, and temperature, eggs become infective in about 3 weeks. Eggs remain infective for a relatively short period, a few months at most under usual environmental conditions.

Early development of *T. trichiura* in man has not been described. In *Trichuris* species of animals (*T. vulpis* of dogs and *T. suis* of pigs), the larvae hatch from the egg in the lower small intestine and the large intestine and penetrate the mucosa of the

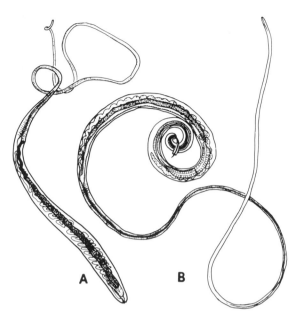

Fig. 11–8. *Trichuris trichiura. A,* Female, showing characteristic whiplike body, convoluted ovary and oviduct, straight uterus, and vagina leading to vulva near junction of intestine and stichosome. *B,* Male, showing characteristically coiled stout hindbody filled with reproductive organs, including convoluted testis, straight genital tube, and extruded spicule. (× 7.) (From Beaver, P.C. 1952. The detection and identification of some common nematode parasites of man. Am. J. Clin. Pathol., *22*:481–494.)

cecum and colon, first in the mucosal epithelium of the crypts, and eventually they work their way to the mucosal surface, with the thin anterior part of the body securely threaded into the epithelium (Fig. 11–10) and the hindbody free in the lumen (Fig. 11–11). All stages of development occur in the intestine. Development of *T. trichiura* to the egg-laying adult stage requires approximately 3 months.

Pathogenesis and Symptomatology. Light infections produce no appreciable symptoms. Larger

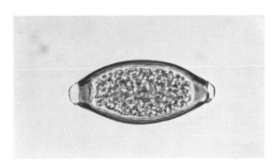

Fig. 11–9. *Trichuris trichiura.* Egg. (× ca. 650.) (By M.D. Little.)

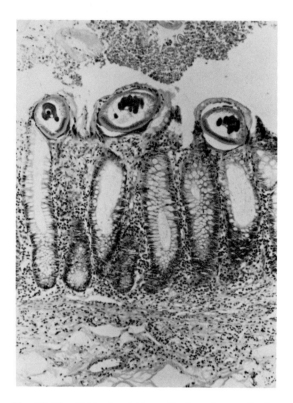

Fig. 11–10. *Trichuris trichiura.* Section of appendix from 1-year-old child showing three sections of thin anterior part of adult worm; as it threads itself into the surface epithelium of the mucosa, the worm induces the formation of a fibrous tunnel that supports it. (× 70.) (By P.C. Beaver.)

numbers cause a corresponding degree of intestinal damage. In heavy infections the mucosa of the entire large bowel may be covered with the worms, matted together in bloody feces; the mucosa itself is hyperemic, at times bleeding and superficially eroded, accompanied by intense eosinophilic inflammation. Irritation produced by these worms in the wall of the lower colon and rectum may eventually provoke prolapse of the rectum (Fig. 11–11).

Children with more than 30 eggs per mg of feces generally have chronic diarrhea or dysentery. The most heavily infected children tend to be between 1 and 5 years of age and have chronic dysentery, rectal prolapse, loss of weight or failure to gain, and anemia. The anemia, microcytic in type, is not caused by sucking of blood by the parasites but by malnutrition and chronic bleeding from the friable intestinal mucosa. Moderate peripheral eosinophilia is often present, and eosinophils and Charcot-Leyden crystals usually are abundant in the dysenteric stools (Fig. 11–12). *Entamoeba histolytica* infection is frequently found in association with trichuriasis.

Diagnosis. Whipworm infection is detected by finding characterstic eggs in the feces (Fig. 11–9). In addition to eggs, diarrheal and dysenteric stools of whipworm patients contain eosinophils and Charcot-Leyden crystals, which may be present several weeks before the worms mature and eggs appear in the stools (Fig. 11–12). Adult or im-

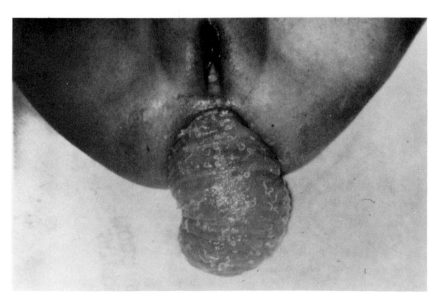

Fig. 11–11. *Trichuris trichiura.* Numerous adult worms attached to mucosal epithelium of prolapsed rectum of 2-year-old child; only the stout posterior end of the worm is evident on the surface. (From Jung, R.C., and Beaver, P.C. 1951. Clinical observations on *Trichocephalus trichiurus* (whipworm) infestation in children. Pediatrics, 8:548–557.)

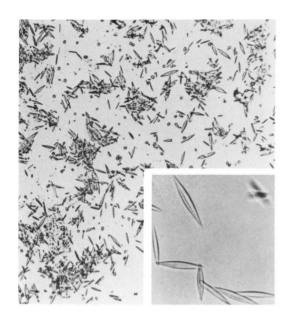

Fig. 11–12. *Trichuris trichiura.* Charcot-Leyden crystals from dysenteric stool of child with heavy worm burden. The crystals are dipyramidal and hexagonal, with each of 6 sides tapering from the base at an angle of 80° and meeting at the apex to form a 20° angle. (× ca. 100; *inset* × 400.) (From Hornung, M. 1962. Preservation, recrystallization and preliminary biochemical characterization of Charcot-Leyden crystals. Proc. Soc. Exp. Biol. Med., *110*:119–124.)

mature worms may be seen attached to the prolapsed rectum (Fig. 11–11) or at sigmoidoscopy.

Treatment. Mebendazole is effective and safe, in a dosage of 100 mg twice daily for 3 days. Light whipworm infections do not require treatment.

Prognosis. For lightly infected persons prognosis is good, but it is poor for those with heavy infections unless the worms are removed.

Epidemiology. Whipworm eggs are evacuated in the stool in an unembryonated condition and require a period of development in soil to reach the infective stage. Conditions favorable for development consist of warm, moist, and shaded soil. After a period of about 4 weeks an active larva is coiled inside the eggshell. The egg is then infective when ingested with contaminated food or taken into the mouth by a dirt-eating child. In endemic foci small children often develop heavy infections by eating contaminated dooryard soil. Yet the highest prevalence characteristically occurs in children of early school age. In countries where trichuriasis is endemic, adults also have high rates of infection. Since there are no important reservoir hosts, human infections are acquired exclusively by ingesting infective-stage eggs derived from human feces.

Control. Whipworm infection can be controlled only by maintaining a high standard of environmental sanitation. Mass treatment may be feasible as a control measure when effective drugs become inexpensive.

Capillaria hepatica
(Hepatic capillariasis)

Capillaria hepatica (Bancroft, 1893) Travassos, 1915, a relative of the whipworm, is a tissue parasite in the liver of domestic and wild mammals, mostly rats. The adult worms are small (about 20 mm long) and more delicate than *Trichuris*. Their eggs, measuring 51 to 67 μm by 30 to 35 μm, resemble those of *T. trichiura* but have a distinctive outer shell (Fig. 11–13*B*). Eggs are deposited and retained in the hepatic parenchyma. When the infected liver is eaten by a predator or scavenger, the eggs are liberated by tissue digestion, passed in the feces, and embryonate in damp shaded soil. Infection results from ingesting the infective-stage eggs. The larva hatched from the egg in the duodenum of the new host enters the intestinal wall and migrates *via* mesenteric-portal blood to the liver; there it penetrates into periportal tissues and matures in about 28 days.

From time to time eggs of this parasite have been found in human feces. Such spurious infection results from eating cooked livers of infected animals. About 20 human cases with liver involvement have been reported, mostly in children. The clinical picture is similar to that of visceral larva migrans. Diagnosis is made by liver biopsy (Fig. 11–13). There is no established therapy. A man with massive infection in Brazil survived after treatment with prednisone, disophenol, and pyrantel tartrate (Pereira and Franca, 1983). Prevention consists of avoiding ingestion of soil and prohibiting dirt-eating by children.

Capillaria philippinensis
(Intestinal capillariasis)

Capillaria philippinensis Chitwood, Velasquez and Salazar, 1968 is the cause of outbreaks of a severe and often fatal sprue-like diarrheal disease in west-central Luzon. An exceptional feature of the infection is that the worm reproduces by internal autoinfection, building up large populations of adult worms and larvae in the intestinal mucosa. Both sexes are small, the female being about 4 mm in length, the male about 3 mm. The esophageal region, with a stichosome characteristic of the genus, extends to the midbody level. Two kinds of eggs, with and without outer shells but of equal size (up to 45 by 21 μm), can be observed in the same worm. The infection also is known to occur in Thailand. The mode of transmission has not been demonstrated, but experimental studies in monkeys suggest that infection is acquired by eating small, uncooked fish. Therapy with mebendazole is effective.

DIOCTOPHYMA AND RELATED SPECIES

Dioctophyma renale

Dioctophyma renale (Goeze, 1782) Stiles, 1901, the giant kidney worm, is rather widely distributed throughout the world in fish-eating mammals, including the dog, wolf, *Canis jubatus*, cat, puma, glutton, raccoon, coati, mink, marten, skunk, weasel, otter, seal, ox, and horse. Thirteen or more human infections with the adult worm are on record. An immature worm was found in a subcutaneous nodule on the chest of a man in California and, likewise, in a boy in Thailand (Beaver and Khamboonruang, 1984).

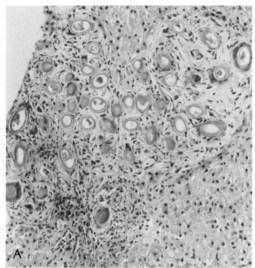
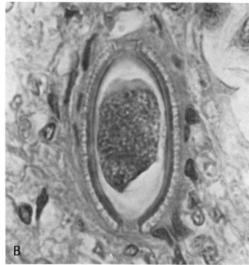

Fig. 11–13. *Capillaria hepatica.* Eggs in punch biopsy of liver from 19-month-old South African child with hypereosinophilia and hepatomegaly. *A,* Cut at various angles. (× 130.) *B,* Cut longitudinally, showing nature of shell and polar plugs. (× 900.) (*A* by P.C. Beaver; *B* by M.D. Little.)

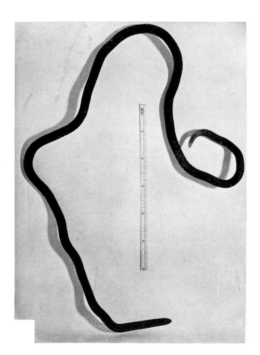

Fig. 11–14. *Dioctophyma renale.* Small, mature female from kidney of naturally infected dog. (Scale is 6 cm.) (Courtesy of T.B. Magath.) (From Beaver, P.C., Jung, R.C., and Cupp, E.W. 1984. *Clinical Parasitology,* 9th ed. Philadelphia, Lea & Febiger, p. 248.)

The adult worms are large cylindrical nematodes, blood-red in color. Males measure 14 to 20 mm in length by 4 to 6 mm in diameter and at their posterior extremity have a bell-shaped copulatory bursa that is not supported by rays. Females measure up to 100 cm in length by 5 to 12 mm in diameter (Fig. 11–14).

The eggs are ellipsoidal, brownish-yellow in color, have deep pittings in the shell except at the poles, and measure 60 to 80 μm by 39 to 46 μm. The normal habitat of adults is in the capsule of a destroyed kidney, but they may be found in the peritoneal and thoracic cavities.

Unembryonated eggs are passed in the urine to water, where development takes place. Aquatic oligochaetes serve as intermediate hosts, and mink and other animals can acquire infection by ingesting infected oligochaetes. However, infective larvae are usually passed through one or more paratenic hosts (tadpoles, frogs, or fish) before reaching the final host.

In the kidney, the worms gradually destroy the parenchyma, finally leaving only the renal capsule. At times a worm migrates into the ureters and may escape through the urethra. All human infections with adult worms have involved the kidneys. Diagnosis is made on microscopic demonstration of typical eggs passed in the urine or on the spontaneous discharge of a worm. No chemotherapy has been developed for this disease.

Eustrongylides

Species of *Eustrongylides,* parasites of the esophagus and proventriculus of fish-eating birds, develop to the infective larval stage in small fish and amphibians. The larvae are red and generally are large, up to 10 cm or more in length. When three fishermen in Maryland (United States) swallowed live bait minnows, all developed severe abdominal pain. Two required abdominal surgery to remove larvae that were migrating through the intestinal wall (Gunby, 1982).

PINWORMS

Members of the Oxyuroidea usually are small worms with a long filamentous tail in the female, a strong muscular esophagus, and a simple life cycle involving transmission of infection through direct transfer of thick-shelled eggs containing the infective larvae, which are highly host-specific.

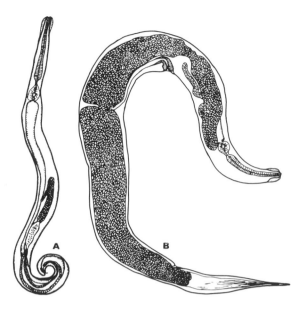

Fig. 11–15. *Enterobius vermicularis*. A, Mature male. B, Gravid female. (× 25.) (From Beaver, P.C. 1952. The detection and identification of some common nematode parasites of man. Am. J. Clin. Pathol., 22:481–494.)

Enterobius vermicularis
(Enterobiasis, oxyuriasis)

The pinworm of man, *Enterobius vermicularis* (Linnaeus, 1758) Leach, 1853, has been known since ancient times. It has a cosmopolitan distribution but is more common in cool or temperate zones than in tropical areas.

Morphology, Biology, and Life Cycle. The mouth of adult *E. vermicularis* has three lips and the anterior end of the worm bears dorsal and ventral bladderlike inflations that can be thrust forward to form a vestibule around the mouth.

The male worm (Fig. 11–15A) measures up to 5 mm long and has a maximum width of 0.1 to 0.2 mm. With its strongly curved posterior end, the lateral view of the worm forms an inverted question mark. The female worm (Fig. 11–15B) is considerably larger than the male, having a length of up to 13 mm and a maximum width of 0.3 to 0.5 mm. The sharply pointed postanal portion is nearly a third of the total length. The characteristic habitat of these worms is the cecum and appendix. When gravid, females migrate down the bowel to the rectum, and during the host's sleep or relaxation they crawl out of the anus onto the perianal and perineal skin. Eggs *in utero* are not fully embryonated when the female worms migrate to the lower levels of the colon. Eggs laid within

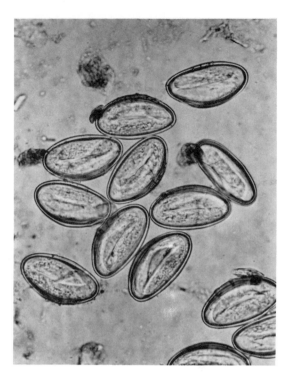

Fig. 11–16. *Enterobius vermicularis*. Eggs on perianal adhesive tape preparation after clearing with toluene. Each contains an infective stage larva and has sides of greater and lesser curvature. (× 400.) (From Beaver, P.C., Jung, R.C., and Cupp, E.W. 1984. *Clinical Parasitology*, 9th ed. Philadelphia, Lea & Febiger, p. 751.)

the bowel are relatively immature. Each female discharges about 10,000 eggs.

The eggs discharged on the skin are essentially mature and within a few hours contain a fully developed infective-stage larva (Fig. 11–16). The eggs are relatively flat on one side and measure 50 to 60 μm by 20 to 30 μm; they have a colorless double shell, an inner membrane, and an outer albuminous layer that causes them to stick to each other and to clothing and other objects. When swallowed the eggs hatch and the larvae, which measure 140 to 150 μm by 10 μm, mature in the cecal area and complete the life cycle in about 1 month or less. It is noteworthy that the prepatent period is not definitely known for man's most common worm parasite.

Pathogenesis and Symptomatology. The first recognizable symptom usually is pruritus as the worms emerge from the anus and crawl over the perianal and perineal skin. Itching is followed by scratching, which adds to the irritation, with scarification or weeping eczema of the area. Because worms in various stages of development are seen in the appendix and occasionally are found deep in the inflamed mucosa, pinworms often are suspected of causing appendicitis (Fig. 11–17). At times worms enter the female genital tract and become encapsulated within the uterus or fallopian tubes or wander into the peritoneal cavity and become encapsulated in the peritoneum. Rarely, they have been found in granulomata in the parenchyma of the lungs and liver (Daly and Baker, 1984). The common symptoms in children, in addition to pruritus ani, consist of restless sleep and tiredness during the daytime. The blood picture in pinworm infection is unremarkable.

Diagnosis. Specific diagnosis may be made on recovery of the worms from the perianal area or following an enema, but more frequently it is made on demonstration of the eggs at the anus. Occasionally eggs are found in the feces. The cellophane tape technique for recovery of pinworm eggs from around the anus has been demonstrated to be the most satisfactory (Fig. 11–16 and Technical Aids, page 252). These preparations are more likely to be positive when perianal impression specimens are taken in the early morning before defecation or a shower or bath.

Treatment. Drugs that are highly effective and without important side-effects are mebendazole, pyrantel pamoate, piperazine hexahydrate, and pyrvinium pamoate. Thiabendazole is also effective but causes nausea and vertigo (see Table 21–1, p. 265). It is often desirable to treat the entire family group at the same time. Treatment should be repeated after about 2 weeks to eliminate worms acquired from eggs persisting in the environment after the initial treatment.

Patients and parents should be made aware of the probability of reinfection, which should not be mistaken for treatment failure. Reinfection may be reduced by hygienic measures described further on under "Control." Individuals constantly exposed in the home, school, or playground and highly susceptible to the annoyances of the infection may require treatment every 5 to 6 weeks. While enterobiasis may be disturbing, it is rarely the cause of serious disease.

Epidemiology. Pinworm infection is often prevalent in large family groups and in schools, asylums, and mental institutions. Eggs contain nearly mature larvae when deposited, and within 6 hours

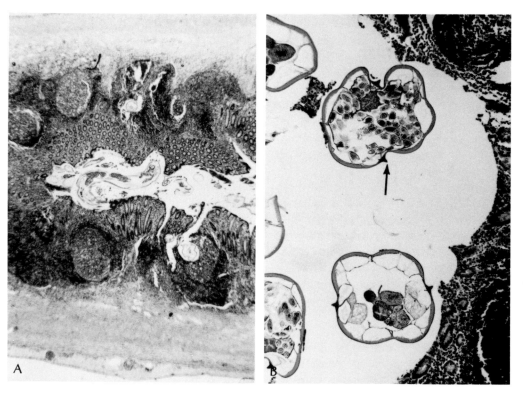

Fig. 11–17. *Enterobius vermicularis.* Section of worms in the appendix of a child. *A,* Numerous immature worms of both sexes in both lumen and deep in mucosa. *B,* Mature nongravid females with eggs in the uterus and characteristic lateral alae *(arrows).* *(A,* × 20; *B,* × 85.) (By P.C. Beaver.)

or less they are fully infective. Exposure may occur in any of three ways: (1) the person harboring the infection may scratch the contaminated skin and transfer the eggs on fingertips to the mouth; (2) individuals sleeping in the same bed or room, using the same toilet, or handling the same objects, such as toys, may be exposed from contaminated fomites; and (3) eggs that become air-borne on floating fibers from soiled undergarments or bed linens may be breathed into the nasopharynx and swallowed by a large number of persons, whose resulting infections usually are light. A cool, moist atmosphere is optimal for survival of infective eggs on fomites; in dry heat and good ventilation they perish rapidly.

Enterobius infection is much more common in children than in adults and is particularly prevalent where several small children sleep together. In any population in which underclothing is worn day after day and bathing is infrequent, a large percentage of the group will be found to be infected. The incidence of infection ranges from saturation to a relatively unimportant figure, depending on environmental conditions and levels of personal and group hygiene. Under similar environmental conditions, infection rates are lower in Negroes than in Caucasians.

Control. Pinworm infection can be controlled by a twofold attack, *viz.,* personal and group hygiene on the one hand and mass chemotherapy on the other. Infection in a family group can be appreciably reduced by providing small children with closed sleeping garments and by keeping the fingernails short. Eggs of pinworms are not killed by chlorination of water in swimming and wading pools.

ASCARIS AND RELATED SPECIES

Members of the *Ascaris* group usually are large and relatively stout, with three fleshy lips bearing sensory papillae around an otherwise simple mouth opening. The life cycles among species living in omnivorous or herbivorous hosts generally tend to differ from those adapted to carnivorous hosts, being more prolonged and complicated in the latter.

Ascaris lumbricoides
(Ascariasis)

Ascaris lumbricoides Linnaeus, 1758, the large intestinal roundworm of man, has been known to physicians since the dawn of history. Davaine in 1863 first discovered that fully mature *Ascaris* eggs

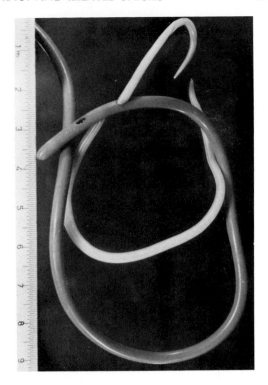

Fig. 11–18. *Ascaris lumbricoides.* Young, 15-cm sexually mature female threaded through the openings of a decompression tube withdrawn from a child under treatment for intestinal obstruction. By its probing tendency, an *Ascaris* occasionally finds its way into the biliary channels, causing abscesses in the liver and less frequently intrahepatic calculi. (Courtesy of R.K. Spillmann.)

hatch in the small intestine, and Stewart in 1916 showed that the hatched larvae require migration to the lungs before final development in the intestine.

With the possible exception of *Enterobius*, *Ascaris lumbricoides* is the most prevalent of all human roundworms and occurs endemically in all parts of the world except in cold, dry climates. Although the highest frequencies are found in tropical areas, ascariasis is also common in many temperate regions of the world.

Morphology, Biology, and Life Cycle. *Ascaris* is the largest roundworm parasitizing the human intestinal tract (Fig. 11–18). It is elongated, cylindrical, and tapers both anteriorly and posteriorly to relatively blunt conical ends. The head is provided with three fleshy lips.

The sexually mature male worm measures 12 to 31 cm in length by 2 to 4 mm in greatest diameter. Its posterior end is somewhat curved ventrally. The female measures 20 to 35 cm in length by 3 to 6 mm in greatest diameter, but specimens up to 45

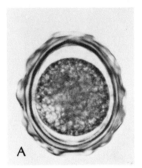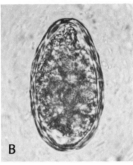

Fig. 11–19. *Ascaris lumbricoides* eggs. *A*, Fertilized. *B*, Unfertilized. (× 500.) (By M.D. Little.)

cm are occasionally observed. The daily egg production per female averages about 200,000.

The fertilized egg of *A. lumbricoides* (Fig. 11–19A) at the time of oviposition is spherical or subspherical, measures 65 to 75 μm by 35 to 50 μm, and consists of the following observable structures: (1) a coarsely granular, spherical ovum that usually does not completely fill the shell; (2) a thin, innermost membrane that is highly impermeable; (3) a relatively thick, colorless middle layer that is smooth on both inner and outer surfaces; and (4) an outermost, coarsely mammillated, albuminoid layer, laid down *in utero,* serving as an auxiliary protective membrane.

Female worms without males produce infertile eggs that are markedly subspherical (88 to 93 μm by 38 to 44 μm). Internally they contain a mass of disorganized granules and globules that completely fill the shell (Fig. 11–19B). Both fertile and infertile eggs usually become tanned by the time they are evacuated in the feces. Fertile eggs are passed in the one-cell stage. They survive putrefaction and can withstand considerable desiccation and cold. At 22° to 33°C, development to the infective stage larva usually occurs in 3 to 4 weeks. Eggs may remain viable in soil for more than a year.

When ingested, the infective larvae hatch in the duodenum and penetrate the intestinal wall, enter mesenteric venules or lymphatics, and *via* the liver, and inferior vena cava, or the thoracic duct reach the right side of the heart and pass through the pulmonary vessels to the lungs. On about the 9th day of infection, after doubling their length in the tissues of the lung (Fig. 11–20A), they begin migration *via* the trachea (Fig. 11–20B) to the intestine, where they become sexually mature 8 to 12 weeks after exposure. The adult worms may live up to 16 months or possibly 20 months, but usually they are passed spontaneously in about 12 months.

Pathogenesis and Symptomatology. In the *stage of larval migration,* unless hundreds of larvae are migrating simultaneously, passage through the liver and lungs in the initial infection provokes no remarkable pathologic changes (Fig. 11–20A). Migrations in subsequent infections may cause intense tissue reaction in the liver and lungs, even when relatively few larvae are involved. The liver changes in man, not fully described, probably are much the same as those in animals, *viz.,* focal eosinophilic infiltration and granuloma formation around and in the paths of migrating larvae and general inflammation along the portal tracts where eosinophils are conspicuous in the acute phase. In later stages there is more or less fibrosis of the periportal and interlobular spaces. More significant is the intense local reaction around the larvae in the tissues, with infiltration of eosinophils, epithelioid cells, and macrophages, and the production of a distinctive type of pneumonitis. Heavy infections causing near-fatal disease attributed to malicious contamination of food with infective eggs of *Ascaris suum* have been reported (Phills *et al.,* 1972).

The cardinal symptoms associated with *Ascaris* pneumonitis consist of dyspnea, often of the asthmatic type; a productive cough; rales, frequently musical and wheezing or coarse and less often crepitant; fever, moderate to 40°C; high but transient peripheral eosinophilia; and x-ray findings showing scattered, shifting mottling of the lungs. This picture of pulmonary infiltration, which is often variable from day to day and spontaneously clears after a few days to 2 weeks, along with high eosinophilia, which persists somewhat longer than the pulmonary changes, is called *Löffler's syndrome.* During the period of productive cough, the sputum characteristically contains many eosinophils and at times abundant Charcot-Leyden crystals (Fig. 11–21). Migrating larvae may also be seen in the sputum, but they can be recovered more easily in gastric washings taken in the early morning (Fig. 11–22). Although Löffler's syndrome is also caused by other agents in areas where ascariasis is endemic, it and other nematode infections (hookworm, *Strongyloides*) are most frequently responsible. However, pulmonary ascariasis appears to be most common and severe in endemic areas where transmission is sharply seasonal. Occasionally it is fatal, even in adults (Fig. 11–21). Sig-

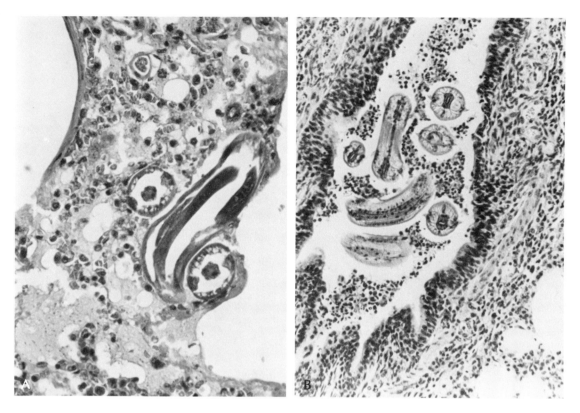

Fig. 11–20. *Ascaris* larvae in sections of lung. *A,* Developing *A. lumbricoides* larva in the interalveolar tissues of the lung of a 1-year-old child. Numerous other larvae were seen in the tissues and in the air passages; death occurred during the third day of illness. (× 300.) *B,* A coiled *A. suum* larva on the ninth day of experimental infection in a pig, having completed its development in the tissues, has entered a bronchiole en route to the intestine via the trachea. Transverse sections of larva show conspicuous lateral alae and intestine with patent lumen. (× 175.) (By P.C. Beaver.)

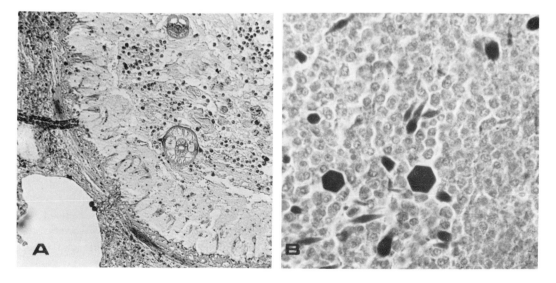

Fig. 11–21. *Ascaris lumbricoides.* *A,* Larva in the stage of migration from lung to intestine, cut at levels of esophagus and midintestine, in human autopsy section of a 1-mm bronchiole filled with mucopurulent exudate. (× 145.) *B,* Charcot-Leyden crystals in a different bronchiole in the same case. (× 550.) (From Beaver, P.C., and Danaraj, T.J. 1958. Pulmonary ascariasis resembling eosinophilic lung. Autopsy report with description of larvae in the bronchioles. Am. J. Trop. Med. Hyg., 7:100–111.)

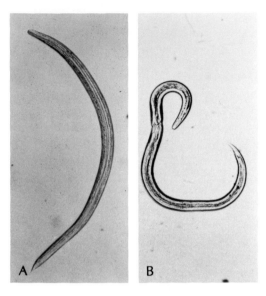

Fig. 11–22. *Ascaris lumbricoides.* Larvae recovered from gastric washings *(A)* and sputum *(B)* of patients with severe seasonal pneumonitis and hypereosinophilia in Saudi Arabia. The larvae are 1.2 mm long and have lips and other features characteristic of the advanced third stage. (× 50.) (By P.C. Beaver. Larvae received from A.P. Gelpi.)

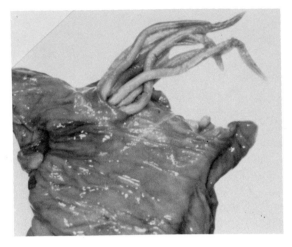

Fig. 11–23. *Ascaris lumbricoides.* Adult worms impacted in the bile duct at the ampulla of Vater. Worms also were found in the liver parenchyma. (Slightly reduced.) (Courtesy of D.E. Wykoff.) (From Beaver, P.C., Jung, R.C., and Cupp, E.W. 1984. *Clinical Parasitology,* 9th ed. Philadelphia, Lea & Febiger, p. 315.)

nificantly, in highly endemic areas where reinfection is more or less continuous, clinical pulmonary ascariasis is uncommon (Spillmann, 1975).

When present in small numbers, adult worms generally cause no symptoms, although even a single ectopic worm may occasionally produce serious disease. Average infections in children cause intermittent colic, loss of appetite, fretfulness, and at times nervous symptoms. The abdomen is characteristically protuberant. The nutritional demands and space requirements of massive infections may be great, as in the case of a 2-year-old girl seen at autopsy in New Orleans, who weighed only 8 kg after having passed 80 worms in the hospital and an unrecorded number earlier and who still harbored 578 worms which weighed more than 800 g. The estimated volume displacement of the total mass of worms was approximately 1 liter. Heavy *Ascaris* infection can lead to significant nutritional impairment, especially in children whose protein intake is low.

From time to time worms are passed spontaneously, unassociated with illness. These events are of no special significance. If attended by an acute febrile illness of any kind, however, the active movement of worms from the intestine is highly significant and is to be interpreted as a direct consequence rather than the immediate cause of the illness. If disturbed by fever or other abnormal conditions, the worms migrate outward in both directions or congregate in closely packed masses that tend to obstruct the intestine. In their forward excursions the worms occasionally enter and block the biliary and pancreatic ducts (Fig. 11–23), where they may form calculi or, more frequently, penetrate into the parenchyma of the liver and pancreas, where they perish. Liver abscesses in children probably are more frequently caused by *Ascaris lumbricoides* than by *Entamoeba histolytica*. Worms leaving the intestine may enter the lungs *via* the trachea (in cases of deep coma) or move into the nasopharynx, where they emerge from the nares. On rare occasions immature worms have been seen coming from the lacrimal duct. Worms may also become lodged in the appendix or may perforate ulcerated and gangrenous areas of the intestinal wall (Fig. 11–24). In the peritoneal cavity the worms die and are resorbed within a few days. The eggs remain, however, and generally become widely scattered before being enclosed in granulomatous reaction. These complications of intestinal ascariasis give rise to a variety of symptoms, depending on the organs and tissues involved.

Worms occasionally are found in the heart, pulmonary arteries, ventricles of the brain, and elsewhere, apparently having migrated, before or after death of the host, through the biliary channels or

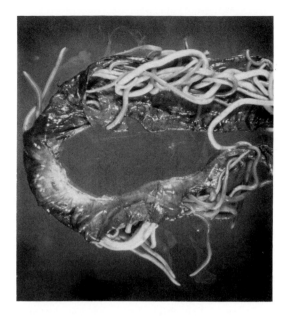

Fig. 11–24. *Ascaris lumbricoides.* Bolus of worms causing obstruction and necrosis of a segment of the ileum of a child. (× ca. 0.5.) (Courtesy of W.H. Sternberg.) (From Beaver, P.C., Jung, R.C., and Cupp, E.W. 1984. *Clinical Parasitology,* 9th ed. Philadelphia, Lea & Febiger, p. 316.)

hepatic and caval venous channels, aided in some cases by abscess formation in the liver.

The survival time of mature *A. lumbricoides* in the human intestine is relatively short, generally not exceeding a year. Yet in hyperendemic communities almost daily exposure is usual, so that new broods of larvae are migrating through the lungs and reaching the intestine to replace the previous mature ones as soon as they are lost.

Ascariasis is frequently associated with whipworm infection as well as diseases due to other causes. These complicate the clinical picture and often lead to inaccurate appraisal of the role played by the ascarids.

Diagnosis. During the prepatent period, unless immature worms are passed, specific diagnosis is not possible, although clinically the syndrome of larval *Ascaris* pneumonitis is relatively pathognomonic. Once in the intestine and mature, the daily egg output of a single female is about 200,000, sufficient to put one to several characteristic eggs in an average direct fecal smear.

Treatment. There is evidence that a benzimidazole—fenbendazole—is lethal to *Ascaris* larvae migrating through the lungs of pigs (Stewart *et al.,* 1984). Its action against human *Ascaris* has not been tested.

The standard treatment for intestinal ascariasis consists of the administration of mebendazole or pyrantel pamoate. Piperazine also is effective and has a wide margin of safety (see Table 21–1, p. 265).

Surgical Considerations. The development of signs and symptoms of ileus in a child who is passing *Ascaris* by mouth or anus indicates obstruction caused by a bolus of worms. In such cases, (1) a search should be made for the cause of the febrile illness that usually precipitates the complication; (2) fluid and electrolyte balance should be restored; (3) antipyretic measures should be taken, (4) decompression should be carried out by intestinal catheter with constant suction, and (5) after rehydration, a single dose of piperazine citrate should be administered through the catheter and the tube clamped for 2 hours. In the majority of instances the obstruction will be spontaneously resolved. If the bolus persists in spite of these measures, laparotomy is indicated. The bowel is opened at the bolus and the worms are removed with sponge forceps. Liver abscess due to *Ascaris* must be treated by drainage and administration of antibiotics.

Prognosis. The prognosis usually is excellent following appropriate treatment. It is grave when there is massive larval invasion of the lungs, in cases of hypersensitization, or when complications requiring surgery develop.

Epidemiology. Endemicity of ascariasis is maintained by fecal contamination of soil. In most hyperendemic areas promiscuous defecation by small children in and around the home provides the major source of infection. Eggs are relatively resistant to desiccation, and embryonation takes place in clay soil as well as in loam. Infective-stage eggs remain viable for weeks, months, or even years, but desiccation, freezing, heat, and direct sunlight are detrimental. Infective eggs are transported from soil to mouth by various means. Dirt-eating is generally responsible for heavy infection in small children. The action of rainfall on the transport and concentration of infective eggs in play areas is an important factor in heavy infections.

Hogs infected with *Ascaris suum* probably constitute an occasional source of intestinal ascariasis in man. *A. suum* larvae do make the lung migration, however, and in some instances develop to the adult stage in man (Shoemaker-Nawas *et al.,* 1982). *Ascaris* of human origin, *i.e., A. lumbricoides,* may develop to the adult stage in pigs.

Control. Anthelmintic medication constitutes

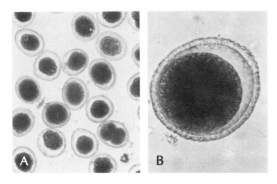

Fig. 11–25. *Toxocara canis.* Eggs washed from feces of an infected pup, showing typical pitting of the outer shell membrane. Those shown in *A* were in a water culture for several days and some are in early stages of cleavage. (*A,* × 90; *B,* × 324.) (By P.C. Beaver.)

only a temporary measure for the great majority of infected individuals, since with relatively few exceptions persons living in *Ascaris* environments are subject to repeated exposure. The problem of control is therefore concerned directly with home and community sanitation or mass treatment repeated at intervals of 2 months to 1 year, depending upon the climate and seasons of transmission. There is no practical method by which soil in and around the dooryard contaminated with *Ascaris* eggs can be rendered safe.

An additional control problem is presented in countries where human feces constitute the essential fertilizer for field crops or truck gardens. Eggs of helminths in feces can be destroyed by composting, which raises the temperature to killing levels and does not appreciably lower the fertilizing qualities of the feces, but except in special circumstances the process is too expensive or for other reasons is impractical.

Toxocara species
(Toxocariasis)

Toxocara canis. *Toxocara canis* (Werner, 1782) Johnston, 1916 is a cosmopolitan ascarid of dogs. It is a human parasite only in the larval stage. The males are 4 to 6 cm, the females 6.5 to 10 cm long. Both sexes bear lateral cervical alae that are much longer than broad and extend distally an appreciable distance from the anterior end. The eggs are subglobose, densely granular internally, superficially pitted, and measure roughly 85 by 75 μm (Fig. 11–25). In moist shaded soil infective larvae develop within the eggs in about 3 weeks. Infection in dogs is acquired by (1) ingesting infective-stage eggs from soil; (2) indirectly, by eat-

ing infected paratenic hosts; (3) receiving larvae through the placenta or in the mother's milk; (4) ingesting larvae passed in the feces of suckling pups. Although adult dogs suffer little harm from this infection, larvae in the mother's tissues are transmitted to their young, which may die of the infection. Pups rarely fail to acquire infection. Larvae of *T. canis* have a remarkably long period of survival in the tissues of the adult dog and in the tissues of other animals (paratenic hosts).

Toxocara cati. *Toxocara cati* (Schrank, 1788) Brumpt, 1927, the common ascarid of cats, has been reported 19 times as a human intestinal infection. In the light of present knowledge of visceral larva migrans, most of these records may be questioned, though some are well documented (von Reyn *et al.*, 1978). Mature males have a length of approximately 6 cm and the females are 10 to 12 cm long. The cervical alae are broader at the posterior margin than are those of *T. canis*. Eggs are subglobose and densely granular internally, with the shell more delicately pitted than that of *T. canis* and somewhat smaller (75 by 65 μm). After at least 3 weeks of embryonation on damp shaded soil, the eggs are infective. Upon being swallowed, they hatch in the duodenum and after a migration route to the lungs mature in the lumen of the small intestine. Prenatal infection apparently does not occur, but transmission through the mother's milk usually does.

The genus *Toxocara* contains nine valid species besides *T. canis* (the type species) and *T. cati*. All are parasites of terrestrial mammals, and as several of them occur in hosts that are associated with people, other species besides *T. canis* and *T. cati* may eventually be recognized as causing disease in man. Human infections with larval *Toxocara canis* and *T. cati* are considered under the heading Larva Migrans (page 165).

Lagochilascaris
(Lagochilascariasis)

Lagochilascaris minor was described by Leiper in 1909 from collections of small worms, 1.0 to 1.5 cm in length, found in subcutaneous abscesses in two patients in Trinidad. Worms identified as *L. minor* have been reported from other cases in Trinidad, Surinam, Tobago, Costa Rica, Venezuela, Mexico, Colombia, and Brazil (Botero and Little, 1984). The worms were recovered from abscesses in the region of the ear, neck, jaw, tonsils, or mastoid bone, or passed from the nose. The life history pattern of *Lagochilascaris minor* is unknown. *Lagochilascaris sprenti*, a species common in opossums in Louisiana, has an obligate mammalian intermediate host. When infective eggs are ingested by small mammals, larvae hatch and migrate to the muscles, where they grow and become encapsulated. When ingested by an opossum, the larvae mature in the gastric mucosa. Human infections with *L. minor* probably are acquired either by eating meat (muscle) from wild animals or by ingesting infective eggs from soil. *L. minor* has keel-like lateral alae that extend practically the length of the body. There are three conspicuous lips, each with a vertical cleft (hence the generic name ''hare-lipped ascaris''), and the entire labial structure is set off from the cervical region by a deep, circumscribing postlabial groove (Fig. 11–26*B*). The eggs are oval or spherical and around 65 μm in diameter, with the surface sculptured in a reticulate pattern of variously shaped pits, somewhat as in *Toxocara* (Fig. 11–26*A*).

Infections in humans produce deep subcutaneous abscesses located on the neck (Fig. 11–26*C*) or in the wall of the pharynx, in which both adult worms and developmental stages are found or can be observed in discharged pus. Untreated infections may persist for years. Treatment with levamisole was effective in recent cases (Botero and Little, 1984).

Anisakids

In parts of Europe where marine fish are eaten lightly salted or smoked, and in Japan where large quantities of fish from the ocean are eaten raw, surgical operations for suspected peptic ulcer, tumor, or other lesions of the stomach or small intestine often reveal an eosinophilic granuloma or abscess containing a large ascaridoid larva that may reach 3.5 cm in length and 0.6 mm in diameter. Though it may protrude from the mucosal surface, the worm usually is deep in the wall of the organ (Fig. 11–27*B,C*). The stomach is affected twice as often as the intestine. Rarely, a worm having migrated through the wall of the intestine may be found in the abdominal cavity (Rushovich *et al.*, 1983). *Anisakis simplex* is the species involved in Europe (Smith, 1983). In Japan, *Anisakis* is the larva involved in most cases, but a second type, *Terranova*, is also involved, more commonly in the acute cases in which severe epigastric pain appears within a few hours of eating raw sea fish (Yoshimura *et al.*, 1979). In the United States, two cases of intestinal anisakiasis due to *Anisakis* have been reported, but most cases have been transient infections in which larvae of *Terranova* or *Phocanema* were coughed up, vomited, or removed from the mouth (Kliks, 1983). The source of all infections was raw or undercooked marine fish. In the adult stage anisakids are parasites of fish-eating marine mammals. They normally live in the stomach in aggregates of up to a hundred or more; with the forebody deeply inserted in a craterlike tumor induced by the worms in the gastric mucosa (Fig. 17–27*A*). Eggs laid by the worms and passed in the host's feces embryonate and hatch as microscopic free-living larvae which, when eaten by small, shrimplike crustaceans (Euphasiidae), develop into infective third-stage larvae. These in turn, when eaten by fish or squid, develop further; when eaten by whales, porpoises, or dolphins, they penetrate the gastric mucosa and develop to maturity, completing the cycle (Smith, 1983).

HOOKWORMS AND OTHER BURSATE NEMATODES

The hookworms and related species have the following characteristics: they lack distinct lips; the posterior end of the male bears a copulatory bursa that is typically supported by seven pairs of rays; and the female internal reproductive organs usually are paired, one set extending anteriorly, the other posteriorly, from the vagina and vulva. Eggs are in an early stage of embryonation when laid and the shell is thin and transparent.

With few exceptions, the adult worms live in the digestive tract. Eggs are discharged in the feces and complete their development in the soil. Larvae hatch from the egg, feed, grow, and after two molts (to third stage) become infective. In some species

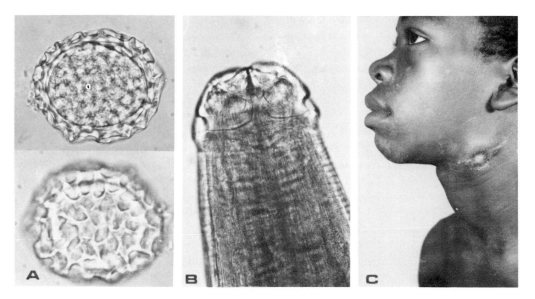

Fig. 11–26. *Lagochilascaris minor. A,* Eggs as seen with microscope focused at the equator *(above)* and at the surface. (× 500.) *B,* Head of worm that was removed, along with many others, from a fibrous nodule in an excised tonsil of a 26-year-old woman with a history of recurrent attacks of tonsillitis for 3 years. (× 105.) *C,* Surinam boy with neck lesion from which pus, adult worms, larvae, and eggs had drained. (*A,* and *B,* by M.D. Little. *C,* Courtesy of B.F.J. Oostburg.) (From Beaver, P.C., Jung, R.C., and Cupp, E.W. 1984. *Clinical Parasitology,* 9th ed. Philadelphia, Lea & Febiger, p. 323.)

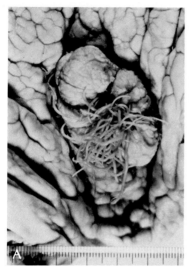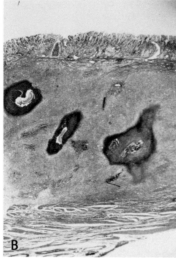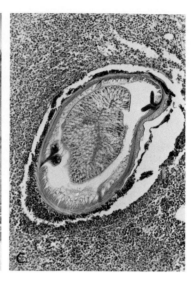

Fig. 11–27. *Anisakis. A,* Adult worms in stomach of blue-white dolphin, *Stenella coeruleo alba.* (Millimeter scale.) *B,* Sections of a larva surrounded by eosinophilic fibrinoid material in large inflammatory lesion in stomach wall of 47-year-old man in Kyushu, Japan. (× 7.5.) *C,* Larva in large submucosal eosinophilic granuloma in resected segment of ileum of 46-year-old man in Kyushu, Japan. (× 75.) (*A,* Courtesy of Akio Kobayashi; *B* and *C* by P.C. Beaver; sections courtesy of Ichiro Miyazaki.)

the larva is infective by the oral route; in others infection is acquired percutaneously. Many of these worms are important parasites of domestic animals and only incidentally infect man, but hookworms are among the most extensive disease-producing agents of mankind.

Hookworms

Human hookworms belong to two genera—*Necator,* in which the buccal capsule is provided with cutting plates, and *Ancylostoma,* in which the capsule contains paired toothlike processes. It is the buccal capsule bearing cutting plates or teeth that sets the hookworms apart most distinctly from the other bursate nematodes.

Necator americanus
(Uncinariasis, necatoriasis)

History and Distribution. *Necator americanus* (Stiles, 1902) Stiles, 1903 is the "New World hookworm." Hookworms recovered from patients in the Americas were first regarded as *Ancylostoma duodenale,* described by Dubini in Italy in 1843, but in 1902 Stiles recognized that they belonged to a new species which he designated *Uncinaria americana,* and a year later he placed it in a new genus, *Necator* (the "killer"). Soon the "American hookworm" was found to be the prevailing species throughout the hookworm belt of the southern United States, Mexico, Central America, the West Indies, and South America east of the Andes.

Some years later *Necator americanus* was discovered to be the important autochthonous species in the Eastern Hemisphere south of 20°N latitude. This hookworm was introduced into the Western Hemisphere with the importation of African slaves. Minimum temperature is an important limiting factor in the geographic distribution of the human hookworms, for whereas the eggs of *N. americanus* quickly die at temperatures below 7°C, those of *Ancylostoma duodenale* do not.

Morphology, Biology, and Life Cycle. *Necator* is strongly flexed dorsally at the anterior end (Fig. 11–28). The small buccal capsule is provided with two ventral cutting plates, two poorly developed dorsal plates, a median dorsal tooth, and in the depth of the mouth cavity a pair of short triangular lancets (Fig. 11–29A). Opening into the buccal capsule are a pair of long cephalic (amphidial) glands that secrete an anticoagulant. A powerful, muscular esophagus bears a dorsal gland and paired ventrolateral glands, which secrete proteolytic enzymes. A pair of unicellular excretory (cervical) glands with a common midventral pore lie between the esophagus and upper intestine and the body wall ventrally.

The male measures 7 to 9 mm in length by 0.3 mm in breadth. The copulatory bursa (Fig. 11–30A) is symmetrical. The supporting rays for each half consist of a small distinctly separated dorsal, bifurcated at the tip; a slender, unbranched externodorsal; three laterals arising from a large

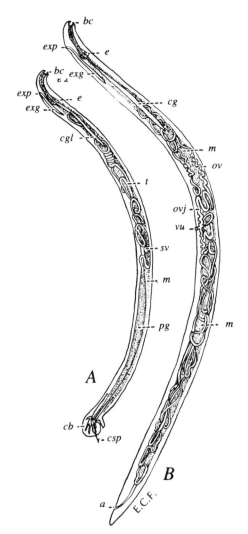

Fig. 11–28. *Necator americanus*, adults, lateral view. *A*, Male. *B*, Female. *a*, Anus. *bc*, Buccal capsule. *cb*, Copulatory bursa. *cg*, Cephalic gland. *csp*, Copulatory spicules. *e*, Esophagus. *exg*, Excretory gland. *exp*, Excretory pore. *m*, Midgut. *ov*, Ovary. *ovj*, Ovejector. *pg*, Prostate gland. *sv*, Seminal vesicle. *t*, Testis. *vu*, Vulva. (× 18.) (Adapted by E.C. Faust from Lane, C. 1932. *Hookworm Infections*. London, Oxford University Press, p. 4.)

fleshy trunk; two ventrals fused half-way or more to the tip; and an inconspicuous short prebursal ray. The two copulatory spicules are long delicate bristles that are fused at their outer ends, terminating in a barb. The female (Fig. 11–28*B*) measures 9 to 11 mm in length by 0.4 mm in breadth. The posterior tip is rather sharply conical. The vulvar opening is midventral, somewhat anterior to the equatorial plane.

The eggs (Fig. 11–31) are thin-shelled, transparent, broadly ovoid, and measure 64 to 76 μm by 36 to 40 μm. They are in an early stage of cleavage when laid. In a freshly passed stool they range in development from 4-celled to a morula stage; in feces stored at room temperature for several hours they may reach the early larval stage. *Necator americanus* normally is attached to the upper levels of the small intestine, but in heavy infections some of the worms may move far down into the ileum and occasionally into the cecum.

When feces bearing hookworm eggs are deposited on moist, sandy loam, in a warm, shaded location, or are spread on the land as fertilizer, embryonation of eggs usually proceeds rapidly and hatching takes place in 24 to 48 hours. Optimal conditions include good aeration, moisture but not flooding, protection from the direct rays of the sun, and a temperature of approximately 30°C. The larva emerging from the egg is *rhabditoid* (Fig. 11–32*A*) and measures 0.25 to 0.3 mm in length by about 17 μm in maximum diameter. It feeds on bacteria and organic debris, grows, sheds its cuticula, and continues to feed and increase in size up to 0.5 to 0.6 mm in length while retaining its rhabditoid form. After 5 to 8 days it stops feeding, becomes relatively inactive, and transforms within the old cuticular sheath into a more slender filariform larva, which has a closed mouth, an elongated esophagus, and a sharply pointed tail (Fig. 11–33*A*). On contact with exposed human skin, the larvae penetrate under epidermal scales or into hair follicles. The most common area of invasion is the feet, but other areas can be penetrated as well. Swallowing the filariform larvae on leafy vegetables or otherwise does not establish infection with *Necator* as it does with *Ancylostoma*. The filariform larvae may remain viable in the soil for days to weeks, depending on environmental conditions.

The filariform larvae penetrate the epidermis, where they remain relatively inactive for 1 or 2 days before moving deeper to the cutaneous blood vessels and on through the right side of the heart to the lungs. After about 1 week, during which there is considerable growth and development, they ascend the respiratory tree to the epiglottis and descend to the upper levels of the small intestine; meanwhile, they have undergone a third molt and acquired a temporary buccal capsule. The young worms now become attached to the mucosa, grow, shed the fourth cuticula, including the temporary buccal capsule, and develop into adult worms. A minimum of 6 weeks is required from the time filariform larvae enter the skin until the worms

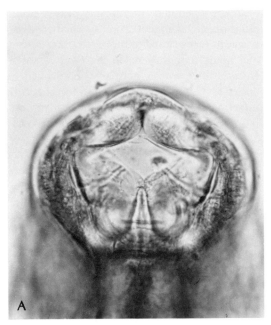

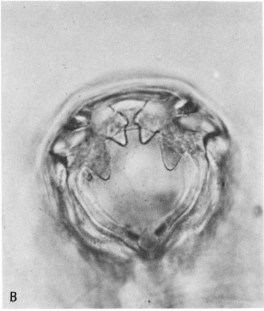

Fig. 11–29. Hookworm, *en face* view. *A, Necator americanus,* showing ventral cutting plates. (× 400.) *B, Ancylostoma duodenale,* showing ventral teeth. (× 250.) (By M.D. Little.)

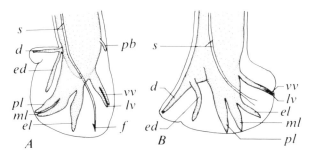

Fig. 11–30. Hookworm, posterior end of male, lateral view from right side, showing bursal rays and spicules. *A, Necator americanus. B, Ancylostoma duodenale. d,* Dorsal ray. *ed,* Externodorsal ray. *el,* Externolateral ray. *f,* Fused tips of spicules. *lv,* Lateroventral ray. *ml,* Mediolateral ray. *pb,* Prebursal ray. *pl,* Posterolateral ray. *S,* Spicules. *vv,* Ventroventral ray. (By M.D. Little.)

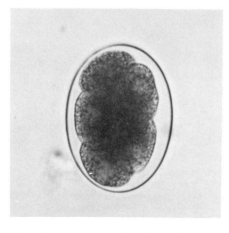

Fig. 11–31. Hookworm egg from human feces. (× 480.) Eggs of *Necator americanus* and *Ancylostoma duodenale* are indistinguishable. (By P.C. Beaver.)

become mature in the intestine, copulate, and begin to lay eggs. Under favorable conditions each female *Necator americanus* produces more than 5,000 eggs daily. Although these worms may remain in the human intestine up to 14 years or longer, most are eliminated much earlier.

For pathologic and clinical aspects of infection with *Necator americanus,* see Hookworm Infection and Hookworm Disease (page 151) and Larva Migrans (page 162).

Ancylostoma duodenale
(Ancylostomiasis)

History and Distribution. Although *Ancylostoma duodenale* (Dubini, 1843) Creplin, 1845, the "Old World hookworm," probably was referred to in the Ebers papyrus (1600 B.C.), the first description was based on worms obtained at autopsy of a Milanese woman in 1838. In 1878 Grassi and Parona demonstrated that the presence of hookworms in the intestine could be diagnosed from

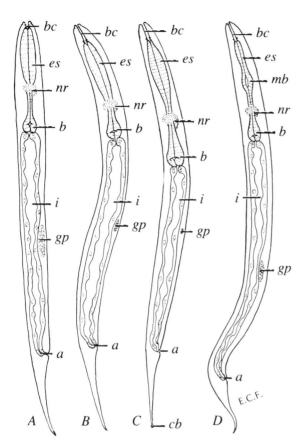

Fig. 11–32. Rhabditoid nematode larvae. *A, Strongyloides. B,* Hookworm. *C, Trichostrongylus. D, Rhabditis.* (× ca 300.) *a,* Anus. *b,* Bulb of esophagus. *bc,* Buccal canal. *cb,* Caudal beadlike knob. *es,* Esophagus. *gp,* Genital primordium. *i,* Intestine. *mb,* Midesophageal bulb. *nr,* Nerve ring. (Adapted from Beaver, P.C., Jung, R.C., and Cupp, E.W. 1984. *Clinical Parasitology,* 9th ed. Philadelphia, Lea & Febiger, p. 263.)

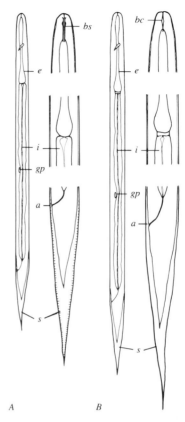

Fig. 11–33. Filariform hookworm larvae. *A, Necator americanus. B, Ancylostoma duodenale.* (× 300.) *a,* Anus. *bc,* Buccal canal. *bs,* Buccal spear. *e,* Esophagus. *gp,* Genital primordium. *i,* Intestine. *s,* Sheath. (By M.D. Little.) (Adapted from Little, M.D. 1981. Differentiation of nematode larvae in coprocultures; Guidelines for routine practice in medical laboratories. W.H.O. Tech. Rep. Ser. No. 666. Intestinal Protozoan and Helminth Infections, 144–150.)

their eggs in the stool, and in 1880 Perroncito hatched the eggs and studied the free-living stages in the soil. In 1896 Looss found that the infective-stage filariform larvae enter the body through the skin.

The original distribution of *A. duodenale* was probably limited to the north temperate and subtropical regions of the Eastern Hemisphere, and its range was extended through the Middle East into the Mediterranean area of Europe and Africa at an early period. Migrations of people carried the infection to more tropical regions, so that today it is mixed with *Necator americanus* in southeastern Asia, the South Pacific and Southwest Pacific islands, and Indonesia. *A. duodenale* is present in numerous localities of Mexico and South America, where it was introduced by the early southern European explorers and colonizers. It is noteworthy

that this did not occur to a significant extent in the United States.

Morphology, Biology, and Life Cycle. Adults of *A. duodenale* in the living state are pinkish in color. The body is narrowed anteriorly, with the head curved dorsally (Fig. 11–34). The cup-shaped mouth capsule is heavily reinforced and is provided on the forward (ventral) side with two pairs of conspicuous, slightly curved, subequal teeth and a third pair that is rudimentary, on either side of the median ventral line (Fig. 11–28*B*). In the depth of the capsule there is a pair of small teeth. Dorsally there is a plate with a median cleft.

The male (Fig. 11–34*A*) measures 8 to 11 mm in length by 0.4 to 0.5 mm in breadth. Its copulatory bursa (Fig. 11–30*B*) is considerably broader than it is long and is supported by rays having the following pattern for each half: a dorsal, single at its root but bifurcated at the tip; externodorsal,

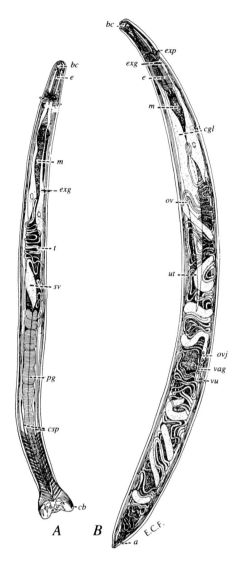

Fig. 11–34. *Ancylostoma duodenale*, adults. *A*, Male, ventral view. *B*, Female, lateral view. *a*, Anus. *bc*, Buccal capsule. *cb*, Copulatory bursa. *cgl*, Cephalic (amphidial) gland. *csp*, Copulatory spicules. *e*, Esophagus. *exg*, Excretory (cervical) gland. *exp*, Excretory pore. *m*, Midgut. *ov*, Ovary. *ovj*, Ovejector. *pg*, Prostate gland. *sv*, Seminal vesicle. *t*, Testis. *vag*, Vagina. *vu*, Vulva. (× 16.) (Adapted by E.C. Faust from Looss, A. 1905. The anatomy and life history of *Ancylostoma duodenale* Dub. A. monograph. Part I. The anatomy of the adult worm. Rec. Egypt. Gov't. School Med., *3*:1–158, Plate I, figs. 1 and 2.)

arising from the root of the dorsal; three laterals, outwardly well separated from one another; and two ventrals, close to each other. The female (Fig. 11–34*B*) measures 10 to 13 mm in length by 0.6 mm in breadth and tapers rather bluntly at the posterior end. The anus lies ventrally near the caudal tip and the vulvar opening is situated midventrally at the beginning of the posterior third of the body. Under favorable conditions, each female lays up

to around 20,000 eggs daily. Man is probably the only normal host of *A. duodenale*.

The broadly ovoid eggs (Fig. 11–31) average 60 by 40 μm, have a thin, transparent shell, and are in the 2- to 8-cell stage of cleavage when evacuated. Embryonation to the first rhabditoid larval stage takes place in 24 to 48 hours on moist sandy loam in a shaded environment at an optimal temperature of about 25°C. The free-living larval stages on the soil are similar to those of *Necator americanus* (page 147), with the infective filariform larva (Fig. 11–33*B*) developing in 5 to 8 days.

Except that the filariform larvae are adapted to entering the body by the oral route as well as by the skin, and there apparently is no inactive period in the skin or essential development in the lungs, infection with filariform larvae of *A. duodenale* and their development to mature male and female worms in the intestine parallel these phases of the life cycle of *Necator* (page 146). On penetration of the skin larvae of *A. duodenale* make a lung migration but may do so and reach maturity in the intestine only after an extended period in the tissues. Thus, the prepatent period in *A. duodenale* infection is highly variable, ranging from 4 or 5 weeks to several months. In view of the fact that *Ancylostoma* infection in animals can be acquired through the mother's milk, it is expected that *A. duodenale* infection can be acquired in this way by human infants.

Ancylostoma ceylanicum

Ancylostoma ceylanicum (Looss, 1911) closely resembles *A. braziliense*, and apparently these species have been confused frequently. *A. ceylanicum* is typically a parasite of cats in Southeast Asia (reported from Malaysia and Taiwan), Surinam, and Brazil, but it also occurs in dogs and man. It has been reported in man in India and in carnivores in Madagascar. The two species chiefly differ in the buccal cavity and the bursa. In *A. braziliense* the inner denticles arising from the large ventral teeth are smaller and more internal, the lateral bursal rays are more curved, the mediolateral and externolateral rays are more divergent, and the externodorsal rays arise much nearer to the origin of the dorsal ray. Observations on experimental infections in man have shown that the prepatent period for *A. ceylanicum* is about 3 weeks and that infection is acquired more readily by oral than by percutaneous inoculation.

Ancylostoma braziliense

Ancylostoma braziliense Gomez de Faria, 1910 was first described from the intestine of cats and dogs in Brazil and subsequently from these hosts in other warm areas of the world. Though it occasionally is mistaken for *A. ceylanicum* and is reported as such, *A. braziliense* in the adult stage probably does not occur in man.

A. braziliense is smaller than *A. duodenale* (males 7.7 to 8.5 mm long, females 9 to 10.5 mm long). The most easily recognized morphologic difference between these species is the buccal capsule; that of *A. braziliense* has a smaller aperture, and the dental plate on each side of the midventral line is provided with a very small inner tooth and a larger outer one. Eggs of this species are indistinguishable from those of other hookworms. The stages of larval development are also similar.

Clinical interest in *A. braziliense* is concerned primarily with human exposure to the filariform larvae derived from canine and feline hosts, causing a dermatitis referred to as "cutaneous larva migrans" or "creeping eruption." This topic is considered under Larva Migrans (see page 162).

Ancylostoma caninum

Ancylostoma caninum (Ercolani, 1959) Hall, 1913, a common hookworm of dogs in temperate climates, has been reported on rare occasions as an incidental intestinal parasite of man. *A. caninum* is appreciably larger than *A. duodenale* (males 10 mm long by 0.4 mm wide, females 14 mm long by 0.6 mm wide). The buccal capsule is wide and has a large orifice. Each of the two upper (ventral) dental plates is provided with three teeth, of which the innermost is the smallest and the outermost the most fully developed. The eggs resemble those of *A. duodenale* but are larger (64 by 40 μm). The life cycle is similar to that of *A. duodenale*. Transmammary infection is common in the dog.

A. caninum has been employed experimentally for many years in studies on the biologic, immunologic, and clinical aspects of hookworm infection in the dog. Occasionally creeping eruption in humans is caused by *A. caninum*.

Clinical Aspects of Hookworm Infection and Disease

The Skin Lesion. At the site of entry on the feet, arms, or other surface areas, the larvae of *Necator americanus* or *Ancylostoma duodenale* usually produce a papular eruption. Persons infected with *N. americanus* frequently give a history of dermatitis, consisting typically of initial intense itching and burning, followed by edema and erythema, and then the appearance of a papule that transformed into a vesicle. This is the uncomplicated "ground itch" of hookworm infection. Occasionally *Necator* produces a "creeping eruption" in the skin similar to that of *A. braziliense* but of shorter duration.

Larval Migration Through the Lungs. Characteristically, the migrating larvae of *Necator americanus* and *Ancylostoma duodenale* reach the pulmonary capillaries almost immediately after entry into the cutaneous venules, though they tend to remain in the skin for 1 or 2 days after penetration. As they penetrate into the air sacs, they produce tissue damage, but only in the case of simultaneous massive migration of larvae is a pneumonitis of a clinical grade produced. Another item of clinical interest is that during transit through the lungs, hookworm larvae do not typically produce the high degree of sensitization characteristic of *Ascaris* (page 140) or *Strongyloides* (page 157).

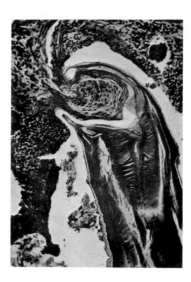

Fig. 11–35. *Necator americanus*. Adult worm attached to human jejunum, with mucosal tissues drawn into the buccal cavity. (Army Medical Museum Collection.) (From Beaver, P.C., Jung, R.C., and Cupp, E.W. 1984. *Clinical Parasitology,* 9th ed. Philadelphia, Lea & Febiger, p. 279.)

However, *A. duodenale* in Japan is described as causing cough, dyspnea, high eosinophilia, and frequently nausea and vomiting one to several days following the ingestion of larvae on green vegetables. The onset and duration of the reactions, known as "Wakana disease," appear to coincide with the period of larval development in the intestinal mucosa and are not always caused by the presence of larvae in the lungs.

Intestinal Infection. Once the larval hookworms have migrated to the small intestine, they soon acquire a mouth capsule and become attached to the mucosa (Fig. 11–35). Little blood is sucked out of the tissues, but large amounts may be lost by hemorrhage at sites of attachment. Abdominal symptoms and eosinophilia, with Charcot-Leyden crystals in the feces, appear during the late prepatent period.

Etiology of Hookworm Disease. The essential damage produced in hookworm infection is hemorrhage from the intestinal wall. In general this is proportional to the number of attached worms, but blood loss is disproportionately great where the worms are crowded. Thus, counts of less than 5 *Necator* eggs per mg of feces are seldom of clinical grade, while people with counts of more than 20 eggs per mg generally develop a significant hookworm anemia. In massive *Necator* infections, egg counts often exceed 50 per mg of feces. Corresponding egg count classes for *A. duodenale* infections generally are reported at markedly lower levels, average counts as low as 5 eggs per mg feces being classified as heavy (Koshy *et al.*, 1978).

The type of anemia produced by hookworms is typically microcytic and hypochromic. In light and moderately heavy infections, the blood loss can be compensated for by an adequate, well-balanced diet containing iron, other minerals, rich animal proteins, and vitamin A. In severe hookworm disease, however, even with a highly fortified diet, the hematopoietic mechanism is unable to produce new supplies of normal red blood cells as rapidly as they are lost. Moreover, underlying protein deficiency in the diet, even with adequate absorbable iron intake, may contribute measurably to the anemia of hookworm patients, a majority of whom subsist essentially on carbohydrates. Nutritional repletion does not cause hookworm infections to be diminished or lost. In hookworm areas, exposure begins fairly early in childhood and is repeated throughout life. Heavy infections may be fatal in infants.

Symptomatology. In *acute cases* resulting from single heavy exposure, there is characteristically a prodromal syndrome of nausea, headache, and irritating cough (during lung migration of the larvae). In the middle to late prepatent and early patent periods (29 to 38 days), there frequently are severe colicky pains, flatulence, diarrhea, loss of weight, dyspnea, dizziness, and marked pallor (Cline *et al.*, 1984). During this period there is an eosinophilic leukocytosis that may persist at a significantly high level for several months.

In *chronic* hookworm disease, the signs and symptoms are essentially those of iron-deficiency anemia. Present in varying degrees are pallor, facial and pedal edema, dull expression, and listlessness. Hemoglobin levels may be reduced to 5 g per dl or lower, and the heart is greatly enlarged. In children, mental and physical development may be markedly retarded.

Diagnosis. Hookworm disease is indistinguishable from the anemia and edema of malnutrition by physical examination alone, and blood chemistry studies indicating a hypoproteinemia will fail to provide a differential diagnosis. On the other hand, by determining the presence and roughly the number of hookworm eggs in the feces, a rapid and relatively accurate diagnosis can be made. In severe cases of hookworm anemia caused by *Necator*, the eggs are numerous (more than 20 eggs per mg feces) and readily detected by the direct smear technique. It is generally held that *A. duodenale* lays twice as many eggs as *N. americanus* and is several times more injurious to the host.

Treatment. In light to moderate hookworm infections in which the anemia is not severe, specific treatment can usually be undertaken without a preliminary period of supportive treatment. For individuals with low hemoglobin levels, it is desirable to prescribe a diet rich in animal protein for a week to 10 days before specific chemotherapy. Iron must also be administered to replace that lost through intestinal hemorrhage caused by the worms. Rarely, whole blood transfusion may be needed. The most effective drug without significant side-effects probably is mebendazole (see Table 21–1, page 265). Pyrantel pamoate is also effective. One or 2 weeks after treatment, a follow-up stool examination should be made. If necessary, retreatment may be undertaken in a week to remove remaining worms.

Prognosis. In uncomplicated hookworm infections, prognosis is good to excellent following removal of the worms and correction of the anemia and hypoproteinemia. Nevertheless, if treatment of heavy infection is delayed, some degree of stunting may persist in spite of eventual cure.

Epidemiology. Hookworm infection constitutes one of the most prevalent of all helminthic parasitoses of man in warm climates. For practical purposes only two causal agents of intestinal infection need to be considered, namely, *Necator americanus* and *Ancylostoma duodenale*. *N. americanus* is typically adapted to a warmer climate, although *A. duodenale* likewise thrives in the tropics. Wherever these infections are endemic, they result from unsanitary disposal of human feces. Defecation on favorable soil or the spreading of the egg-laden feces in the form of nightsoil on the land provides opportunity for the eggs to complete embryonation and for the larvae that emerge from the egg to feed, grow, and transform into the infective filariform stage. These larvae tend to remain near the surface and close to the site where eggs were deposited. The longevity of infective larvae depends on the amount and frequency of rainfall as well as temperature and the character of the soil.

The continued propagation of hookworm infection depends largely on frequency of contact with contaminated soil. People working in fields that have been recently fertilized with untreated human nightsoil are exposed wherever the hands or feet touch the soil, while miners in unsanitary underground tunnels may become infected on practically any area of the skin. There is no marked sex, age, or race difference in susceptibility to infection, although the highest prevalence usually is found in young adult males.

Data on the prevalence of hookworm infection in an area must be supplemented by an estimate of the intensity of the infection in each infected individual, *i.e.,* the worm burden. This can be done by estimating the output of eggs per mg or per g of feces (see Chapter 18, p. 251). Correlation of egg counts with hemoglobin level will indicate the significant levels of egg output, which differ somewhat depending on age, dietary habits, and species of hookworms prevalent in the area.

Another measure for studying hookworm epidemiology is related to the sites on the soil polluted with human excreta and the degree of soil infestation with hookworm larvae. Recovery of larvae from the soil and their separation from free-living nematode larvae are accomplished by special techniques (see Technical Aids, page 255).

Control. Two major lines of attack are indicated for the control of hookworm disease: (1) anthelmintic treatment of all infected individuals to reduce to a minimum the sources of soil infestations, and (2) selective treatment of individuals showing evidence of hookworm disease and those whose egg counts indicate heavy worm burdens. Equally important is the sanitary disposal or sterilization of human feces to prevent infestation of the soil.

Control also entails improvement in the diet of hookworm communities to reduce the effects of malnutrition. Thus, it is evident that hookworm control must be made an integral part of comprehensive health programs, including medical care, sanitary improvements, health education, nutrition, and improved agricultural practices. With economic and social development of communities, there is a general decline in infections with hookworm and other intestinal parasites without specific control programs.

Other Bursate Nematodes

Bursate nematodes that normally occur in other animals but have been reported in man include *Ternidens, Oesophagostomum, Mammomonogamus, Trichostrongylus,* and *Angiostrongylus.* When found in man, these worms are usually present in small numbers or in an immature stage and a specific diagnosis is often difficult.

Ternidens
(Ternidensiasis)

Ternidens deminutus (Railliet and Henry, 1905) Railliet and Henry, 1909 has been diagnosed in man in Zimbabwe, Malawi,

and Mozambique. In size and shape *Ternidens* resembles human hookworms, but it is distinguished from them by a terminal buccal capsule that is subglobose and is guarded internally by a double crown of stout bristles. The eggs are also like those of hookworms but larger, averaging 84 by 51 μm. The third-stage larva is semirhabditoid rather than filariform and is not capable of penetrating the skin; hence it enters the body only by the oral route.

T. deminutus is found in the colon with its head inserted into the wall. It produces cystic nodules or small, circumscribed, craterous ulcers and at times causes perforation with peritonitis. Pyrantel pamoate and thiabendazole are effective in eliminating *T. deminutus.*

Oesophagostomum
(Oesophagostomiasis)

Species of *Oesohagostomum* are frequently found in monkeys and apes in Asia, Africa, and South America. They resemble hookworms in size and general appearance but, as in *Ternidens* species, the buccal capsule opens forward and has a crown of bristles or setae (sometimes double) around the opening. The buccal capsule is cylindrical rather than globose. There is a transverse groove on the ventral side at the esophageal level, and the cuticula between it and the mouth is somewhat inflated. The bursa is symmetrical and of medium size; the spicules are long and equal. Two uterine branches extend forward from the vulva and ovejector located near the anus. The eggs resemble those of hookworms in size and appearance.

Adult worms live attached to the mucosa of the cecum and colon. As in hookworms, there are three free-living larval stages, the third being infective. Infection is acquired by the oral route. Ingested larvae invade deeply into the cecal mucosa and induce development of a large, firm encapsulating nodule in which development is completed, after which the adult emerges and attaches to the mucosa.

In man, the larval stages produce tumorlike masses and abscesses, usually 1 to 2 cm in diameter, in the abdomen, abdominal wall, other organs of the abdomen, and in the wall of the intestine, at times requiring surgical removal. The species involved in human infection usually is presumptively identified, most often as *Oesophagostomum apiostomum,* although several other species are known to occur in man. Tumors containing several worms may exceed 5 cm in diameter, requiring surgical intervention. The disease may resemble appendicitis, carcinoma of the colon, ileocecal tuberculosis, or ameboma. No anthelmintic is known to be effective against the larvae in nodules.

Mammomonogamus
(Syngamiasis)

Species of the genus *Mammomonogamus* (formerly *Syngamus*) are relatively small nematodes in which the male and female worms are joined in permanent copula. They have a thick-walled, cavernous buccal capsule, armed at its base with a number of small teeth. The male is only about one third as long as the female. The outer shell of the eggs consists of a large number of truncated prisms cemented together. Eggs of related species (*Syngamus* spp.) parasitizing birds have a pair of polar caps; eggs of *Mammomonogamus* species parasitizing mammals lack these caps.

Several species have been described from mammals. Human infection, probably for the most part with *M. laryngeus* but possibly also with *M. nasicola,* has been reported from Puerto Rico, Brazil, Martinique, St. Lucia (West Indies), Guiana, Trinidad, and the Philippines.

These worms live in the upper respiratory tract, causing asthma, hemoptysis, and paroxysms of coughing and sneezing, during which the worms may be expelled from their attachment

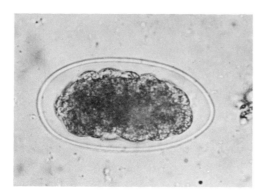

Fig. 11–36. *Trichostrongylus orientalis*. Egg from feces of Korean student. (× 500.) (By M.D. Little.)

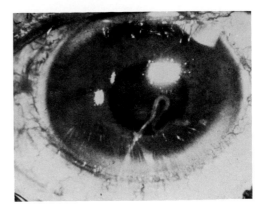

Fig. 11–37. *Angiostrongylus cantonensis*. Young male worm in the eye of a man in Bangkok. The worm was removed, described, and identified specifically. (Courtesy of Kobchai Prommindaroj.) (From Beaver, P.C., Jung, R.C., and Cupp, E.W. 1984. *Clinical Parasitology*, 9th ed. Philadelphia, Lea & Febiger, p. 293.)

to the respiratory mucosa. Life history data have not been reported for species of *Mammomonogamus*. Human infection is incidental; since the worms are often expelled during paroxysms of coughing, special therapeutic measures may not be indicated.

When worms are attached in a location that is beyond the reach of a bronchoscope, a diagnosis may nevertheless be made by the recognition of characteristic eggs (unembryonated, about 85 × 50 μm, shell with surface layer striated) in feces, sputum, or gastric washings. In a case of infection requiring treatment, recovery was rapid and examinations for eggs were negative after the third day of an 8-day course of treatment with thiabendazole.

Trichostrongylus
(Trichostrongyliasis)

Species of *Trichostrongylus* are delicate threadlike nematodes that lack a buccal capsule and have a relatively large copulatory bursa in the male. They are typically threaded into the mucosa of the small intestine of ruminants and usually are incidental parasites of man. However, in some countries *T. orientalis* is more commonly found in man than in other hosts. Eggs of these worms (Fig. 11–36) measure 70 to 90 μm by 40 to 50 μm, depending on the species, and are usually in the morula stage of development when evacuated in the stool. Under favorable conditions, eggs become fully embryonated and hatch in about 24 hours. The first- and second-stage larvae are rhabditoid in type like those of hookworms but can be readily distinguished by a minute beadlike knob at the tip of the tail (Fig. 11–32C). Transformation to the infective pseudofilariform larva usually occurs on the 3rd or 4th day. This stage is resistant to desiccation and is unable to penetrate skin. When ingested, it burrows into the intestinal mucosa. About 4 days later it emerges, and without a migration to the lungs develops into an adult. The prepatent period is about 3 weeks.

Generic diagnosis is made on finding the characteristic eggs (Fig. 11–36) in stools and differentiating them from hookworm eggs (Fig. 11–31). Specific diagnosis depends on study of the differential features of the copulatory bursa and spicules in the male.

Trichostrongylus colubriformis (Giles, 1892) Ransom, 1911, cosmopolitan in distribution, has been recovered from sheep, goats, gazelles, antelopes, deer, camels, baboons, apes, squirrels, and rabbits, and from man in Egypt, Iran, Iraq, India, Armenia, Indonesia, Australia, and once from a surgically removed appendix in New Orleans, U.S.A. Other species reported from man include *T. probolurus* in Egypt, Armenia, and Siberia; *T. vitrinus* in Egypt, Armenia, and Siberia; *T. orientalis* in Japan, Korea, China, Taiwan, and Armenia; *T. brevis* in Japan, and others. Seven species are common in man and an-

imals in Iran. In parts of Japan and Korea, *T. orientalis* is endemic. This species normally lives in the duodenum, but worms have been found in the wall of the pyloric stomach and jejunum. Males measure 3.8 to 4.8 mm in length and females 4.9 to 6.7 mm; the delicate heads measure only 7 and 9 μm in diameter, respectively. Eggs of *T. orientalis* (Fig. 11–36) measure 75 to 91 μm by 39 to 47 μm.

Clinical Notes. Light infections usually produce no symptoms, but large numbers of worms can cause intestinal disturbances. Transient eosinophilia has been observed, and severe diarrhea and high eosinophilia (up to 81%) have been reported. Pyrantel pamoate has been successfully used for treatment.

Angiostrongylus

Angiostrongylus cantonensis (Chen, 1935) Dougherty, 1946 is a metastrongyle lungworm of rats acquired through eating land snails and slugs, which are the intermediate hosts. The adult worms live in the pulmonary arteries, and the eggs are held and develop to the first-stage larvae in the tissues of the lungs. Larvae migrate from the lungs *via* the trachea and eventually are passed in the feces. Snails acquire infection by eating the feces of infected rats, and the larvae develop to the infective third stage in about 3 weeks. When snails are eaten by rats, the larvae migrate to the brain and meninges, where they become young adult worms in about 4 weeks, then migrate to the pulmonary arteries and begin laying eggs in about 2 weeks. In man, the larvae and young adults usually die in the brain, meninges, or spinal cord, though migration to the interior of the eye is not uncommon (Fig. 11–37), and adult worms in the pulmonary arteries were observed in one case in Taiwan. Light infections may cause little or no disturbance, but in the usual case signs and symptoms of meningoencephalitis (headache and stiffness of neck and back) develop 1 to 3 weeks after ingestion of infective raw snails. Crabs and fish that have eaten infective snails serve as transport hosts. Infection can be acquired by eating raw vegetables bearing small transport hosts or free larvae shed or passed from snails, slugs, or transport hosts. In symptomatic cases there is a high eosinophilia of the cerebrospinal fluid and, usually, of the blood. The disease is commonly referred to as *eosinophilic meningoencephalitis*. Human infections have been reported from Taiwan, Thailand, the Philippines, Indonesia, numerous islands of the Pacific, and Cuba (Pascal *et al.*, 1981). Since the disease usually is self-limiting and chemotherapy is potentially hazardous, administration of anthelmintic drugs is not recommended. In patients with severe headache, the most common symptom, relief may be obtained by spinal puncture and withdrawal of about 10 ml of cerebrospinal fluid. This may be repeated if necessary.

A related species, *Angiostrongylus costaricensis,* is a parasite of wild rats in Central America. Except that it develops and lives in the mesenteric arteries of the ileocecal region without invasion of the brain or meninges and its larvae develop in the wall of the intestine, the life cycle of *A. costaricensis* parallels that of *A. cantonensis.* Land molluscs and slugs *(Vaginulus plebeius)* are the intermediate hosts. Larvae become infective in about 3 weeks in the slug, and worms reach maturity during the fourth week of infection in the rat. In most cases of infection in man, the worms are discovered in sections of intestinal wall removed at operation for acute abdomen in preschool-aged children. More than 130 cases have been recorded in Costa Rica. In some cases the worms were found in the liver (Morera *et al.,* 1982). A satisfactory method of chemotherapy has not been definitely established. Administration of thiabendazole in a dosage of 75 mg/kg of body weight daily for 3 days has been recommended, but this dosage is likely to cause side-effects.

STRONGYLOIDES AND OTHER RHABDITOIDEA

The Rhabditoidea is a large group containing mostly small, free-living forms, some of which may be encountered as pseudoparasites in human feces, urine, gastric washings, or sputum. Some species occasionally are found contaminating laboratory reagents and solutions. *Micronema,* normally free-living, has been found to invade and multiply in the tissues of horses and humans. The parasitic members of Rhabditoidea are unique in that they have an alternation of free-living and parasitic generations, the eggs of one generation giving rise to adults of the alternate generation. Adults of the free-living generation are dioecious, the males and females resembling those of the nonparasitic genus *Rhabditis,* while in the parasitic generation the adult is a relatively robust hermaphroditic female, as in *Rhabdias;* a small filariform parthenogenetic female, as in *Strongyloides;* or small filariform males and females, as in *Parastrongyloides.* The genus *Strongyloides* contains a large number of species in birds, amphibians, reptiles, and mammals. *S. stercoralis* occurs endemically in man throughout the warm regions of the world, and *S. fuelleborni,* a natural parasite of monkeys and apes in Africa and Asia, is also endemic in man in Central and East Africa. Transient infections in man with other zoonotic species of *Strongyloides* are also known to occur.

Strongyloides stercoralis
(Strongyloidiasis)

Strongyloides stercoralis (Bavay, 1876) Stiles and Hassall, 1902, first observed in diarrheal stools of French troops who had served in North Vietnam, is primarily a parasite of warm climates, but it has been found sporadically in temperate and even cold regions.

Morphology, Biology, and Life Cycle. The slender parasitic female (Fig. 11–38*A*) measures up to 2.7 mm in length by 30 to 40 μm in diameter. The normal habitat is the mucosal epithelium of the upper small intestine (Fig. 11–39). Reproduction is parthenogenetic. Thin-shelled, ovoid eggs, 50 to 58 μm by 30 to 34 μm, are laid in the epithelium, each female producing relatively few, probably less than 50 per day. The eggs, after undergoing development, are sloughed into the lumen of the crypts of Lieberkühn, where the first-stage rhabditoid larva hatches. Larvae then migrate into the intestinal lumen and are evacuated in the stool (Figs. 11–38*D* and 11–40). If deposited in a warm, moist, shaded site, *direct development* to the filariform third-stage larva (Fig. 11–38*E*) may occur in 24 to 36 hours in the fecal mass or in soil. This larva, measuring 500 to 630 μm in length by 15 to 16 μm in diameter, is the infective stage and initiates infection by skin penetration.

Under certain conditions there may be an abbreviated type of direct development in which the first-stage larva develops to the infective stage within the intestinal tract, and the larvae can reinfect the host by penetrating the mucosa of the colon without leaving the body *(internal autoinfection)* or by penetrating the perianal or perineal skin after being passed in the stool *(external autoinfection).* Autoinfection possibly may occur at a low level in relatively healthy individuals, which could account for the reports of infections persisting in individuals for several decades after they had left an endemic area. In individuals with an induced or acquired immunodeficiency, autoinfection may occur at an accelerated rate, resulting in a disseminated, fatal infection.

The interpolation of a free-living generation may occur when the first-stage larvae, after reaching the external environment in feces, develop to free-living rhabditoid adults in 2 to 4 days *(indirect development).* The male is about 0.9 mm long by 40 to 50 μm in diameter, with the caudal end curved conspicuously to the ventral side (Fig. 11–38*C*). The female is about 1.2 mm long by 50 to 85 μm in diameter and contains up to 28 eggs in its two uteri (Fig. 11–38*B*). After the eggs are deposited by the female, they rapidly develop, in most cases, to the infective, filariform larval stage.

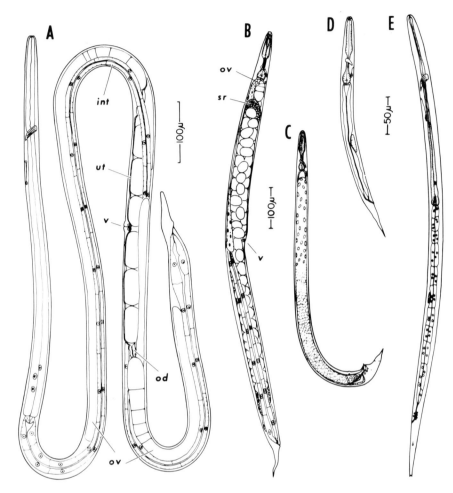

Fig. 11–38. *Strongyloides stercoralis. A,* Parasitic female. *B,* Free-living female. *C,* Free-living male. *D,* First-stage (rhabditoid) larva from fresh feces. *E,* Third-stage (filariform) larva from surface of fecal specimen 24 hours after collection. *int,* Intestine. *od,* Oviduct. *ov,* Ovary. *sr,* Seminal receptacle. *ut,* Uterus containing eggs. *v,* Vulva. (From Little, M.D. 1966. Comparative morphology of six species of *Strongyloides* (Nematoda) and redefinition of the genus. J. Parasitol., *52*:69–84.)

Rarely, these eggs have been observed to develop to second generation free-living adults, but continuing cycles of free-living generations are not known to occur.

On contact with skin, the filariform larvae (either direct or indirect mode of development) penetrate the epidermis to the small blood vessels and are carried to the lungs. When they reach the pulmonary capillaries, they break out into the alveoli and proceed *via* the trachea to the intestine, where they invade the epithelium of the glands, molt twice, and reach maturity in about 2 weeks. The most common level of the intestine parasitized by *S. stercoralis* is the duodenum, followed by the jejunum.

Pathogenesis. No skin lesion has been described comparable to the "ground itch" of hookworm infection. Usually *Strongyloides* larvae proceed rather rapidly from the sites of entry to the cutaneous blood vessels. Similarly, passage through the lungs is rapid and, except in cases of internal autoinfection, pulmonary lesions caused by larvae are minimal. In the intestine, the adult worms cause relatively little irritation unless large numbers are present. There may be a moderate infiltration of eosinophilic leukocytes and other inflammatory cells.

While infections are usually mild or asymptomatic, chronic relapsing infections that persist for several decades or rapidly developing, potentially fatal hyperinfections may develop through the process of internal autoinfection. This may occur when the host has an impaired immune system resulting from a debilitating condition such as malnutrition, hypogammaglobulinemia, or a concurrent chronic infection such as tuberculosis, or from

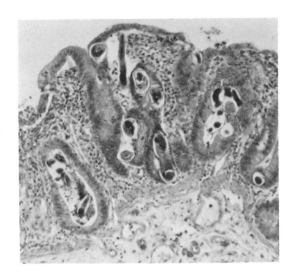

Fig. 11–39. *Strongyloides stercoralis.* Parasitic female and eggs in intestinal mucosal epithelium and rhabditoid larvae in lumen of glands. (× 150.) (By M.D. Little. Tissue courtesy of P. Hartz.)

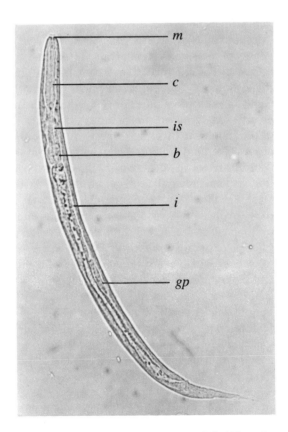

Fig. 11–40. *Strongyloides stercoralis.* Rhabditoid larva from feces. *b,* Bulb of esophagus. *c,* Corpus of esophagus. *gp,* Genital primordium. *i,* Intestine. *is,* Isthmus of esophagus. *m,* Mouth. (× ca. 400.) (By M.D. Little.)

receiving immunosuppressive or corticosteroid therapy.

In disseminated infections due to internal auto-infection, the invasion of large numbers of filariform larvae into the wall of the colon and their migration by blood routes through various organs on their way to the lungs produce various degrees of damage to these organs. In fatal cases, moderate to severe lesions may be found in the colon, liver, kidneys, heart, lymph nodes, central nervous system, and other organs. The migration of large numbers of larvae through the lungs produces alveolar hemorrhage and edema and pneumonitis. Chronic bronchitis or an asthmalike condition may also be produced. In some cases, the infective larvae develop to the adult stage within the lungs, primarily in the bronchial or bronchiolar mucosa, resulting in additional pulmonary irritation. In the sputum or bronchial washings from these patients, filariform larvae, rhabditoid larvae, eggs, and even parasitic females may be found. In the intestine, damage to the mucosa results from the migration of the females within the epithelium, the deposition and sloughing of eggs, and the penetration of juvenile worms newly arrived from the lungs. As the infection becomes heavier, the affected intestinal tissues become increasingly nonfunctional, with intense infiltration of inflammatory cells in the submucosa, atrophy of villi, and sloughing of large areas of the mucosa.

Symptomatology. Entry of larvae into the skin and cutaneous blood vessels produces relatively mild needling sensations. In transit through the lungs, the young worms may cause symptoms resulting from pneumonitis.

The symptoms of the uncomplicated intestinal infection are typically abdominal pain, usually localized in the right upper quadrant and resembling peptic ulcer, and diarrhea (Midler *et al.,* 1981). The blood picture is typically one of leukocytosis with a moderate to high eosinophilia ranging up to 85%. As the infection becomes chronic, the eosinophilia generally decreases.

Chronic infections of mild to moderate severity tend to develop in people with an associated chronic illness and may persist for several decades. The complaints are primarily gastrointestinal, including nausea, vomiting, diarrhea, and pain, and there is usually a peripheral eosinophilia (Midler *et al.,* 1981). A form of chronic strongyloidiasis seen in American, British, and Australian ex-prisoners of war who were in labor camps in Burma

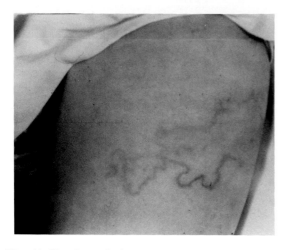

Fig. 11–41. *Strongyloides stercoralis.* Rapidly advancing linear lesion referred to as "larva currens" on the thigh of a Texas oil-field worker whose stool and that of his wife contained larvae reported as *Strongyloides stercoralis.* (From Stone, O.J., Newell, G.B., and Mullins, J.F. 1972. Cutaneous strongyloidiasis: Larva currens. Arch. Dermatol., *106*:734–736.)

and Thailand during World War II is characterized by the presence of urticarial creeping eruptions of the skin of the buttocks, abdomen, and thighs in addition to gastrointestinal complaints (Pelletier, 1984). *Larva currens* is the term applied to the distinctive cutaneous lesions observed in chronic strongyloidiasis (Fig. 11–41). They are broad, rapidly developing urticarial trails, often starting at or near the anus.

In hyperinfections, patients commonly have a combination of respiratory and gastrointestinal complaints, including nausea, vomiting, diarrhea, abdominal pain, bloating, anorexia, dyspnea, wheezing, cough, hemoptysis, low-grade fever, malaise, and weakness. Concurrent bacterial infections resulting in septicemia, septic meningitis, brain abscess, or pneumonia are common. Protracted diarrhea and loss of electrolytes may cause dehydration and marked hypokalemia and lead to paralytic ileus, respiratory muscle paralysis, or cardiac arrest (da Silva *et al.*, 1981).

For the relationship of *S. stercoralis* to "creeping eruption" see Larva Migrans, page 162.

Diagnosis. Although in endemic areas the diagnosis of strongyloidiasis should be suspected in persons with symptoms of peptic ulcer and peripheral eosinophilia, proof of the infection depends on demonstration of the organism. Routine diagnosis is made by finding active rhabditoid larvae (Figs. 11–38*D*, 11–40) in fecal films examined microscopically, but filariform larvae (Fig.

11–38*E*) may be found when the feces have stood at laboratory temperature for a day or more before examination is made. The Baermann larval extraction technique is the most sensitive procedure for detecting larvae in feces and should be used when the infection is suspected but routine stool examination is negative. Examination of duodenal aspirates may occasionally be positive when the fecal examination is negative. Occasionally larvae of *S. stercoralis* are found in the sputum, urine, or in aspirates from body cavities.

Treatment. Thiabendazole in a dosage of 25 mg per kg of body weight twice daily (maximum of 3 g per day) for 2 or 3 days is the drug of choice at present. Repetition after 1 or 2 weeks may be necessary. In cases of hyperinfection, the drug may need to be given for a longer period, and in some immunodeficient patients a prolonged low-dose course may be required (Shelhamer *et al.*, 1982). Albendazole has also been reported to be effective in treating strongyloidiasis when given at a dosage of 800 mg per day for 3 days (Coulaud *et al.*, 1982) and can be used when the patient cannot tolerate thiabendazole.

Prognosis. Prognosis is generally good except in cases of massive hyperinfection. In general, the absence of eosinophilia in such patients is a poor prognostic sign. Electrolyte and fluid imbalance, anemia, and bacterial infections, if present, should be corrected during treatment.

Epidemiology. In some respects *S. stercoralis* behaves like human hookworms; in other ways it is quite different. In *S. stercoralis* infections, rhabditoid larvae rather than eggs are passed in the feces, and these can mature rapidly, in 24 to 36 hours, to the infective filariform stage by direct development in feces, soil, or water. These larvae are able to swim, whereas hookworm larvae are not. Under suitable conditions indirect development through the free-living adult generation may occur instead, and since the progeny of each free-living female is about 30 to 50, this will result in the development of a greater number of infective larvae in the soil. Reports of continuous free-living generations in the soil that serve as constant sources of infective larvae have not been confirmed. Infection is by skin penetration, as in the hookworm. Strongyloidiasis tends to parallel hookworm infection in some geographic areas, being found in moist warm areas along rivers, streams, and coasts, and is related to poor sanitation. It generally has a lower prevalence than hookworm infection, but in some tropical areas, such as in parts of Brazil and Colombia, strongyloidiasis is the more prevalent and serious disease. It is generally more prevalent in adults than in young children. It tends to be common in institutional groups, such as in mental hospitals, prisons, and homes for retarded children, even in temperate regions. Dogs are readily susceptible to human strains of *S. stercoralis* and may serve as a source of human infection through fecal contamination of the environment.

Control. Control of human strongyloidiasis is concerned primarily with reduction of the sources of exposure, both extrinsically and in the individual. Since contaminated soil and *Strongyloides*-positive human stools will frequently contain infective-stage larvae in 1 to 2 days, special attention must be given to prompt and proper disposal of feces.

Zoonotic Strongyloidiasis

Strongyloides fuelleborni is a common parasite in Old World monkeys and apes. It can also develop to patency in man, and in many areas of Africa, from Zambia northward through central African countries, it has become endemic (Hira and Patel, 1980). In many of these areas, *S. fuelleborni* and *S. stercoralis* are found together. *S. fuelleborni* differs from *S. stercoralis* in that the stage passed in the feces is an egg containing a larva; it differs as well in the distinctive morphology of the parasitic and free-living adults. In studies in Zaire, *S. fuelleborni* was shown to be transmitted to infants by the passage of infective larvae in the milk of the mother (Brown and Girardeau, 1977). In western Papua New Guinea an *S. fuelleborni*-like species is endemic in people living in scattered isolated villages (Kelly *et al.*, 1976: Ashford *et al.*, 1981). In one area, an acute, commonly fatal disease of infants—''swollen belly disease''—is attributed to this parasite. *S. procyonis*, a parasite of the raccoon, can develop to patency in man (Little, 1965) and, along with other zoonotic species, it can cause cutaneous larva migrans (see Larva Migrans, page 162).

Other Rhabditoid Nematodes

Species of the genus *Rhabditis* and related free-living forms that are coprophagous or saprophagous in their mode of nutrition are seen in human stools from time to time and may be diagnostically confused with the rhabditoid larvae and free-living adult stages of *Strongyloides*, although some have a long acuminate tail. These pseudoparasites can be readily distinguished from the rhabditoid stages of *Strongyloides*, hookworms, and *Trichostrongylus* by the presence of a median esophageal swelling (Fig. 11–31*D*) that is lacking in the others (Fig. 11–31*A–C*).

The recovery of such forms in fecal smears usually indicates contamination of the specimen after it was passed, but occasionally these nematodes may be ingested and survive passage through the digestive tract (*Rhabditis, Rhabditoides, Pelodera* spp.). *Diploscapter coronata*, a species that resembles *Rhabditis* and inhabits soil and decaying vegetation, occasionally is seen in gastric washings and less commonly in sputum and urine. As all stages of development up to mature females occur together, it appears that the worms are able to live temporarily and multiply in the body. Both larvae and young adults are extremely small (less than 1 mm in length) and are easily mistaken for *Strongyloides*.

Pelodera strongyloides has a resistant larval stage, the "dauer larva," that is commonly found in the orbit of burrowing wild rodents. This species has also been reported to cause skin lesions in dogs, horses, cattle, and sheep, and in an 11-year-old girl in Poland and an infant in Alabama (Ginsburg *et al.*, 1984).

Rhabditoid nematodes of the genus *Micronema* are normally saprophagous, living in decaying plants, manure, and soil, but under certain conditions these minute worms can invade and multiply in mammalian tissues. They apparently enter the body through skin lesions and then spread to various organs, especially the central nervous system. Disseminated infections, mostly fatal, have been reported in horses in Egypt, Europe, and the United States. Three fatal human infections due to *Micronema*, two in the United States and one in Canada, have also been reported (Gardiner *et al.*, 1981). Meningoencephalitis due to invasion of the brain by the worms was the cause of death in each case.

DRACUNCULUS AND RELATED SPIRURIDS

The spirurid roundworms vary remarkably in appearance; some are delicate and filiform, others are relatively stout, and still others are very long and wiry. In all, the esophagus is divided into a short anterior muscular part and a longer posterior glandular part. The worms generally occur in the esophagus or stomach or in tissues or tissue spaces. All use an arthropod as an intermediate host.

Dracunculus medinensis
(Dracontiasis, dracunculiasis)

The guinea worm, *Dracunculus medinensis* (Linnaeus, 1758) Gallandant, 1773, has been known since the days of antiquity. The ancient Egyptians, Hebrews, Greeks, and Romans were all familiar with it. In 1869 Fedtschenko first provided evidence that the infection required a copepod (*Cyclops*) intermediate host.

Guinea worm infection is present in the Nile Valley, northern Uganda and Kenya, central equatorial Africa, the west coast of Africa, Saudi Arabia, Yemen, Iraq, Iran, Afghanistan, Pakistan, and semiarid parts of western India. Infections reported from Indonesia and Singapore apparently were acquired in India. The parasite is not endemic in the Western Hemisphere nor has it ever been acquired by man in the United States. However, a species closely resembling *D. medinensis* is found in fur-bearing mammals in North America.

Morphology, Biology, and Life Cycle. Although the adult worms resemble the filariae, they are morphologically and biologically distinct. The adult male, rarely recovered from humans, is best known from specimens obtained from experimentally infected dogs and monkeys. It measures up to 40 mm in length, with a maximum diameter of 0.4 mm. The mature female is much larger, measuring 70 to 120 cm in length by 0.9 to 1.7 mm in diameter. In the gravid female, the vulva, located near the midbody, atrophies and the vagina disintegrates; the uterus becomes a distended sac containing first-stage, rhabditoid larvae.

The worms of both sexes develop to maturity in deep somatic and visceral connective tissues. Near the end of the prepatent period of development, *i.e.*, at about 12 months, the female migrates to the subcutaneous tissues near the skin surface where a papule is formed, followed by a large blister (Fig. 11–42*A*). Eventually, on immersion in water, the blister sloughs, the anterior end of the worm ruptures, the uterus prolapses and bursts, and a swarm of motile first-stage larvae is discharged into the water. Over the course of a few weeks, the process may be repeated until all the larvae have been discharged and the worm itself is sloughed. The larvae measure 500 to 750 μm in length and have a long filiform tail that constitutes almost one third of the total body length. Their stiff movement in the water apparently attracts the copepods that ingest them. In the hemocoel of the copepod the larvae undergo two molts to become infective (third-stage larvae) in about 2 weeks. When the infected copepod is ingested and digested by a suitable host, the larvae migrate through the intestinal wall into deep somatic tissues, where they grow to the adult stage in about 12 months.

Pathogenesis and Symptomatology. Characteristically, no symptoms are produced in the infected person during the biologic incubation period. A few hours preceding the appearance of the skin lesion, there may be pronounced systemic symptoms, including erythema and urticarial rash with intense pruritus, nausea, vomiting, diarrhea, dyspnea, giddiness, and syncope. The focal lesion appears as a reddish papule with a vesicular center and an indurated margin measuring roughly 15 to 20 mm in diameter. The lesion most frequently is on the feet and ankles (Fig. 11–42) but may develop on the hands or arms, trunk, buttocks, scrotum, knee joint, shoulders, and even the face. When the blister ruptures, the symptoms abate. However, attempts to remove the worm by traction may reactivate the symptoms. Secondary infection of the lesion is a common occurrence and seriously aggravates the condition. If the worm fails to reach the body surface, it dies and disintegrates, at times producing a sterile abscess, or it may become calcified.

Although infections with several worms are by no means rare, relatively few individuals have more than a few and the majority have only one. However, in highly endemic areas reinfection is common.

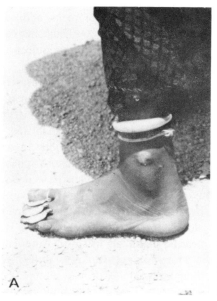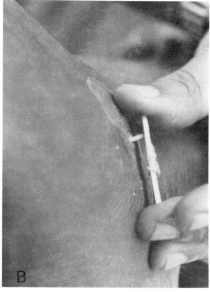

Fig. 11–42. *Dracunculus medinensis*. *A*, Bleb on ankle of woman in Rajasthan, India, produced by gravid worm in preparation for emerging to discharge larvae into water. (By P.C. Beaver.) *B*, Extruded worm being drawn onto match stick from ankle of a man in Singapore. (Courtesy of J.F. Schacher.)

Diagnosis. A diagnosis of dracontiasis is possible only with the onset of systemic symptoms followed by development of the cutaneous lesions. Most frequently, patients appear for treatment after the infection becomes patent. Dead, calcified worms may be detected by x-ray examination.

Treatment. Allergic reactions may be relieved with antihistamines or corticosteroids. Thiabendazole, niridazole, and metronidazole have been shown to be active in relieving the symptoms of dracontiasis (see Table 21–1, p. 265). The administration of these drugs relieves the pain and pruritus associated with the appearance of the worm and facilitates its removal by traction (Fig. 11–42B).

Prognosis. Dracontiasis is temporarily disabling and occasionally results in chronic invalidism, but prognosis usually is good.

Epidemiology and Control. *Dracunculus medinensis* is acquired by drinking water containing the infected *Cyclops*. Customs of bathing and washing clothes in ponds and drawing water from open wells are responsible for propagation of this disease (Fig. 11–43). The only effective method of control developed thus far is to provide piped water or wells that are curbed or covered to prevent transfer of larvae from infected persons to the water pool. All other methods have been ineffective, although treatment of pond water with an insect larvicide, temephos (Abate), to kill the copepods has been recommended and apparently is effective and safe.

Gongylonema

Gongylonema pulchrum Moli, 1857 is a cosmopolitan parasite of ruminants and has also been found in pigs, bears, hedgehogs, monkeys, and occasionally in man, with human cases diagnosed chiefly in Europe, Morocco, the U.S.S.R., China, New Zealand, Sri Lanka, and the U.S.

In ruminants, the male worms reach a length of 62 mm and a diameter of 0.15 to 0.30 mm, and the female worms grow to 145 mm and 0.2 to 0.5 mm, respectively. The female lays fully embryonated eggs that are transparent, thick-shelled, broadly ovoid, and measure 50 to 70 μm by 25 to 37 μm.

When ingested by various species of dung beetles and cockroaches, the eggs hatch and the larvae burrow into the hemal cavity and become encapsulated. The definitive host is infected by swallowing the insect; the larvae are freed and migrate up to the esophagus or mouth cavity, in the mucous and submucous membranes of which they develop into adult worms and in which the females lay eggs.

In the reported human cases worms have been extracted from or have spontaneously emerged from the lips, gums, hard and soft palate, tonsil, and angle of the jaw, but never from the esophagus. The symptoms in human infection consist primarily of local irritation, and in one case pharyngitis and stomatitis. These manifestations disappear on mechanical removal of the worm. No chemotherapy is indicated.

Thelazia

Thelazia callipaeda Railliet and Henry, 1910 and *Thelazia californiensis* Kofoid and Williams, 1935 live in the conjunctival sac of the host. *T. callipaeda* is Oriental in distribution and commonly parasitizes the dog, while *T. californiensis* from California, New Mexico, Oregon, and Nevada parasitizes the cat, fox, coyote, dog, horse, rabbit, sheep, black bear, and two species of deer. Human infection with the former species has been described from China, Korea, Thailand, Japan, Russia, and India. Seven human infections with *T. californiensis* have been reported, all from California.

The adult worms are wiry, creamy-white threads that measure 4.5 to 13 mm by 0.25 to 0.75 mm (males) and 6.2 to 17 mm by 0.3 to 0.85 mm (females). The female lays hyaline, thin-shelled ovoid eggs containing a larva. Intermediate hosts in California are flies (*Fannia* sp.).

Thelazia causes considerable damage to tissues of the eye, including inflammation of the conjunctival sac, excess lacrimation, and superficial scarification as the worms migrate out of the conjunctival sac across the front of the eye and back again. They may be removed with fine forceps after the introduction of a few drops of procaine into the conjunctival sac.

Physaloptera

Physaloptera caucasica von Linstow, 1902 occurs in African monkeys but the species has a considerably wider geographic range than tropical Africa. Infection or pseudoinfection with *Physaloptera* in the human intestinal tract has been reported from southern Russia, tropical Africa, southern Rhodesia, India, Israel, Panama, and Colombia.

The worms are relatively large, stout, and creamy-white. Males measure 14 to 50 mm long by 0.7 to 1.0 mm in diameter and females 24 to 100 mm long by 1.14 to 2.8 mm in diameter. Although they have a superficial resemblance to young ascarids, they may be distinguished by a cuticular collarette, a pair rather than three lips surrounding the mouth, and distinctive dental processes and papillae just inside the mouth. The smooth, hyaline thick shelled eggs are broadly ovoid, measure 44 to 65 μm by 32 to 45 μm, and are fully embryonated when laid. Various insects serve as intermediate hosts. Infection may be revealed by the discovery of worms in vomitus as well as eggs in feces.

The adult worms live with the head buried in the wall of the digestive tract from the level of the stomach to the midlevel of the ileum. The liver may at times be parasitized. Epidemiologic, clinical, and preventive aspects of human infection have not been studied.

Gnathostoma

Gnathostoma spinigerum Owen, 1836 and *Gnathostoma hispidum* Fedtschenko, 1872 are natural parasites of certain mammals that feed on fish, snakes or other cold-blooded vertebrates. Adults of *Gnathostoma spinigerum* are found in tumors of the stomach of the cat, wildcat, leopard, lion, tiger, and dog from Japan to Indonesia and India. Human infection with this species, almost invariably in an advanced larval stage in extraintestinal sites, has been reported from Thailand, Malaysia, Vietnam, China, Japan, Indonesia, and India. Adults of *G. hispidum* have been obtained from gastric tumors of wild and domestic hogs in Japan, China, India, and other parts of Asia, and from Europe and Australia. Human infections with immature worms of this species in extraintestinal sites have been described once each from Japan and China and twice from India.

Adult worms of both species are robust, with rounded ends. In the tiger, the adult males of *G. spinigerum* reach a length of 11 to 25 mm and the females grow to 25 to 54 mm. They have a subglobose cephalic swelling separated from the body proper by a distinct cervical constriction. Both ends are curved

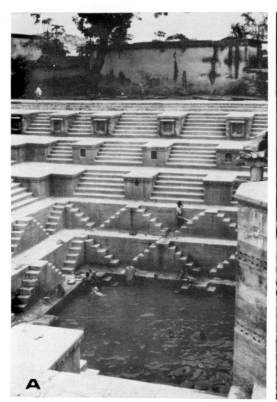
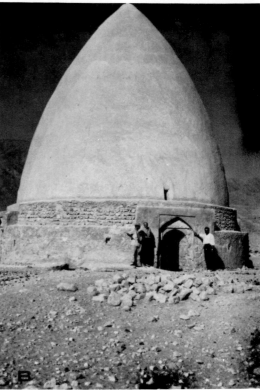

Fig. 11–43. Step well and *berkeh*, major sources of infection with *Dracunculus medinensis*. A, Step well in Rajasthan, India, illustrating a form of public water supply used in semiarid regions of India, Pakistan, and contiguous areas; the water level, very low in the illustrated well, fluctuates with the water table. The plankton flora and fauna, including *Cyclops* species, are rich during the warmer months, the season of guinea-worm transmission. *B, Berkeh* in the Lar region of Iran. This is a type of cistern adapted to near-desert conditions. Where rains are relatively light and are limited to one period of only a few days annually, surface water is channeled into the berkeh where, although densely turbid with soil and feces of man and animals at first, it becomes clear and potable through sedimentation and biologic conditioning. The heavy roof and wall provide insulation against heat, evaporation, and sunlight, yet enough direct sunlight is admitted (through small window above entrance) to sustain a stable, moderately dense population of algae and zooplankton, including *Cyclops*. Berkehs range in size up to 20 m in diameter, with the depth being generally approximately equal. As they must provide water for all needs, a community of 200 people must maintain a dozen or more berkehs. (By P.C. Beaver.)

ventrally, and in the digestive tract the worms are tightly coiled within a tumor cavity. The head portion of adults is provided with eight encircling rows of sharp curved hooklets. The third-stage larvae have four rows of cephalic hooklets (Fig. 11–44). The eggs deposited by the females in the tumor cavities are transparent and ovoid, with a pitted outer shell and a mucoid plug at one end. They measure 65 to 70 μm by 38 to 40 μm and are essentially unembryonated when evacuated in the feces of the cat.

In the life cycle of *G. spinigerum*, eggs in water become fully embryonated and hatch within 1 week at temperatures of 27° to 31°C. Free-swimming first-stage larvae, when eaten by freshwater copepods *(Cyclops)*, bore into the hemocoel and in 10 to 14 days transform into second stage, then third stage, larvae. When the infected *Cyclops* is ingested by a freshwater fish, frog, snake, bird, or mammal, the larvae migrate into the tissues. When one of these infected animals is eaten by another animal that is not the natural final host, the third-stage larvae are unable to complete their development; they merely migrate to the tissues of these transfer *(paratenic)* hosts and remain infective. Even in the appropriate final host there is a period of normal migration and development in the liver before the worms enter the stomach wall, which apparently always is invaded from the serosal surface. Development to the adult stage takes about 6 months.

Species of *Gnathostoma* are not well adapted to man as the definitive host and hence rarely, if ever, reach maturity in tumor cavities of the digestive tract. Instead, the excysted third-stage larva digested out of the flesh of the fish host (Fig. 11–44) or the early third-stage larva in the copepod accidentally swallowed in water migrates from the intestinal canal to cutaneous and subcutaneous and somatic muscular tissues, where it produces a picture of larva migrans, a granulomatous lesion or a stationary abscess. The worms have been observed in tissues from practically all surface areas, including the breast and occasionally the eye (see Larva Migrans, page 162).

The only effective treatment is removal of the worms by excision. Thorough cooking of fish or other second intermediate hosts intended for human consumption will prevent infection.

LARVA MIGRANS

Larva migrans is a term applied to the migration of larval helminths in hosts that are suitable for

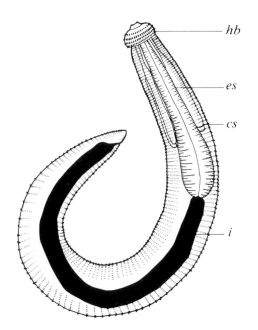

Fig. 11–44. *Gnathostoma spinigerum.* Third-stage larva. *cs,* Cervical sac. *es,* Esophagus. *hb,* Head bulb with four rows of hooklets. *i.* Intestine. (× 40.) (Adapted by M.D. Little from Miyazaki, I. 1960. On the genus *Gnathostoma* and human gnathostomiasis, with special reference to Japan. Exp. Parasitol., 9:338–370.)

long survival but are unsuitable for their development to the mature adult stage. The larval worms wander for a time in the host's tissues, but in most instances they eventually are encapsulated.

Larval nematodes that develop to the infective stage in soil and are adapted to the cutaneous mode of entry into the body (*e.g.,* hookworms and *Strongyloides* species) are responsible primarily for *cutaneous larva migrans.* Those that hatch from eggs in the small intestine and normally require a migration to the lungs (ascarids) are responsible primarily for *visceral larva migrans.* A third type, those that are ingested in an advanced larval stage in host tissues and are adapted for transmission through intermediate hosts (*i.e.,* spiruroid nematodes), may migrate through the viscera or the subcutaneous tissues. The types of worms whose larvae are most typically involved in *larva migrans* are those which in nature are transmitted through paratenic (transport) hosts, *i.e.,* smaller animals in whose tissues the infective larvae migrate and persist for long periods without essential development and are transmitted to the final host (predator) when the paratenic host (prey) is eaten. The behavior and persistence of these larvae in man are essentially the same as in the paratenic host.

Cutaneous Larva Migrans Caused by Hookworm Larvae

Historical and Geographical Notes. The clinical manifestations of cutaneous larva migrans, also referred to as "creeping eruption," have been known since 1874, when Lee described a linear cutaneous eruption with an advancing end, but the etiology was not definitely demonstrated until 1926 when Kirby-Smith, Dove, and White proved experimentally that a common causative agent in the southern United States is *Ancylostoma braziliense,* a hookworm of dogs and cats.

Cutaneous larva migrans resulting from exposure to *A. braziliense* has a widespread distribution throughout the sandy coastal areas of the United States, from southern New Jersey to the Florida Keys on the Atlantic Coast and along the entire littoral of the Gulf of Mexico, extending inland in Texas as far as Dallas and San Antonio. The largest number of cases has been found in the vicinity of Jacksonville, Florida. Creeping eruption has also been reported from many other subtropical and tropical coastal regions, including Mexico, southern Brazil, Uruguay, and northern Argentina, Spain, southern France, South Africa, India, the Philippines, and Australia.

Other species of hookworms are also capable of producing cutaneous larva migrans in man, *viz.,* the cosmopolitan hookworms of dogs, *Ancylostoma caninum,* the European dog hookworm *Uncinaria stenocephala,* and the hookworm of cattle, *Bunostomum phlebotomum.* However, cases resulting from natural exposure to the infective stage of these worms other than *A. caninum* apparently are very few compared with cases resulting from exposure to *A. braziliense.* Transient creeping eruption can be caused by larvae of the human hookworms, *Necator americanus* and *Ancylostoma duodenale.* Since larvae in skin cannot be recovered for identification, the species involved in the individual infection usually is unknown.

Pathogenesis and Symptomatology. At each point at which the larva of *A. braziliense* invades the skin, it produces an itching, reddish papule. In 2 or 3 days the larva has developed a serpiginous tunnel between the stratum germinativum and the corium. The lesion is at first erythematous and soon becomes elevated and vesicular (Fig. 11–45). As the larva proceeds through the skin at a rate of several millimeters a day, the older portion of the tunnel becomes dry and crusty. The progressive

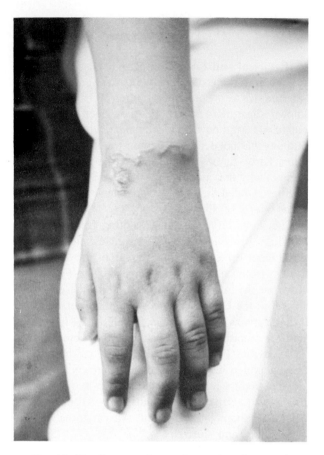

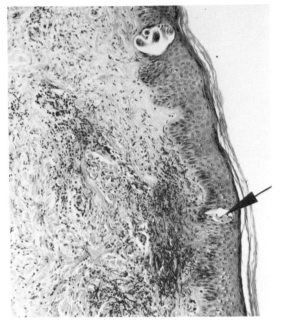

Fig. 11–46. *Ancylostoma braziliense.* Larva presumed to be *A. braziliense* in section of skin biopsy from a man with creeping eruption in Florida. (× 100.) Because the area around the larva in the epidermis above has no inflammatory infiltrate, whereas the trail behind the migrating larva *(arrow)* is marked by acute inflammatory reaction, attempts to obtain a biopsy specimen containing the larva are rarely successful. (By P.C. Beaver. Section courtesy of Harvey Blank.)

Fig. 11–45. Cutaneous larva migrans (creeping eruption). Typical lesion produced by unidentified hookworm larva, probably *Ancylostoma braziliense,* on wrist of child in Merida, Mexico. (Courtesy of A. Muhlfordt and A. D'Alessandro.) (From Beaver, P.C., Jung, R.C., and Cupp, E.W. 1984. *Clinical Parasitology,* 9th ed. Philadelphia, Lea & Febiger, p. 282.)

movement of the worm and the tissue irritation that it produces cause intense pruritus, which almost invariably leads to scratching. This opens the lesion to pyogenic organisms. Activity of the larva may continue for several weeks or months, resulting in extensive skin involvement (Fig. 11–46) and at times serious systemic illness.

Potentially both small mammals and insects may serve as paratenic hosts of *Ancylostoma* species. *A. caninum* larvae and probably those of most other species of *Ancylostoma* infect at least as readily by mouth as by the cutaneous route. If true, then it could be expected that hookworm larvae will invade the deep tissues of man as well as the skin, and those entering the skin and causing creeping lesions will later migrate to the deeper tissues. Creeping eruption frequently is followed by pneumonitis (Guill and Odom, 1978), and occasionally large numbers of the migrating hookworm larvae are found in the sputum. *Ancylostoma* larvae are

also known to invade the cornea. Little *et al.* (1983) observed that after leaving the skin, *Ancylostoma* larvae may enter and persist for long periods in skeletal muscle fibers of man (Fig. 11–47), as they do in mice and other small mammals.

Diagnosis. The classic picture of an advancing serpiginous tunnel in the skin with an associated intense pruritus is readily recognized as pathognomonic of cutaneous larva migrans, but the lesion may be atypical. Furthermore, creeping eruption of hookworm origin must be differentiated from that produced by fly larvae *(Hypoderma, Gasterophilus)* and, in Oriental regions, from that due to *Gnathostoma.*

Treatment. Therapy may be directed toward removing or killing the larva, relieving symptoms, or facilitating the deep migration of the larva. Symptoms may be alleviated by antihistaminics, antipruritics *(e.g.,* trimeprazine), sedatives, and anesthetic or protective coatings. Corticosteroids will inhibit the skin reaction but are recommended only in severe infections. Thiabendazole has now become the drug of choice, rarely failing to cure

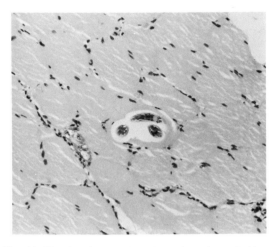

Fig. 11–47. *Ancylostoma* larva in section of muscle biopsy from thigh of pest control worker who had acquired a creeping eruption from soil under a house 3 months earlier. The larva is inside a muscle fiber and no inflammation is evident. (× 175.) (From Little, M.D., Halsey, N.A., Cline, B.L., and Katz, S.P. 1983. *Ancylostoma* larva in a muscle fiber of man following cutaneous larva migrans. Am. J. Trop. Med. Hyg., 32:1285–1288.)

when given either by mouth or applied topically in regular dosage (see Table 21–1, p. 265).

Epidemiology. Exposure results from contact of the skin with warm, moist sandy soil containing filariform larvae of hookworms originating from the feces of dogs and cats. The sites of exposure to *A. braziliense* usually are unprotected sandboxes, bathing beaches, and under houses where workers temporarily lie prone repairing exposed plumbing fixtures. In these situations, extensive body surfaces are exposed to infection.

Control. The hookworms responsible for cutaneous larva migrans are, with few exceptions, intestinal parasites of domestic animals, almost exclusively of dogs and cats. Control of the sources of exposure must therefore be directed toward removal of hookworms from dogs and cats, including periodic deworming of these animals, and elimination of stray animals.

Cutaneous Larva Migrans Caused by *Strongyloides* Larvae

Observations by Napier and of Caplan in 1949 on a type of creeping eruption associated with strongyloidiasis in men who had been prisoners of war in Thailand and Burma, and the reported existence of the same clinical type of dermatitis in Indochina, Iraq, on the Mediterranean Coast, and in the United States, have shown that cutaneous larva migrans results from perianal autoinfection

in people harboring *Strongyloides stercoralis* infection (Pelletier, 1984). Also, it has been shown experimentally that larvae of *Strongyloides* species in wild animals cause creeping eruption in man (Fig. 11–48). The cutaneous lesions caused by *Strongyloides,* whether derived from man or animals, are characteristically somewhat wider and less sharply delineated than those caused by hookworms (Fig. 11–41). However, the most distinctive features are rapid progression (up to 10 cm per hour) and a tendency for the lesions to disappear for several hours or days and reappear at a different location. The rapid advance of lesions caused by *Strongyloides* larvae suggested the term "larva currens" for this type of cutaneous larva migrans.

Visceral Larva Migrans Caused by *Toxocara* Larvae

The visceral type of larva migrans was not recognized until 1952. As in the cutaneous type, the invading larvae are of species that are naturally adapted to hosts other than man, and they remain for long periods in the tissues. These lesions have been found in the liver (Fig. 11–49) and brain and numerous other organs, including the eye (Fig. 11–50). Studies on the larvae in liver biopsies and in tissues obtained at autopsy, as well as experimental studies, have led to the conclusion that the larvae involved most frequently are those of *Toxocara,* in most instances *T. canis*. The diagnostic features of *T. canis* and other tissue-invading larvae were described by Nichols in 1956.

Because *Ascaris lumbricoides* has at times been found as an intestinal infection in association with granulomatous lesions of the viscera, it has commonly been assumed that the latter are necessarily the result of visceral migration of human *Ascaris* larvae. There is no reliable record of *Ascaris* having invaded visceral organs other than the liver and lungs, and in these organs their residence is limited to the period required for essential development.

In visceral larva migrans caused by *Toxocara* larvae, the clinical picture varies from asymptomatic to a syndrome of chronic hypereosinophilia, hepatomegaly, moderate pulmonary infiltrations, fever, cough, and hyperglobulinemia. Numerous cases involving the eye, brain, heart, and other organs, some of them fatal, have now been reported from most parts of the world. Typical cases of visceral larva migrans are now seen so commonly and in so many different localities that case reports are published only when special features are noted.

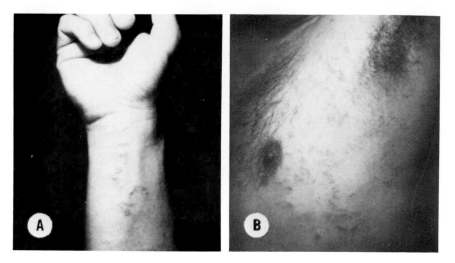

Fig. 11–48. *Strongyloides* species. Dermatitis produced by *(A)* two migrating larvae of *Strongyloides procyonis,* a parasite of the raccoon, and *(B)* 30 larvae of *S. myopotami,* a parasite of the nutria, in a volunteer. (From Little, M.D. 1965. Dermatitis in a human volunteer infected with *Strongyloides* of nutria and raccoon. Am. J. Trop. Med. Hyg., *14*:1007–1009.)

Since the diagnosis is often based on clinical findings only, unusual cases may represent diseases of a different etiology. Invasion of an eye by a *Toxocara* larva not only causes loss of vision but frequently results in enucleation of the eye. The presence of the causative larva can be demonstrated either by examination of histopathologic serial sections of the enucleated eye or by direct ophthalmoscopic examination. Reports involving the eye are of continuing interest, though hundreds of cases have been reported (Molk, 1983).

Specific diagnosis requires demonstration of the

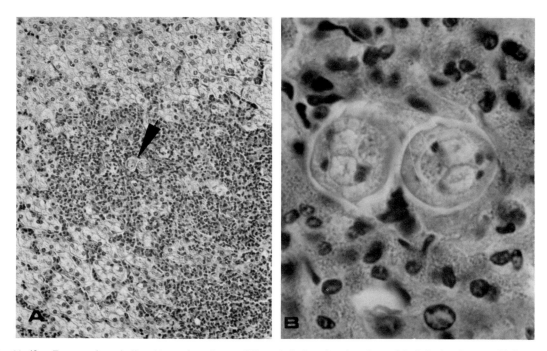

Fig. 11–49. *Toxocara* larva in liver biopsy from 2-year-old boy. *A,* In the migration phase of the infection the area of inflammation is great as compared with the size of the larva (20 by 400 μm), which here is located within the inflammatory area *(arrow),* although it frequently is found in normal tissue a millimeter or more from the lesion. (× 150.) *B,* Two transverse sections of the larva, showing characteristic features (paired excretory columns, lateral alae, and cordlike intestine); most of the cells surrounding the larva are eosinophils. (× 1250.) (By P.C. Beaver. Section courtesy of J.W. Walsh.) (From Beaver, P.C., Jung, R.C., and Cupp, E.W. 1984. *Clinical Parasitology,* 9th ed. Philadelphia, Lea & Febiger, p. 328.)

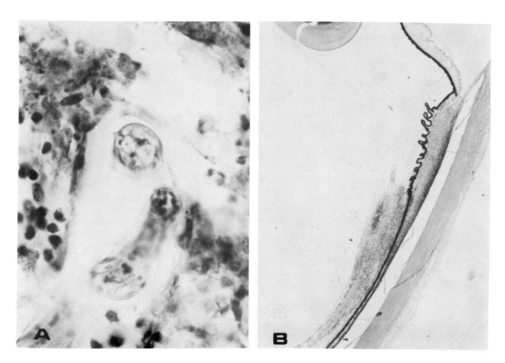

Fig. 11–50. *Toxocara canis,* larva in eye of child. *A,* Transverse and oblique sections showing features that made specific identification possible (× 650.) *B,* Granuloma surrounding larva in ora serrata. (× 17.) (By P.C. Beaver. Section courtesy of A.R. Irvine.)

parasite in specimens obtained by biopsy or at necropsy. In cases with liver involvement, biopsy of a small subcapsular nodule will usually provide the necessary evidence. However, confidence is increasing in serologic tests with antigens prepared from infective stage larvae or their excretion products (van Knapen *et al.,* 1983).

There is no specific therapy of demonstrated efficacy, although thiabendazole has shown some promise. In a majority of cases the prognosis is excellent, with complete recovery. If life is endangered by asphyxia resulting from bronchiolar spasm or allergic pneumonia, corticosteroids may be indicated as a temporary measure, but they should not be used in the usual case.

The high prevalence of *Toxocara* infection in dogs throughout the United States and elsewhere emphasizes a need for ridding household pets of their intestinal parasites at frequent intervals in order to safeguard young children from contracting roundworm infections normally occurring in these animals. Dogs that are allowed to defecate in playgrounds and other public areas in Europe as well as in the United States are often infected with *Toxocara* and *Ancylostoma*.

Larva Migrans Caused by Other Helminths

Larvae of *Gnathostoma* species *(G. spinigerum* and *G. hispidum)* have been recovered from subcutaneous tissues of man (see page 161). In Japan and Thailand, where *G. spinigerum* has been found many times in people, infection usually results from eating uncooked fish that contain the encapsulated third larval stage of the worm. As that stage of development is reached in the copepod, infection possibly can be acquired from ingestion of infected copepods in natural waters. Unable to develop to the adult stage in the wall of the human stomach, the larva undertakes an extraintestinal migration and is discovered in serpiginous tunnels in the skin, in abscess pockets in subcutaneous tissues, or occasionally in the eye, central nervous system, lungs, and other sites (Kagen *et al.,* 1984).

Two other helminths, *Spirometra* and *Alaria,* whose natural life cycles include transmission of larval stages through mammalian paratenic hosts, occasionally are found migrating in the tissues of man. The sparganum (larva) of *Spirometra* and the mesocercaria (larva) of *Alaria* are discussed in the chapters on cestodes and trematodes (see pp. 125 and 84).

Other zoonotic infections are sometimes erroneously regarded as examples of visceral larva migrans. *Capillaria hepatica* (p. 135), *Angiostrongylus cantonensis,* and *Angiostrongylus costaricensis* (p. 154), *Anisakis* and related forms (p. 145), and *Dirofilaria* species (p. 188) are forms whose relationship to the human host is the same as that to their natural final hosts and they often develop to the mature adult stage. Infection with these and other forms that undergo significant development in human tissues cannot be regarded as examples of visceral larva migrans.

SUMMARY

1. Roundworms (nematodes) are covered with a cuticula secreted by a hypodermis, have a somatic muscle layer, a body cavity not lined with mesothelium, and a complete digestive tract. With few exceptions they are dioecious, and the male is smaller than the female.

2. Their life cycle stages include the adult worms, the egg, and four successive larval stages.

3. *Trichinella spiralis* is found in most countries where pork is eaten. Trichinosis is enzootic among rats and some other wild mammals. Human infection results from eating rare or undercooked pork and occasionally from bear or walrus meat. Clinical evidences of the infection are (1) acute diarrhea during the 1st week; (2) symptoms of severe muscular inflammation during larval migration in the 2nd to 4th weeks, and (3) symptoms developing from cumulative traumatic, inflammatory, and toxic damage following encystation of the larvae in muscle fibers. Most cases are asymptomatic. Specific diagnosis is made on discovery of larvae in muscle biopsy or on immuologic tests. There is no standard therapy. Control by thorough cooking or freezing of pork for at least 24 hours is effective.

4. The whipworm, *Trichuris trichiura,* prevalent in warm moist climates, lives with the delicate anterior end threaded into the mucosal epithelium of the large intestine. Eggs, unembryonated when laid, become infective in about 4 weeks on warm, moist, shaded soil. When ingested, the eggs hatch and larvae develop into adult worms in about 90 days. Heavy worm burdens produce diarrhea or dysentery. Diagnosis is based on recovery of eggs in feces. The drug of choice for treatment is mebendazole. Control consists of sanitary disposal of human excreta.

5. The pinworm, *Enterobius vermicularis,* is a cosmopolitan human parasite, particularly prevalent among children. Adult worms normally live free in the appendix and cecum. Gravid females migrate from the anus and deposit nearly infective eggs on the perianal and perineal skin. When ingested, eggs hatch and larvae develop into adult worms in 4 weeks or less. The commonest symptom is perianal itching. Diagnosis is by recovery of eggs on a transparent adhesive tape anal swab. Piperazine, pyrvinium, pyrantel pamoate, and mebendazole are satisfactory for treatment.

6. The large intestinal roundworm, *Ascaris lumbricoides,* is cosmopolitan and is particularly common in small children. Adult worms live in the small intestine. Eggs, unembryonated when laid, become infective within 2 to 3 weeks in favorable soil. When embryonated eggs are ingested, larvae hatch and migrate from intestine to lungs *via* blood or lymphatic vessels; then after 8 to 9 days of growth they move up the air passages, are swallowed, and develop into adults in 8 to 12 weeks after exposure. In the lungs the larvae often produce transient pneumonitis and peripheral eosinophilia (Löffler's syndrome). Later, in the intestine, the infection is commonly accompanied by colicky pains, and heavy infections may cause intestinal obstruction, may block the appendiceal lumen or the common bile duct, or enter the parenchyma of the liver, where the worms die and cause septic abscesses. Effective anthelmintics are mebendazole, pyrantel pamoate, and piperazine. Diagnosis is made on recovery of eggs in the feces. Control consists of sanitary disposal of human feces.

7. The two common human hookworms are *Necator americanus,* more abundant in warm climates including the southeastern United States, and *Ancylostoma duodenale,* more frequent in the north temperate zones of the Mediterranean area and Eastern Hemisphere. Attached to the mucosa of the small intestine, each female lays several thousand eggs daily, in early stages of embryonation. When deposited on warm, moist, sandy soil in a shaded location, eggs soon hatch and in 5 days or more the larvae become infective. On contact with human skin, they penetrate to the cutaneous blood vessels, are carried to the lungs, and *via* the trachea reach the intestine, where they become attached and develop into adults in 5 weeks or more in *Ancylostoma* and 7 weeks in *Necator.* In *Necator* there is essential development in the lungs. *Ancylostoma* may be infective by mouth; *Necator* is not. Loss of blood caused by the hookworms feeding from and laceration of the intestinal mucosa leads to anemia and hypoproteinemia and indirectly to stunted physical and sexual growth and mental retardation. Diagnosis is made on recovery of eggs in the feces. Control of human hookworms requires anthelmintic treatment, together with provision for sanitary disposal of human feces.

8. In certain countries people are exposed to infection with hookworms and related nematodes of domestic animals, including *Ancylostoma ceylanicum, A. caninum, Ternidens deminutus, Mammamonogamus laryngeus,* several species of *Oesophagostomum* and *Trichostrongylus,* and *Angiostrongylus cantonensis* and *A. costaricensis.*

9. *Strongyloides stercoralis* is prevalent in warm, moist climates and occurs sporadically in temperate regions. The infection results from pollution of warm, wet, shaded sites with human feces. The parasitic females live embedded in the epithelium of the intestinal mucosa, usually in the duodenum and jejunum. Eggs hatch in the intestine and the rhabditoid larvae are passed in the feces. In the feces or soil, larvae become infective in 24 hours or may pass through a free-living cycle before producing the infective filariform stage. On contact with human skin, the filariform larva enters the cutaneous blood vessels and migrates through the lungs before reaching the intestine. The prepatent period is about 2 weeks. At times filariform larvae developing in transit down the intestine or at the anus produce autoinfection. The most frequent symptoms of strongyloidiasis are diarrhea and upper abdominal pain. Diagnosis is based on demonstration of larvae in the stool or duodenal aspirate. Thiabendazole is the drug of choice. Control requires sanitary disposal of human feces. *Strongyloides fuelleborni,* a parasite of monkeys and apes, is found in man in parts of Africa and in Papua New Guinea. Human infants can acquire infection through their mother's milk.

10. The guinea worm, *Dracunculus medinensis,* is endemic

in the semiarid regions of tropical Africa, the Middle East, and India. Females up to a meter long when gravid migrate to the skin, form a blister that sloughs to expose the worm, and on contact with water, motile larvae escape and are eaten by minute copepods. People acquire infection by drinking water that contains infected copepods. The life cycle requires about 12 months. Chemotherapy facilitates worm removal by traction. Installation of piped water provides effective control. Spiruroid nematodes that are parasites of domestic and wild mammals occur infrequently in man. Infection is acquired by ingestion of the encysted larva in an intermediate or paratenic host. Species reported from man include *Gongylonema pulchrum, Thelazia callipaeda* and *T. californiensis, Physaloptera caucasica, Gnathostoma spinigerum,* and *G. hispidum.*

11. The giant kidney worm, *Dioctophyma renale,* has a cosmopolitan distribution in fish-eating mammals and also occurs in man.

12. Larva migrans is prolonged migration of larval nematodes in the tissues without development. *Cutaneous larva migrans* (creeping eruption) is produced by filariform larvae of nonhuman hookworms and *Strongyloides. Visceral larva migrans* is produced mainly by larvae of *Toxocara* that hatch from eggs in the small intestine and migrate into liver, lungs, or other organs. Cutaneous larva migrans may occur as a sequela of perianal autoinfection in strongyloidiasis. Certain spirurid nematodes also cause cutaneous and visceral larva migrans. Thiabendazole is relatively effective for treating hookworm-induced cutaneous larva migrans. Control of larva migrans requires primarily the periodic anthelmintic treatment of dogs and cats.

REFERENCES

Ashford, R.W., Hall, A.J., and Babona, D. 1981. Distribution and abundance of intestinal helminths in man in western Papua New Guinea with special reference to *Strongyloides.* Ann. Trop. Med. Parasitol., 75:269–279.

Beaver, P.C., and Khamboonruang, C. 1984. *Dioctophyma*-like larval nematode in a subcutaneous nodule from man in Northern Thailand. Am. J. Trop. Med. Hyg., 33:1032–1034.

Botero, D., and Little, M.D. 1984. Two cases of human *Lagochilascaris* infection in Colombia. Am. J. Trop. Med. Hyg., 33:381–386.

Brown, R.C., and Girardeau, M.H.F. 1977. Transmammary passage of *Strongyloides* sp. larvae in the human host. Am. J. Trop. Med. Hyg., 26:215–219.

Campbell, W.C. 1983. Historical Introduction. In *Trichinella and Trichinosis.* Edited by W.C. Campbell. New York, Plenum Press, pp. 1–30.

Cline, B.L., Little, M.D., Bartholomew, R.K., and Halsey, N.A. 1984. Larvicidal activity of albendazole against *Necator americanus* in human volunteers. Am. J. Trop. Med. Hyg., 33:387–394.

Coulaud, J.P., Deluol, A.M., Cenac, J., and Rossignol, J.F. 1982. L'albendazole dans le traitement de la strongyloidose. A propos de 66 observations. Bull. Soc. Path. Exot., 75:530–533.

Daly, J.J., and Baker, G.F. 1984. Pinworm granuloma of the liver. Am. J. Trop. Med. Hyg., 33:62–64.

Dick, T.A. 1983. Infectivity of isolates of *Trichinella* and the ability of an Arctic isolate to survive freezing temperatures in the raccoon, *Procyon lotor,* under experimental conditions. J. Wildlife Dis., 19:333–336.

Gardiner, C.H. 1976. Habitat and reproductive behavior of *Trichinella spiralis.* J. Parasitol., 62:865–870.

———, Koh, D.S., and Cardella, T.A. 1981. *Micronema* in man: Third fatal infection. Am. J. Trop. Med. Hyg., 30:586–589.

Ginsburg, B., Beaver, P.C., Walson, E.R., and Whitley, R.J. 1984. Dermatitis due to larvae of a soil nematode, *Pelodera strongyloides.* Pediatr. Dermatol., 2:33–37.

Guill, M.A., and Odom, R.B. 1978. Larva migrans complicated by Loeffler's syndrome. Arch. Dermatol., 114:1525–1526.

Gunby, P. 1982. One worm in the minnow equals too many in the gut. JAMA, 248:163.

Hira, P.R., and Patel, B.G. 1977. *Strongyloides fuelleborni* infections in man in Zambia. Am. J. Trop. Med. Hyg., 26:640–643.

Kagen, C.N., Vance, J.C., and Simpson, M. 1984. Gnathostomiasis. Infestation in an Asian immigrant. Arch. Dermatol., 120:508–510.

Kelly, A., Little, M.D., and Voge, M. 1976. *Strongyloides fuelleborni*-like infections in man in Papua New Guinea. Am. J. Trop. Med. Hyg., 25:694–699.

Kliks, M.M. 1983. Anisakiasis in the western United States: Four new case reports from California. Am. J. Trop. Med. Hyg., 32:526–532.

Koshy, A., Raina, V., Sharma, M.P., Mithal, S., and Tandon, B.N. 1978. An unusual outbreak of hookworm disease in North India. Am. J. Trop. Med. Hyg., 27:42–45.

Kotula, A.W., Murrell, K.D., Acosta-Stein, L., Lamb, L., and Douglass, L. 1983. *Trichinella spiralis:* Effect of high temperature on infectivity in pork. Exper. Parasitol., 56:15–19.

Kozek, W.J. 1971. The molting pattern in *Trichinella spiralis.* II. An electron microscope study. J. Parasitol., 57:1029–1038.

Little, M.D. 1965. Dermatitis in a human volunteer infected with *Strongyloides* of nutria and raccoon. Am. J. Trop. Med. Hyg., 14:1007–1009.

———, Halsey, N.A., Cline, B.L., and Katz, S.P. 1983. *Ancylostoma* larva in a muscle fiber of man following cutaneous larva migrans. Am. J. Trop. Med. Hyg., 32:1285–1288.

Midler, J.E., Walzer, P.D., Kilgore, G., Rutherford, I., and Klein, M. 1981. Clinical features of *Strongyloides stercoralis* infection in an endemic area of the United States. Gastroenterology, 80:1481–1488.

Molk, R. 1983. Ocular toxocariasis: A review of the literature. Ann. Ophthalmol., 15:216–231.

Morera, P., Perez, F., Mora, F., and Castro, L. 1982. Visceral larva migrans-like syndrome caused by *Angiostrongylus costaricensis.* Am. J. Trop. Med. Hyg., 31:67–70.

Pascual, J.E., Bouli, R.P., and Aguiar, H. 1981. Eosinophilic meningitis in Cuba, caused by *Angiostrongylus cantonensis.* Am. J. Trop. Med. Hyg., 30:960–962.

Pawlowski, Z.S. 1983. Clinical aspects in man. In *Trichinella and Trichinosis.* Edited by W.C. Campbell. New York, Plenum, pp. 367–398.

Pelletier, L.L., Jr. 1984. Chronic strongyloidiasis in World War II Far East ex-prisoners of war. Am. J. Trop. Med. Hyg., 33:55–61.

Pereira, V.G., and Mattosinho Franca, L.C. 1983. Successful treatment of *Capillaria hepatica* infection in an acutely ill adult. Am. J. Trop. Med. Hyg., 32:1272–1274.

Phills, J.A., Harrold, A.J., Whiteman, G.V., and Perelmutter, L. 1972. Pulmonary infiltrates, asthma and eosinophilia due to *Ascaris suum* infestation in man. N. Engl. J. Med., 286:965–970.

Rushovich, A.M., Randall, E.L., Caprini, J.A., and Westenfelder, G.O. 1983. Omental anisakiasis: A rare mimic of acute appendicitis. Am. J. Clin. Pathol., 80:517–520.

Seawright, G.L., Despommier, D., Zimmermann, W., and

Isenstein, R.S. 1983. Enzyme immunoassay for swine trichinellosis using antigens purified by immunoaffinity chromatography. Am. J. Trop. Med. Hyg., *32*:1275–1284.

Shelhamer, J.H., Neva, F.A., and Finn, D.R. 1982. Persistent strongyloidiasis in an immunodeficient patient. Am. J. Trop. Med. Hyg., *31*:746–751.

Shoemaker-Nawas, P., Frost, F., Kobayashi, J., and Jones, P. 1982. *Ascaris* infection in Washington State. West. J. Med., *137*:436–437.

Silva, O.A. da, Amaral, C.F.S., Silveira, J.C.B. da, Lopez, M., and Pittella, J.E.H. 1981. Hypokalemic respiratory muscle paralysis following *Strongyloides stercoralis* hyperinfection: A case report. Am. J. Trop. Med. Hyg., *30*:69–73.

Smith, J.W. 1983. *Anisakis simplex* (Rudolphi, 1809, det. Krabbe, 1878) (Nematoda: Ascaridoidea): Morphology and morphometry of larvae from euphausiids and fish, and a review of the life history and ecology. J. Helminthol., *57*:205–224.

Spillmann, R. 1975. Pulmonary ascariasis in tropical communities. Am. J. Trop. Med. Hyg., *24*:791–800.

Stewart, T.B., Bidner, T.D., Southern, L.L., and Simmons, L.A. 1984. Efficacy of fenbendazole against migrating *Ascaris suum* larvae in pigs. Am. J. Vet. Res., *45*:984–986.

van Knapen, F., van Leusden, J., Polderman, A.M., and Franchimont, J.H. 1983. Visceral larva migrans: Examinations by means of enzyme-linked immunosorbent assay of human sera for antibodies to excretory-secretory antigens of the second-stage larvae of *Toxocara canis*. Z. Parasitenkd, *69*:113–118.

Von Reyn, C.F., Roberts, T.M., Owens, R., and Beaver, P.C. 1978. Infection of an infant with an adult *Toxocara cati* (Nematoda). J. Pediatr., *93*:247–249.

World Health Organization. 1983. Trichinosis surveillance. Wkly. Epidemiol. Rec., *58*:395.

Yoshimura, H., Akao, N., Kondo, K., and Ohnishi, Y. 1959. Clinicopathological studies on larval anisakiasis, with special reference to the report of extra-gastrointestinal anisakiasis. Jpn. J. Parasitol., *28*:347–354.

Chapter 12

Filariae

T. C. Orihel

FILARIAE AS A GROUP

The filariae, members of the superfamily Filarioidea, parasitize various vertebrate animals ranging from amphibians to man. These nematodes have a unique stage in their life cycle, the *microfilaria,* which distinguishes them as a group. The adult worms live in various tissues of the definitive host including the body cavities, subcutaneous tissues, and the lymphatic and vascular systems. Each species has a characteristic habitat within its host. The microfilariae produced by the female worm are motile, and those of some species migrate into the bloodstream; others accumulate in the skin. Host-to-host transmission is accomplished when the microfilaria is ingested by a bloodsucking arthropod intermediate host, in whose tissues it develops to the infective stage; when the infected arthropod again takes a blood meal, the larva invades the tissues of the definitive host through the bite site and develops to the sexually mature adult stage (Fig. 12–1).

Although taxonomic determinations are based primarily on the morphologic features of the adult worms, specimens for identification usually are not readily obtained from host tissues. As a consequence, routine diagnosis of filarial infection depends on the detection and identification of microfilariae found in the blood or skin of the host.

Some of the filariae that infect man may produce severe and debilitating disease, while others seem to be relatively innocuous. At least eight species of filariae are endemic in various parts of the world, including *Wuchereria bancrofti, Brugia malayi, Brugia timori, Loa loa, Onchocerca volvulus, Mansonella ozzardi, Mansonella perstans,* and *Mansonella streptocerca.* In addition, several species of filariae that are natural parasites of animals, *i.e.,* enzootic, also occasionally infect man, but these zoonotic infections usually are cryptic and rarely patent; they include species of *Dirofilaria, Dipetalonema,* and *Onchocerca,* among others.

Wuchereria bancrofti
(Bancroftian filariasis)

The dramatic symptoms accompanying bancroftian filariasis were known to the ancient Hindus (600 B.C.) and the Persians. In 1863 Demarquay, in Paris, first found the microfilariae in hydrocoele fluid of a patient from Cuba. In 1866 Wucherer, in Brazil, observed them in chylous urine, and in 1872 Timothy Lewis, in India, discovered them in peripheral blood. Adult females were first seen by Bancroft in 1876–77 and the adult males by Sibthorpe in 1888, both recovered from lymphatic tissues of man in Australia. In 1878 Patrick Manson first demonstrated that a night-biting mosquito, *Culex quinquefasciatus,* was an intermediate host, and a year later he described the nocturnal periodicity of the microfilariae in peripheral blood.

Bancroftian filariasis is widely distributed throughout the tropical regions of the world and may extend well into subtropical areas. Generally, it is endemic from about 41°N to about 28°S in the Eastern Hemisphere and from about 30°N to 30°S in the Western Hemisphere. It is probable that bancroftian filariasis was introduced into the Western Hemisphere from Africa with the slave trade. There is more bancroftian filariasis now than existed 100 years ago, principally because of increases in population of the areas where the disease is endemic.

Morphology, Biology, and Life Cycle. The adult worms, usually found in lymph vessels, are small, threadlike, and have a smooth cuticle; the

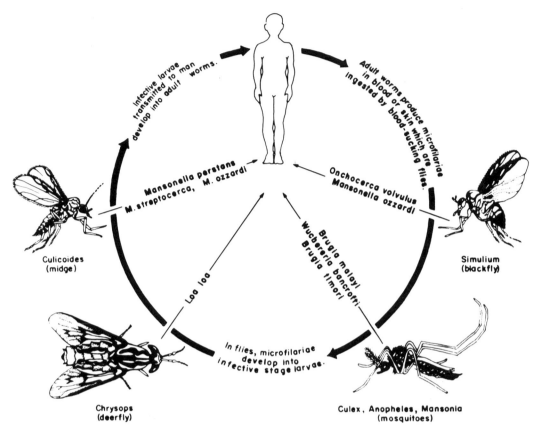

Fig. 12–1. Life cycles of the filariae of man. (Adapted by T.C. Orihel. From Smith, J.W., Melvin, D.M., Orihel, T.C., Ash, L.R., McQuay, R.M., and Thompson, J.H. 1976. *Diagnostic Medical Parasitology: Blood and Tissue Parasites.* Chicago, American Society of Clinical Pathologists, p. 17.)

anterior extremity is slightly bulbous. The male measures about 40 mm in length by 0.1 mm in diameter. The caudal extremity is curved sharply ventrad. There are up to 12 pairs of perianal pedunculated papillae and at least 3 pairs of larger sessile papillae farther caudad. The copulatory spicules are distinctly unequal and dissimilar; the gubernaculum is crescent-shaped (Fig. 12–2). The female measures 80 to 100 mm in length by 0.24 to 0.30 mm in diameter. The vulva opens midventrally about 0.8 to 0.9 mm from the anterior end. The short muscular vagina divides into paired uterine branches that fill the body cavity through most of its length. These in turn open into the muscular oviducts and thence into the highly coiled ovaries. Young embryos fill the uterine tubes and are confined in thin, hyaline, ovoid shells. As the developing microfilaria moves forward toward the vagina, the ''shell'' becomes elongated to accommodate the uncoiling embryo and forms the ''sheath'' of the mature microfilaria that is discharged by the female.

The motile microfilariae make their way from the lymphatics to the bloodstream and, in most regions of the world, *W. bancrofti* microfilariae circulate in the peripheral blood with a marked nocturnal periodicity. The numbers are highest during the period 2 hours before and 2 hours after midnight, and are scant, usually absent, during daylight hours when they tend to accumulate in the viscera and particularly in the lungs. In the South Pacific region, microfilariae show no marked periodicity but tend to circulate continuously, with some increase in numbers during the afternoon and evening hours. This type is referred to as *diurnal subperiodic,* but the term subperiodic when applied to *W. bancrofti* is understood to mean *diurnal.* In general, west of 140°E longitude only nocturnal periodicity occurs, between 140° and 180°E longitude either type may occur, and east of 180°E only the subperiodic type is present. The mechanisms and stimuli involved in the periodicity of microfilariae in peripheral blood are still essentially unknown.

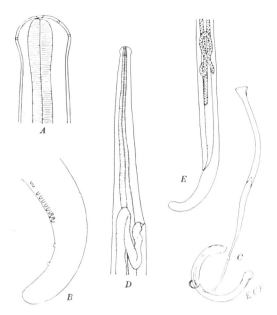

Fig. 12–2. *Wuchereria bancrofti.* *A,* Anterior end, ventral view. (× 300.) *B,* Posterior end of male, lateral view. *C,* Spicules and gubernaculum. *D,* Anterior end of female, lateral view. *E,* Posterior end of female, lateral view. (× 70.) (Adapted by E.C. Faust from York, W., and Maplestone, P.A. 1926. *The Nematode Parasites of Vertebrates,* London, J. & A. Churchill, p. 402.)

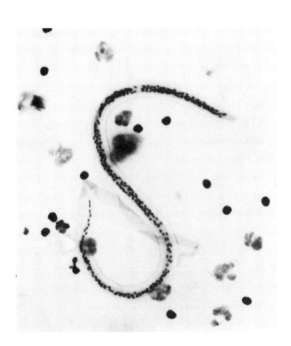

Fig. 12–3. *Wuchereria bancrofti.* Microfilaria in thick blood film stained with hematoxylin, showing graceful curves in the body and the sheath trailing from the posterior end. (× 700.) (By T.C. Orihel.)

The microfilariae of *W. bancrofti* (Fig. 12–3) from the peripheral blood measure 244 to 296 μm in length by 7.5 to 10 μm in diameter. The anterior end is bluntly rounded, the posterior end is tapered, and the body is enclosed in a relatively large sheath. In wet blood films, the microfilariae move slowly and in graceful curves. In stained blood films, they typically lie in smooth, open curves. Although ultrastructural studies reveal that the morphology of the microfilaria is complex and highly differentiated, in stained films the body appears to be composed of no more than a column of dark-staining nuclei that is interrupted along its length by spaces and special cells (Fig. 12–3). In *W. bancrofti,* the column nuclei are discrete and dispersed, the head space is short, the nerve ring is well demarcated, and the excretory pore and cell usually can be seen. Posteriorly the column of nuclei is reduced to a single row, which does not extend to the end of the tail. The *Innenkorper* or "innerbody" may be seen or not, depending on the choice of stains. Likewise, the sheath is conspicuous with certain stains (hematoxylin) and not with others (Giemsa).

The important diagnostic morphologic and behavioral features of the sheathed microfilariae of *W. bancrofti, Brugia malayi, B. timori,* and *Loa loa* are provided in Table 12–1 and Fig. 12–4.

Microfilariae ingested by an appropriate mosquito vector will be found, initially, still ensheathed in the midgut. Very quickly, usually within a few hours, the microfilaria exsheaths and migrates through the midgut wall into the thoracic muscle cells and becomes a quiescent, intracellular parasite (Fig. 12–5A). Within the muscle cell, the microfilaria transforms into a short, thick larva (Fig. 12–5B), molts to the second stage after a period of about 7 to 8 days and then rapidly grows, increasing in length to more than 1.0 mm; it molts for the second time at 12 to 14 days. The new third-stage larva then leaves the thoracic muscles and migrates to the head and mouthparts of the mosquito (Fig. 12–5C). It continues to grow, reaching a length that often exceeds 1.5 mm. When the mosquito takes its next blood meal, the infective (third-stage) larva is released.

After they enter the skin, the route followed by the infective larvae as they migrate to the sites where they develop into adults is not completely known. It is generally accepted that they enter the skin at the puncture site after the mosquito's mouthparts have been withdrawn. The larvae move primarily to the afferent lymph vessels and subcap-

Table 12–1   Characteristics of *Wuchereria*, *Brugia*, and *Loa* Species

Characteristic	W. bancrofti	B. malayi	B. timori	L. loa
Geographic distribution	Cosmopolitan; tropics and subtropics	Asia, Indian subcontinent	Timor, Lesser Sunda Islands	West and Central Africa
Vector	Mosquitoes	Mosquitoes	Mosquitoes	Tabanids
Habitat of				
Adult	Lymphatics	Lymphatics	Lymphatics	Subcutaneous
Microfilaria	Blood	Blood	Blood	Blood
Microfilaria				
Form	Sheathed	Sheathed	Sheathed	Sheathed
Periodicity	Nocturnal*	Nocturnal†	Nocturnal	Diurnal
Length (μm) in smears	244–296(260)	177–230(220)	265–323(287)	231–250(238)
2% formalin	275–317(298)	240–298(270)	332–383(358)	260–300(281)
Width (μm)	7.5–10.0	5–6	4.4–6.8	3–5
Tail shape	Tapered	Tapered	Tapered	Tapered
Tail nuclei	Absent	Terminal and subterminal	Terminal and subterminal, minute	Irregularly spaced

*Subperiodic in Pacific region.
†Subperiodic in parts of Southeast Asia, Indonesia, and the Philippines.

sular sinuses of the regional lymph nodes. Maturation is relatively slow. Although experimental studies indicate that female worms become gravid in about 4 months, microfilariae are not usually seen in the peripheral blood until the 8th month or even later. Observations indicate that in the absence of re-exposure, infections with *W. bancrofti* generally disappear in less than 8 years, suggesting that the life span of the worm or its reproductive period is even shorter. Microfilariae may live and circulate in the blood for more than a year.

Pathogenesis and Symptomatology. In the

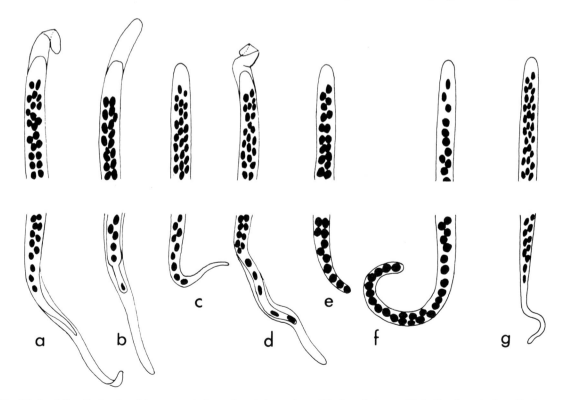

Fig. 12–4.   Microfilariae found in man, anterior and posterior ends. *a, Wuchereria bancrofti, b, Brugia malayi, c, Onchocerca volvulus, d, Loa loa, e, Mansonella perstans, f, Mansonella streptocerca,* and *g, Mansonella ozzardi.* (By T.C. Orihel.)

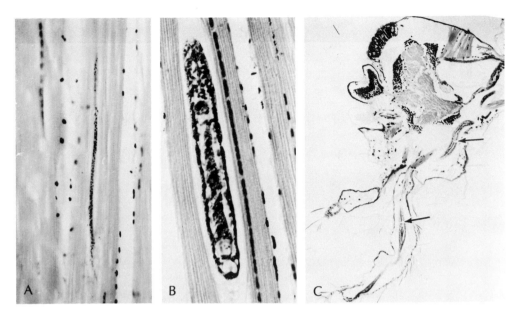

Fig. 12–5. *Wuchereria bancrofti. A,* Typical microfilaria. *B,* First-stage larva in thoracic muscles of *Culex quinquefasciatus. C,* Third-stage larvae in proboscis of the mosquito *(arrows).* (By T.C. Orihel.)

acute stage, symptoms resulting from infection with *W. bancrofti* are caused primarily by local and systemic sensitization and tissue reaction to the parasite. Apparently, immature worms produce relatively little local reaction. However, at times they produce an acute tissue response consisting of an accumulation of histiocytes, epithelioid cells, lymphocytes, plasma cells, giant cells, and eosinophils in the lumen of the vessel around the worms. Hyperplasia of the endothelium and perilymphatic cellular infiltration occur around the worms and proximally along the vessel to the regional lymph nodes in an ascending lymphangitis and lymphadenitis; stenosis of the lymph vessel results.

Whenever such acute inflammatory reaction takes place, there is a reddened, swollen, raised lymphatic tract immediately around and retrograde to the site of blockage (Fig. 12–6). It is exquisitely tender, painful, and at times there is a febrile reaction. It has been stated that the earliest symptoms in young adult males develop 3 to 16 months after exposure and that the cardinal manifestations are lymphangitis, usually with an associated lymphadenitis; only in 20% is there fever of a mild type and of short duration. The lymphangitis may originate in an upper extremity, mostly epitrochlear, but eventually practically all the lesions concentrate in the scrotum and consist of inflammatory involvement of the spermatic cord, epididymis, testis, or

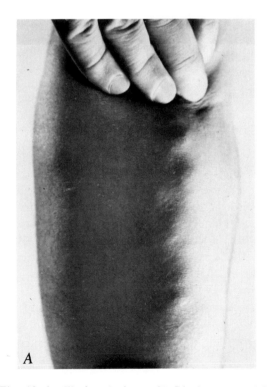

Fig. 12–6. *Wuchereria bancrofti.* Blockage caused by worm(s) in lymph vessel of forearm of man in Singapore. (Courtesy of J.F Schacher.) (From Beaver, P.C., Jung, R.C., and Cupp, E.W. 1984. *Clinical Parasitology,* 9th ed. Philadelphia, Lea & Febiger, 1984, p. 359.)

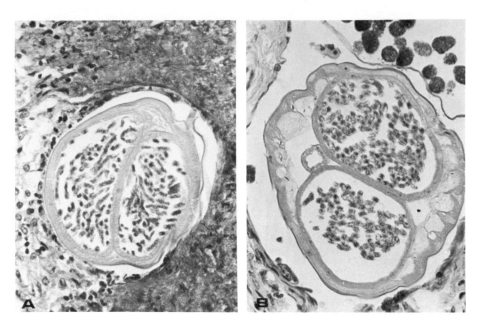

Fig. 12–7. *Wuchereria bancrofti.* Gravid females in lymph vessels of spermatic cord. *A,* Dead worm containing living microfilariae, partially encased in eosinophilic fibrinoid cellular debris. *B,* Living worm in functional vessel, showing typical microstructure. (× 170.) (From Beaver, P.C., Jung, R.C., and Cupp, E.W. 1984. *Clinical Parasitology,* 9th ed. Philadelphia, Lea & Febiger, p. 358.)

entire scrotal organ (Fig. 12–7*a*). Relapses of the syndrome are frequent.

In lightly exposed immigrants in Samoa, it was observed that bouts of lymphangitis with fever occurred annually. In natives of endemic areas, this stage of the infection may be symptomless. Since first exposure is likely to take place early in childhood, the severe, early involvement of the genitalia is usually lacking. In the *chronic stage* of the disease, living worms may be present for years in dilated lymphatic channels without causing remarkable symptoms (Fig. 12–7*b*). These individuals characteristically have microfilariae circulating in the blood and constitute the usual source of infection for the mosquito.

The advanced chronic stage may develop in highly sensitized reactors directly from the acute inflammatory condition of a lymphatic vessel containing the worms or may build up slowly from the milder fibrotic type. Eventually the worms die and are absorbed or become calcified. This may not occur until many years after initial exposure. The organs and tissues in which these changes occur are the groin, with the development of nodular groin-gland varicosities; the lower extremities, one or both of which become elephantoid, with redundant skin (Fig. 12–8) and a dense fibrous subcu-

taneous matrix filled with islands of lymph, and the external genitalia.

Filariasis without microfilaremia may occur in three general forms (Beaver, 1970).

1. Filarial elephantiasis in its extreme form, with enormous enlargement of one or both legs or of the external genitalia, is seldom accompanied by microfilaremia. Since this type of complication of filariasis is characteristically seen only in highly endemic areas and occurs in only a small percentage of the infected population, its pathogenesis is thought to involve a secondary streptococcal or other types of bacterial infection (Bosworth *et al.,* 1973).

2. A second form of filariasis without microfilaremia is *tropical eosinophilia,* also called Weingarten's syndrome and more specifically referred to as eosinophilic lung or tropical pulmonary eosinophilia. Before 1966 it was defined as chronic infiltration of the lungs resembling miliary tuberculosis and hypereosinophilia of the blood, with cough and asthmatic breathing more marked at night and symptoms promptly relieved by treatment with diethylcarbamazine or organic arsenicals. The definition later was expanded to include the presence of microfilariae in the

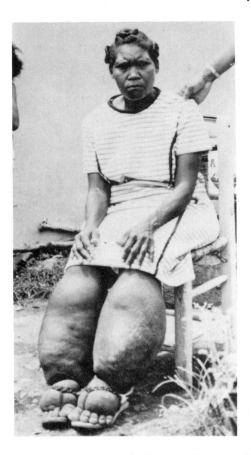

Fig. 12–8. *Wuchereria bancrofti.* Woman in Dominican Republic with filarial elephantiasis. (From Vincent, A.L., de Gomez, M.V., Gonzalvo, A., Nayar, J., and Sodeman, W.A. 1981. Filariasis in the Dominican Republic. Am. J. Trop. Med. Hyg., *30*:739–741.)

affected tissues of the lungs but not demonstrable in the blood (Danaraj *et al.,* 1966). The location of the worms producing the microfilariae that are screened out and destroyed in the lungs is unknown. *W. bancrofti* or *Brugia malayi* probably is the causative agent in most cases, and the pulmonary arteries and the pelvic lymphatics are the most likely locations of the adult worms. *B. malayi* and *W. bancrofti* have been found in pulmonary arterioles. Neva and Ottesen (1978) have attempted to further clarify the clinical concepts of tropical eosinophilia and have provided the criteria for differentiating it from related clinical states with which it may be confused.

3. Cryptic filariasis characterized by eosinophilia, retrograde lymphangitis, lymphedema, lymphadenitis, and general manifestations, with adult worms frequently demonstrable in lymphatic channels and lymph node biopsies but without microfilaremia, was described by Meyers and Kouwenaar in Indonesia in 1939. Because microfilariae were seen in lymph node sections in some cases and pulmonary disease was a prominent finding in others, the Meyers-Kouwenaar syndrome is not sharply differentiated from tropical eosinophilia. Cryptic filariasis with or without pulmonary manifestations was high among the troublesome, nonfatal forms of filariasis acquired by United States military personnel in the Southwest Pacific during World War II and by French servicemen in North Vietnam. The American experience was especially notable, because among many thousands who acquired the infection—over 12,000 in a period of about 1 year—less than 20 developed a detectable microfilaremia. Fifteen years after leaving the area, some of the men continued to have recurrent attacks of acute filarial lymphangitis or swellings and genital symptoms.

Diagnosis. Field surveys to determine the prevalence of bancroftian filariasis in an area are based on demonstration of microfilariae in blood films and signs and symptoms of the disease. In native populations in endemic regions, these two types of findings seldom coincide. A higher percentage of persons in the younger age groups have microfilaremia and a higher percentage in the older age groups have symptoms.

Diagnosis during the prepatent phase of infection must be based on a history of exposure, lymphangitis, and lymphadenitis compatible with bancroftian filariasis, and the occasional demonstration of immature worms by biopsy of an inflamed lymph node.

During the patent phase of infection, microfilariae will be found in blood films characteristically in small numbers. In all areas except the South Pacific Islands, they are present in appreciable numbers in the peripheral blood only at night with the greatest frequency, as stated earlier, occurring between 10 P.M. and 2 A.M. Diagnosis is routinely made with thick films, usually of 20 to 50 μl volume. For the detection of low-level microfilaremia, concentration methods (*e.g.,* Knott, Millipore filtration) can be used (see Technical Aids).

After the adult worms die, microfilariae gradually disappear from the blood over a period of months or a few years. As already noted, microfilariae of some species may live and circulate in the blood for more than 2 years.

Treatment. *Diethylcarbamazine* (1-diethyl-carbamyl-4-methylpiperazine hydrogen citrate) (DEC) is the drug of choice for treating bancroftian filariasis. The advantages of this drug are its oral route of administration, the patient's relatively high tolerance of the drug, and its relatively rapid, beneficial, clinical effects. Generally, excellent results are obtained when the drug is administered in the amount of approximately 6 mg per kg body weight per day (in 1 to 3 doses) for 2 to 3 weeks. It rapidly eliminates circulating microfilariae but acts more slowly on the adult worms; it has been reported that DEC sterilizes the female worm. DEC has been shown to be effective when administered in small doses for long periods mixed in food, drinks, and cooking salt (Sasa, 1976).

Other drugs have been used in the treatment of bancroftian filariasis (suramin, metrifonate, levamisole), but generally they are less effective or more toxic than DEC.

Epidemiology. Man is the only natural definitive host of *Wuchereria bancrofti*, although the silvered leaf monkey (*Presbytis*) will develop patent infection under experimental conditions. A morphologically distinct species of *Wuchereria*, *W. kalimantani*, has been described from *Presbytis cristatus*. Whether it can develop in man is unknown.

Mosquitoes belonging to the genera *Culex*, *Aedes*, *Mansonia*, and *Anopheles* serve as intermediate hosts for the filaria, with *C. quinquefasciatus* being the most common vector of the nocturnally periodic parasite. In the Pacific areas, day-biting species of *Aedes* are the principal vectors. Conditions highly favorable for continued propagation of the infection include a pool of microfilaria carriers in the human population and the appropriate vector mosquitoes breeding near human habitations.

Control. The control of bancroftian filariasis can be effected by (1) treatment of all microfilaria carriers in an endemic area, and (2) elimination of the mosquito vectors. The use of an effective insect toxicant as a residual spray in and around human habitations as well as larvicides will effectively control the vectors. When combined with DEC therapy, these measures can control the disease.

BRUGIA SPECIES

In addition to species of *Wuchereria*, the lymphatic-dwelling filariae include species belonging to the genus *Brugia*. These filariae parasitize man and numerous other mammals. The group is morphologically and biologically similar to *Wuchereria*. Two species, *B. malayi* and *B. timori*, are natural parasites of man; others occasionally infect man and produce cryptic infections.

Brugia malayi
(Malayan filariasis)

The microfilaria of *Brugia malayi* was first seen by Lichtenstein in blood films from natives in Sumatra. It was subsequently studied by Brug, who found that it differed from the microfilaria of *W. bancrofti*, and in 1927 he designated it *Filaria malayi*. Adult worms obtained by Rao and Maplestone in 1940 in India were described as a species of *Wuchereria*, and in 1960 Buckley placed the species in a new genus, *Brugia*.

The geographic distribution of *B. malayi* includes parts of India, Sri Lanka, Burma, Thailand, North Vietnam, the Philippines, Malaysia, Indonesia, South Korea, Japan, and China. In some of these countries, *B. malayi* coexists with *W. bancrofti*.

Extensive investigations by British workers in Malaysia during the 1950s showed that *B. malayi* occurs in cats and monkeys as well as in man and that closely related *Brugia* species that normally occur in these and other mammals occasionally may be transmitted to man.

Brugia timori, a species known for years only as a microfilaria, was fully described in 1977 by Partono *et al.* from residents of Timor. Related species that occur in wild and domestic animals include *B. pahangi* in dogs, cats, and monkeys in Malaysia; *B. patei* in dogs and cats in East Africa; *B. buckleyi* from the hare in Ceylon; *B. ceylonensis* in dogs in Sri Lanka; *B. guyanensis* from the coatimundi *(Nasua)* in Guiana; *B. beaveri* from the raccoon and bobcat in the United States; *B. tupaiae* from tree shrews in Malaysia; and *B. lepori* from the cottontail rabbit in the United States. Generally, the *Brugia* species are smaller than *W. bancrofti* and almost all live in the lymphatics. In all, the microfilaria is sheathed, has a terminal tail nucleus (usually a subterminal one as well), and circulates in the peripheral blood. For all *Brugia* species studied thus far, mosquitoes are the natural vectors.

Morphology, Biology, and Life Cycle. The adults of *B. malayi* (Fig. 12–9) resemble those of *W. bancrofti* in most respects but are specifically

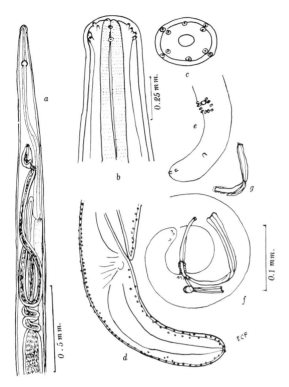

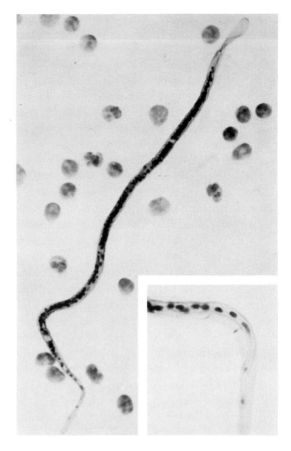

Fig. 12–9. *Brugia malayi. a,* Anterior part of female, ventral view. *b,* Anterior end of female, lateral view. *c,* Head-on view showing pattern of papillae. *d,* Posterior end of female showing cuticular bossing. *e,* Posterior end of male, ventrolateral view showing papillae. *f,* Posterior end of male showing spicules and gubernaculum. *g,* Right spicule enlarged. (Adapted from Buckley, J.J.C., and Edeson, J.F.B. 1956. On the adult morphology of *Wuchereria* sp. *(malayi?)* from a monkey *(Macaca irus)* and from cats in Malaya, and on *Wuchereria pahangi* n. sp. from a dog and a cat. J. Helminthol., *30*:1–20.)

Fig. 12–10. *Brugia malayi.* Microfilaria stained with hematoxylin. (× 250). *Inset,* tail showing subterminal and terminal nuclei. (By T.C. Orihel.)

distinguishable. Males measure 13 to 23 mm in length by 88 μm (maximum) in diameter. The posterior end is tightly coiled. Females vary in length from 43 to 55 mm and range in diameter up to 170 μm.

The microfilaria is readily distinguished from that of *W. bancrofti.* Although both are sheathed, the microfilaria of *B. malayi* is somewhat smaller, measuring about 270 μm in average length; it has a longer head space, a dense column of overlapping nuclei, a rather prominent *Innenkorper,* and a distinctive tail with terminal and subterminal nuclei, the two being separated by a constriction in the tail (Fig. 12–10). In Giemsa-stained blood films, the sheath of *B. malayi* stains a bright pink in contrast to that of *W. bancrofti,* which does not stain at all.

Pathogenesis and Symptomatology. Recurrent fever with acute inflammation of superficial lymph nodes and associated lymphatic vessels is charac-

teristic of the acute stage of Malayan filariasis. Elephantiasis of the limbs is a common sign of Malayan filariasis, but involvement of the genitalia and genitourinary systems (hydrocoele, chyluria, funiculitis, and elephantiasis of the scrotum) generally does not occur.

Diagnosis. The demonstration of microfilariae in night or day blood samples (depending on the area) is the only practical and reliable diagnostic method.

Treatment. Diethylcarbamazine (DEC) is highly effective against the parasite when administered at the rate of 6 mg per kg body weight daily for at least 10 times, at daily, weekly, or monthly intervals so that the total dosage is at least 60 mg per kg. *Brugia malayi* apparently is more susceptible to treatment with DEC than *W. bancrofti,* but the febrile reactions that may occur following administration of the initial dose are more severe in *B. malayi* than in *W. bancrofti* infection.

Epidemiology. There are two distinct types of *B. malayi* that differ in their microfilarial periodicity and vector requirements: the nocturnally periodic and the subperiodic. The former is the more widely distributed in Asia and the Indonesian archipelago and is commonly found in association with coastal rice fields and open swamps and ponds, where species of *Anopheles* serve as natural vectors. The latter (subperiodic) is found in swamp forest areas of Malaysia, Thailand, Indonesia, and the Philippines, where *Mansonia* species are the principal vectors. In India the microfilaremia is nocturnal, and *Mansonia* is the vector.

Control. Control of Brugian filariasis to date has been based primarily on mass chemotherapy with DEC rather than on a combination of vector and parasite control. Although the drug is a potent microfilaricide, side-effects and febrile reactions are frequent and occasionally severe. In endemic areas where species of *Anopheles* are the vectors, antilarval spraying and residual spraying of homes with insecticides provide some control. In localities where *Mansoni* spp. are involved and the infection is rural, the problem is more complicated, since larvae of these mosquitoes obtain oxygen by inserting their breathing tubes into the hanging roots of water plants. In India periodic removal of these aquatic plants as a practical control measure has been applied with some success.

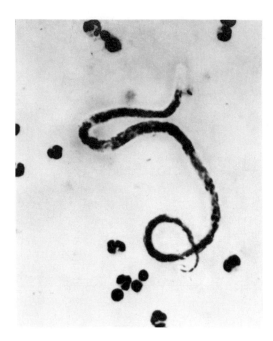

Fig. 12–11. *Brugia timori.* Microfilaria in thick blood film stained with Giemsa. (× 450.) (By T.C. Orihel.)

Brugia timori
(Timoran filariasis)

The microfilaria of *Brugia timori* was discovered in 1965 by David and Edeson during an investigation of filariasis on the island of Timor in the Indonesian archipelago. Eventually, the adult worms were recovered from experimentally infected Mongolian jirds *(Meriones)* and described by Partono and associates in 1977.

Morphology, Biology, and Life Cycle. The adult worms are small, threadlike, and delicate. In humans, they have been recovered from inguinal lymph nodes. The males measure 13 to 23 mm in length by approximately 72 μm in mean diameter; the tail is tightly coiled in a spiral of two or three turns. Females measure 21 to 39 mm in length by 99 μm in diameter. The microfilaria, nocturnal in periodicity, is readily distinguished from that of *B. malayi* on the basis of its greater length, the failure of the sheath to stain with Giemsa, and the inconspicuous bulging of the cuticle over the subterminal and terminal nuclei in the tail. Also, there apparently is a tendency for the microfilaria to shed its sheath in thick blood films (Table 12–1 and Fig. 12–11).

Pathogenesis and Symptomatology. Symptoms of inguinal and femoral lymphadenitis with retrograde lymphangitis are common. There may be suppurating and draining abscesses along the great saphenous vein (Fig. 12–12). Abscess scars are frequently found over the femoral triangle and on the medial aspects of the thigh, knee, and calf. Uncomplicated lymphadenitis and lymphangitis appear often during early childhood;

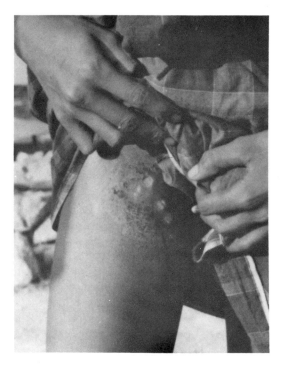

Fig. 12–12. *Brugia timori.* Draining abscesses caused by worms in lymph vessels along saphenous vein. (Courtesy of F. Partono.) (From Beaver, P.C., Jung, R.C., and Cupp, E.W. 1984. *Clinical Parasitology,* 9th ed. Philadelphia, Lea & Febiger, p. 368.)

the prevalence of abscesses and scars increases somewhat later. Elephantiasis most often develops during the third decade of life.

Diagnosis and Treatment. The diagnosis of infection is based on recognition of morphologic characters of the microfilaria. *B. timori* should be distinguished from periodic *W. bancrofti*, with which it may overlap in distribution. Treatment for the two parasites is similar.

Epidemiology and Control. *Brugia timori* apparently is limited to the Lesser Sunda Islands at the eastern end of the Indonesia archipelago. No other species of *Brugia* occurs in the endemic areas of *B. timori*. However, *W. bancrofti* does occur in the same region, and people may harbor both species. The natural vector is *Anopheles barbirostris*, which breeds in rice fields and feeds at night both indoors and out. As far as is known, there are no animal reservoirs. Periodic mass treatment with DEC followed by two annual selective retreatments, together with prompt treatment of individuals with acute clinical manifestations, was highly successful (Partono *et al.*, 1977).

Onchocerca volvulus
(Onchocerciasis)

Onchocerca volvulus was first described in 1893 by Leuckart from specimens removed from a native of Ghana in West Africa. In 1915 Robles found the same worm in a native worker on a coffee plantation in Guatemala and demonstrated that it was a cause of blindness. In 1926 Blacklock reported that a black fly, *Simulium damnosum*, was an essential intermediate host and transmitter of the disease in Africa.

Onchocerciasis is endemic in extensive areas of Africa and in a small area of Yemen. In the Western Hemisphere, to which it probably was introduced from Africa, it is established on the Pacific Coast of Guatemala, the adjacent Mexican states of Chiapas and Oaxaca, in parts of Venezuela, in the Amazonas and Roraima regions of northwest Brazil, in southwestern Colombia, and in northwestern Ecuador. Human infections with zoonotic *Onchocerca* have been reported in residents of the Crimean region of the U.S.S.R., Switzerland, eastern Canada, and the United States.

Morphology, Biology, and Life Cycle. The adults of *O. volvulus*, frequently a mated pair, are intricately coiled up in the midst of a dense fibrous, subcutaneous tumor but occasionally females have been found free in connective tissue. The nodules may develop on any part of the body but are frequently located near the junction of long bones, on the pelvic arch, or on the head. In most instances they can be seen or palpated (Fig. 12–13), but there are cases in which microfilariae are present in the skin without evidence of nodules.

The worms themselves are long, slender, and highly coiled (Fig. 12–14). Males measure 19 to

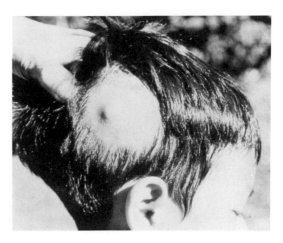

Fig. 12–13. *Onchocerca volvulus.* Nodules on scalp of Guatemalan boy. (From Smith *et al.* 1976. *Atlas of Diagnostic Medical Parasitology: Blood and Tissue Parasites*. Chicago, The American Society of Clinical Pathologists. Used by permission.)

42 mm in length by 0.13 to 0.21 mm in diameter. Females, in contrast, are very large, measuring 33 to 50 cm in length by 0.27 to 0.40 mm in diameter. The cuticle is modified to form annular thickenings in the female and a corrugated surface in males.

The microfilaria lacks a sheath, measures about 309 μm in average length, and has a diameter of 5 to 9 μm. The tail is attenuated and characteristically flexed. The column of cells does not extend to the end of the tail (Figs. 12–4, 12–15, and Table 12–2). The microfilariae are typically found in the upper layers of the dermis (Fig. 12–16), frequently in urine, occasionally in cytologic smears, and rarely in blood.

Simulium flies ingest blood and tissue juices in the feeding process and thereby pick up microfi-

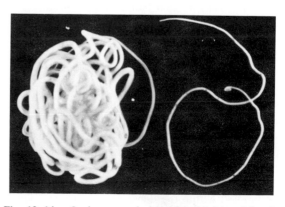

Fig. 12–14. *Onchocerca volvulus.* Male *(right)* and female digested out of a nodule. (× ca. 3.5.) (From Beaver, P.C., Jung, R.C., and Cupp, E.W. 1984. *Clinical Parasitology*, 9th ed. Philadelphia, Lea & Febiger, p. 370.)

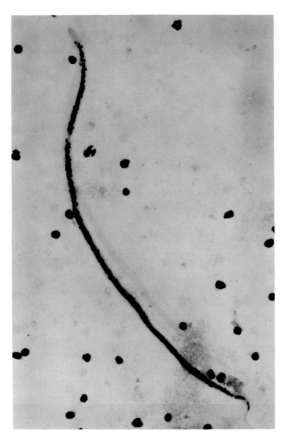

Fig. 12–15. *Onchocerca volvulus.* Microfilaria from skin, stained with Giemsa. (× 400.) (By T.C. Orihel.)

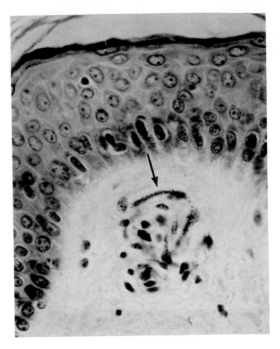

Fig. 12–16. *Onchocerca volvulus.* Microfilaria *(arrow)* in superficial dermal tissue. (× 450.) (By T.C. Orihel.)

lariae of *O. volvulus*. The microfilariae migrate from the alimentary tract to the thoracic muscles, where they undergo development to the infective stage over a period of 5 to 7 days. The infective larvae move to the mouthparts of the fly, and from there they may invade the tissues of man when the black fly takes its next blood meal. It is estimated that the worms require up to 1 year to reach sexual maturity and for microfilariae to appear in the skin. The females live for as long as 15 years, during which time they may produce thousands of microfilariae each day. Microfilariae have a life span in the human host of 1 to 2 years.

Pathogenesis and Symptomatology. With a still undetermined frequency of exceptions, the presence of the maturing or adult *O. volvulus* causes a local cellular reaction of a fibrotic nature; this results in encapsulation of the worms, which lie tangled within the dense fibrous matrix. There may be only a single nodule or many. In Africans, the nodules are more common about the pelvis and especially on the iliac crests, trochanters, and the

lateral chest wall. Less frequently, they may occur on the extremities. In contrast, in the Americas, particularly in Mexico and Guatemala, more than half the nodules are found on the head, 15% on the chest wall, and only 25% around or below the pelvis. It is generally accepted that in large part the biting habits of the main vectors determine the location of nodules.

The dispersal of microfilariae into the dermal layers of the skin throughout the body causes various types of acute and chronic skin lesions. The most common is an intense pruritic dermatitis. There may be diffuse changes of a chronic nature, including atrophy, hypertrophy, and abnormal pigmentation. Papular eruptions associated with itching can appear within a few days and may disappear spontaneously in a few weeks or months. In Africa, these typically affect the trunk and legs.

"Sowda," from an Arabic word meaning black, is the name of an important manifestation of localized onchocerciasis in Yemen. Usually the affected area of skin is markedly pruritic, dark, and thickened, and shows a papular or pustular eruption. Sowda occurs predominantly in young adult males and usually is localized and limited to a lower limb. However, in females and in children it tends to occur on the arms or back, probably due in part

Table 12–2. Characteristics of *Mansonella* and *Onchocerca* Species

Characteristic	M. ozzardi	M. perstans	M. streptocerca	O. volvulus
Geographic distribution	South and Central America, Caribbean	Africa, South and Central America	West and Central Africa	Africa, Central and South America
Vector	*Culicoides, Simulium*	*Culicoides* (midge)	*Culicoides* (midge)	*Simulium* (black fly)
Habitat of				
Adult	Subcutaneous	Body cavities	Dermis	Subcutaneous*
Microfilaria	Blood	Blood	Skin	Skin
Microfilaria				
Form	Unsheathed	Unsheathed	Unsheathed	Unsheathed
Periodicity	Aperiodic	Aperiodic	Aperiodic	Aperiodic
Length (μm) in smears	163–203(183)	190–200(195)	—	—
2% formalin	203–254(224)	183–225(203)	—	—
Skin snips	—	—	180–240(210)	304–315(309)
Width (μm)	4–5	4–5	5–6	5–9
Tail shape	Tapered, curved	Blunt, straight	Blunt, hooked	Tapered, flexed
Tail nuclei	Absent	Present	Present	Absent

*Subcutaneous and deeper tissues.

to the different styles of dress and exposure to biting black flies.

Lymphadenopathy is commonly associated with onchocerciasis. In some areas of Africa, individuals may have "hanging groin," a saclike projection of loose, atrophied skin containing a mass of large, fibrotic lymph glands. High rates of genital elephantiasis have been observed in endemic foci of onchocerciasis in regions of Zaire, where bancroftian filariasis is absent.

Ocular complications are the most serious and dreaded consequences of onchocerciasis in some areas of Africa and Central America. The microfilariae of *O. volvulus* invade all tissues of the eye, producing congestion, hemorrhage, and degeneration of the tissues as well as degenerative changes in the optic nerve. Extensive studies of the causes of blindness in Africa and Central America have demonstrated that the inflammatory lesions of onchocerciasis result from the death of microfilariae in the tissues. Microfilariae in the cornea, causing little or no damage while alive, later produce cellular infiltrates in the form of fluffy opacities. These may progress to dense infiltrations which usually start in the lower half of the cornea.

Diagnosis. Specific diagnosis usually depends on the demonstration of microfilariae in the skin. The generally accepted method is to examine a skin snip. A small snip of skin can be taken from any location on the body, although the scapular region and iliac crest are preferred. The skin snip is placed on a slide in water or saline for about 30 minutes

and may be teased to facilitate escape of microfilariae. Microfilariae, if present, tend to migrate out of the tissues where they can be counted and, if desired, stained for more detailed study. Skin snips may be obtained with a corneal-scleral punch such as the Holth, which results in uniform snips that usually are bloodless. Microfilariae in the anterior chamber of the eye and cornea can be demonstrated with an ophthalmoscope. When microfilariae cannot be demonstrated otherwise, their presence can be revealed by the urticarial reaction that follows the oral administration of a single dose of diethylcarbamazine (Mazzotti test).

Treatment. Surgical removal of nodules (nodulectomy) has been widely practiced in Mexico and Guatemala for more than 50 years. Removal of nodules reduces the risk of eye disease but does not appear to affect the prevalence of infection in a population. Nodulectomy is rarely practiced in Africa because nodules are scattered over various parts of the body.

Diethylcarbamazine is an effective microfilaricide even in smaller doses than are used in bancroftian filariasis patients, but it produces significant side-effects, including severe pruritus, urticaria, and some visual problems (e.g., conjunctivitis, photophobia). Concurrent administration of antihistamines or corticosteroids may relieve these severe allergic symptoms.

Suramin administered by intravenous injection is an effective macrofilaricide but also produces serious side-effects, including exfoliative dermatitis and renal complications. By reducing the dosage, toxicity may be decreased without significant loss of efficacy (Rougemont *et al.*, 1980). It has been suggested that DEC be given initially to reduce the microfilaria load, followed by suramin to kill the adult worms, and then DEC again to kill the residual microfilariae. The treatment requires practiced medical supervision.

Mebendazole and flubendazole have been shown to be effective microfilaricides and may prove to be useful alternatives to DEC in the treatment of onchocerciasis.

In Yemen, the removal of enlarged, regional lymph nodes is the traditional treatment for sowda.

Epidemiology. Man is the only natural definitive host of *O. volvulus* and species of *Simulium* are the natural vectors. The flies breed in fast-flowing streams above coastal plains, and the adults usually bite man close to their breeding sites; but the flies have a long flight range or may be carried by air currents and thus pick up, incubate, and transmit the infection many kilometers from where they breed.

Control. At present the control of onchocerciasis is directed at the vector. In West Africa a larvicide, Abate, is employed in long-term control programs. Aerial application of the compound has been successful, although it is evident that control rather than eradication of the vector is all that can be hoped for. Such control must be maintained over very large areas in order to combat peripheral invasion by flies coming from outside the control area.

In Mexico and Guatemala where vectors tend to breed in small, often inaccessible streams, the main effort has concentrated on nodulectomy. However, experience has shown that while routine nodulectomy reduces ocular disease, it has little or no effect on transmission. No drug is available that is sufficiently safe to use for mass treatment of heavily infected populations. The maximum life span of *O. volvulus* adults is about 15 years. Microfilariae may live in the skin for as long as 30 months (Duke, 1977).

Loa loa
(Loiasis)

Loiasis is endemic in the rain forest belt of West and Central Africa. The first African record of this infection was made by Guyot in Angola in about 1777, although "eyeworm" infections were recorded earlier, in 1770, in West African slaves

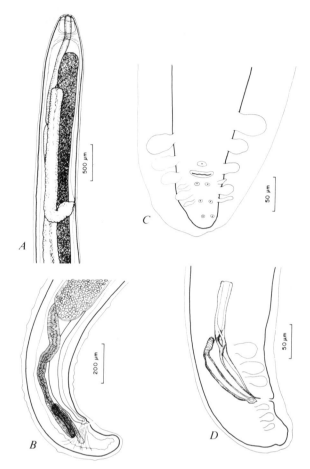

Fig. 12–17. *Loa loa*, adult worms. *A*, Anterior end of female, lateral view. *B*, Posterior end of female, lateral view. *C*, Tail of male worm, ventral view showing arrangement of papillae. *D*, Posterior end of male showing spicules and papillae. (Adapted from Eberhard, M., and Orihel, T.C. 1981. Development and larval morphology of *Loa loa* in experimental primate hosts. J. Parasitol., *67*:556–564.)

brought to the West Indies. The adult worms were specifically described by Cobbold in 1864. Connal and Connal in 1921 conclusively demonstrated that the mango fly, *Chrysops dimidiata*, is the natural vector of the filaria.

Morphology, Biology, and Life Cycle. The adult worms (Fig. 12–17*A–D*) inhabit and migrate freely through the subcutaneous tissues. They are rather robust worms that have conspicuous cuticular bosses. The male measures 30 to 34 mm in length by 0.35 to 0.43 mm in diameter. Its caudal end is curved ventrally. The female measures about 50 to 70 mm in length by 0.5 mm in diameter.

The microfilariae of *Loa loa* are sheathed and exhibit a diurnal periodicity in the peripheral blood. They measure 260 to 300 μm in length by 6 to 8

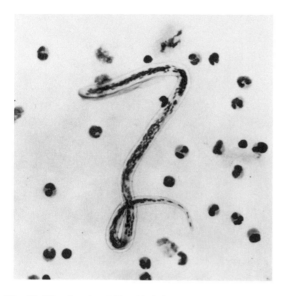

Fig. 12–18. *Loa loa.* Microfilaria in thick blood film stained with hematoxylin. (× 400.) (By T.C. Orihel.)

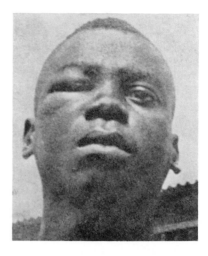

Fig. 12–19. Unilateral palpebral edema in *Loa loa* infection at the time a female worm is migrating across the front of the right eye. (From Dubois, A., and van den Berghe, L. 1948. *Diseases of Warm Climates.* New York, Grune & Stratton, p. 323.)

μm in diameter; the column cells (nuclei) extend to the tip of the tail (Fig. 12–18*a*). The morphologic features that distinguish the microfilaria of this species from those of *W. bancrofti, B. malayi,* and *B. timori* are provided in Table 12–1 and Figs. 12–4 and 12–18.

Species of day-biting *Chrysops, C. dimidiata,* and *C. silacea* are the natural vectors. Microfilariae ingested with the blood meal migrate from the midgut to the fat body of the fly, where they develop to the third stage in about 1 week. The infective stages that invade the human subcutaneous tissues develop there to sexually mature adults in approximately 5 months. The adult worms migrate freely through the subcutaneous tissues and often enter the orbit and conjunctiva. The human *Loa* has been observed to live for more than 8 years in experimentally infected monkeys. The maximum recorded life span of the adult worms in man is 17 years.

Pathogenesis and Symptomatology. In their migrations through various parts of the body, adult worms may appear in the extremities, trunk, or head. The worms are more of a nuisance than a cause of severe local tissue reaction, although characteristically there are recurrent swellings ("fugitive swelling" or "Calabar swelling") in the areas invaded by the worm. Swellings develop rapidly, may be painful, reach a diameter of 5 cm or more, and last for 2 or 3 days. Moreover, migration through the bulbar conjunctivae is always trouble-some and is attended by considerable pain and edema (Fig. 12–19). An associated eosinophilia may reach levels of over 50% of the leukocytes. At times loiasis produces periods of allergic reaction, particularly in Caucasians, with reddened giant urticarial swellings of skin and mucous membranes, an associated fever, and high eosinophilia.

Diagnosis. Loiasis may be suggested by the presence of "fugitive swellings" in association with high eosinophilia in persons who have visited or lived in endemic areas. Infection can be specifically diagnosed by the demonstration of microfilariae in peripheral blood during the day or by removal of the adult worms from the skin or conjunctiva.

Treatment. The annoyance of migrating worms can be eliminated by their surgical removal at the time they are migrating through the corneal conjunctiva (Fig. 12–19) or across the bridge of the nose. *Diethylcarbamazine* (DEC) is the drug of choice for treatment and is effective against both adult worms and microfilariae. An adult dosage of 200 mg per day for 20 days is recommended. Treatment should begin with low doses, especially in patients with high microfilaremia because of the allergic reaction associated with the death of large numbers of microfilariae. Simultaneous administration of steroids may also be necessary, especially during the first 2 or 3 days of treatment. DEC treatment is especially effective against light infections. In heavily parasitized persons, some of the worms may resist several courses of treatment.

Chemoprophylaxis apparently is possible with *Loa*. The recommended dose is 200 mg DEC twice a day, on 3 consecutive days, given once a month.

Epidemiology and Control. The distribution of *L. loa* corresponds to that of the mango flies *Chrysops dimidiata* and *C. silacea*. They breed in relatively clear, flowing streams in high-canopied rain forests and come out to nearby clearings to feed. North American species of *Chrysops*, such as *C. atlanticus* and others, will support development of human *Loa* to the infective stage (Orihel and Lowrie, 1975). Several species of monkeys are naturally infected with a related species of *Loa*, but the microfilariae exhibit a nocturnal periodicity and are transmitted by different species of *Chrysops*.

Reduction in the infection rate in native populations in endemic areas depends on (1) chemotherapeutic destruction of the microfilariae in the human host, and (2) the utilization of larvicides to kill the breeding stages of the *Chrysops* vectors. Bites of these flies may be avoided for short periods of time by application of various chemical repellants to exposed areas of the skin.

MANSONELLA SPECIES

Recent experimental studies have added considerably to knowledge of *Mansonella ozzardi*, its biology, taxonomic status, and its relationships to other filarial parasites of man (Orihel and Eberhard, 1982; Eberhard and Orihel, 1984). It has been concluded that *Tetrapetalonema* (=*Dipetalonema*, *Acanthocheilonema*) *perstans*, *T. streptocerca*, and *M. ozzardi* are congeneric and should be placed together in the genus *Mansonella*. These filariae inhabit the subcutaneous tissues or body cavities and produce small, unsheathed microfilariae that are found in the blood or skin. Bloodsucking gnats or black flies are natural vectors.

Mansonella ozzardi
(Ozzardiasis)

Mansonella ozzardi was first obtained by Ozzard as a microfilaria from Carib Indians in Guiana near the turn of the century. As very few adult worms have been recovered from man, present knowledge is based primarily on specimens removed from experimentally infected monkeys. The filaria is indigenous to Latin America, extending from northern Argentina to the Yucatan, and is widely distributed in the West Indies. Prevalence among Amerindians in some localities approaches 100%.

Morphology, Biology, and Life Cycle. Experimental studies indicate that the adult worms live in the subcutaneous tissues, where their small size and threadlike form make them difficult to find. Female worms obtained from experimentally infected monkeys measure 32 to 62 mm in length and have a diameter of 0.13 to 0.16 mm; males are 24 to 28 mm long and 70 to 80 μm in diameter. Morphologic features are illustrated in Fig. 12–20. The microfilaria, which circulates in the blood without periodicity, is small, delicate, and unsheathed; it has an average length of 224 μm and a diameter of 4 to 5 μm. The tail is long and slender and, when fixed in 2% formalin, has a "buttonhook" appearance (Table 12–2; Figs. 12–4 and 12–21). Di-

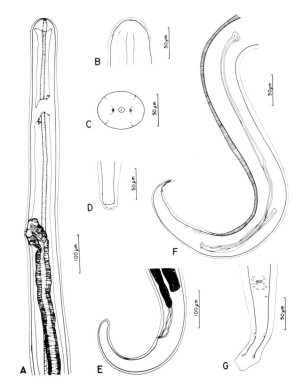

Fig. 12–20. *Mansonella ozzardi. A,* Anterior part of female, lateral view. *B,* Cephalic structures of female, lateral view. *C,* Cephalic structures, en face view. *D,* Tail of female, ventral view. *E,* Posterior end of female, lateral view. *F,* Posterior end of male, lateral view. *G,* Posterior end of male, ventral view. (From Orihel, T.C., and Eberhard, M.L. 1982. *Mansonella ozzardi.* A redescription with comments on taxonomic relationships. Am. J. Trop. Med. Hyg., *31*:1142–1147.)

agnosis depends on the identification of the characteristic microfilaria in blood. Because microfilaremias tend to be in low concentrations in the blood, Knott's method is especially useful in diagnosis. *Culicoides* species are the natural vectors in the Caribbean islands, whereas species of *Simulium* are the principal vectors in the Amazon basin. It is possible that *Culicoides* also are vectors in parts of the Amazon region. Development of the microfilaria to the infective stage in the vector occurs in the thoracic muscles. The prepatent period in monkeys is approximately 5 months and, based on the frequently observed presence of microfilariae in young infants, it probably is the same in humans.

Pathogenesis and Treatment. There are no characteristic symptoms in infected individuals, since the adult worms apparently do not produce any reactions in the tissues. No effective treatment is known. Diethylcarbamazine has no lethal or sterilizing effect on any stage of this filaria.

Mansonella perstans
(Perstans filariasis)

The adult stages of *Mansonella perstans* were first found by Daniels in 1898 in Amerinds in Guiana. The worms were identified by Manson as the adult that produced the same microfilariae that he had previously described from blood films of natives from the Congo and for which in 1891 he had proposed the species name "*perstans*." Because of the meager numbers of adult worms recovered from man and the chaotic taxonomy

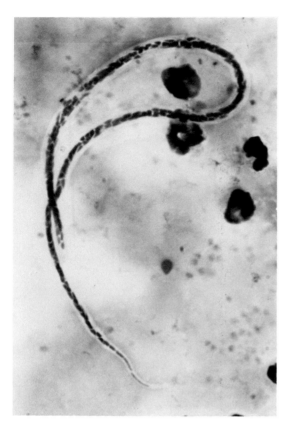

Fig. 12–21. *Mansonella ozzardi*. Microfilaria in thick blood film from Amerindian in Venezuela near Brazil border. Giemsa stain. (× 650.) (From Beaver, P.C., Jung, R.C., and Cupp, E.W. 1984. *Clinical Parasitology*, 9th ed. Philadelphia, Lea & Febiger, p. 382.)

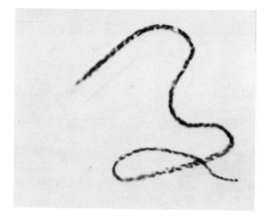

Fig. 12–22. *Mansonella perstans*. Microfilaria in thick blood film stained with hematoxylin, showing the blunt tail filled with nuclei. (× 450.) (Photo by T.C. Orihel.)

Mansonella streptocerca
(Streptocerciasis)

Mansonella streptocerca (Macfie and Corson, 1922) Orihel and Eberhard, 1982 was named and described from the microfilarial stage found in skin biopsies from natives of West Africa. It is restricted in its distribution to the rain forest belt of West and Central Africa.

Morphology, Biology, and Life Cycle. The adult worms and microfilariae live in the dermis of the skin (Fig. 12–23), the latter being somewhat concentrated near the epidermis. The microfilariae are small, slender, and unsheathed; they measure 180 to 240 μm in length by 3 to 5 μm in diameter. They are readily recognized in tissue sections as well as in teased and stained skin snips by the pattern of nuclear distribution in the

of the dipetalonematid filariae, this filaria has been variously listed as a species of *Acanthocheilonema*, *Dipetalonema*, and *Tetrapetalonema*. Experimental studies indicate that it belongs to the genus *Mansonella* as redefined by Orihel and Eberhard in 1982.

Mansonella perstans is widely distributed throughout the tropical regions of Africa and is found in northern, coastal South America, the Amazon region, and Trinidad.

Morphology, Biology, and Life Cycle. The adult worms are found in the body cavities, the connective tissues of the viscera, and possibly in small lymphatic vessels in the liver. They are small and delicate. Females measure 70 to 80 mm by approximately 120 μm; males, about 45 mm by 60 μm. The microfilariae, which circulate in the peripheral blood day and night, are small and unsheathed, measuring 183 to 225 μm by 4 to 5 μm, and are easily recognized by their short, blunt tail bearing nuclei to the extreme tip (Table 12–2 and Figs. 12–4 and 12–22). *Culicoides* (*C. austeni* and *C. grahami*) are the natural vectors.

Pathogenesis and Treatment. Disease manifestations attributed to *M. perstans* include transient abdominal pain, subcutaneous swelling, rashes, pain in the limbs and serous cavities, and fatigue, especially in persons not indigenous to endemic areas. Apparently, diethylcarbamazine has no microfilaricidal action but may temporarily sterilize the adults. There are reports of successful treatment with mebendazole, given in a dosage of 100 mg twice daily for 30 days.

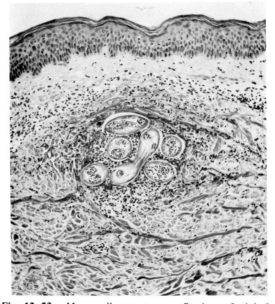

Fig. 12–23. *Mansonella streptocerca*. Sections of adult female in upper dermis. (× 100.) (From Neafie, R.C., Connor, D.H., and Meyers, W.M. 1975. *Dipetalonema streptocerca* (Macfie and Corson, 1922): Description of the adult female. Am. J. Trop. Med. Hyg., 24:264–267.)

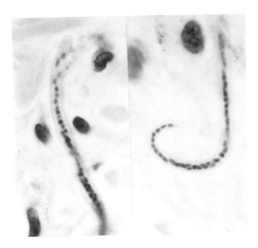

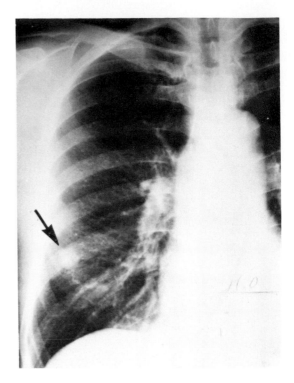

Fig. 12–24. *Mansonella streptocerca.* Microfilariae in tissue sections, showing characteristic pattern of nuclei at anterior *(left)* and posterior ends, and curved, "shepherd's-crook" configuration of tail. (× 1080.) (From Neafie, R.C., Connor, D.H., and Meyers, W.H. 1975 *Dipetalonema streptocerca* (Macfie and Corson, 1922): Description of the adult female. Am. J. Trop. Med. Hyg., *24*:264–267.)

anterior and posterior ends. Anteriorly, the column begins as a single row of 10 to 12 elongated, staggered nuclei; posteriorly, the nuclei tend to be quadrate in shape, and form a single row extending to the end of the tail (Figs. 12–4, 12–24). The latter typically is bent into a shepherd's crook curve.

A biting gnat, *Culicoides grahami,* is regarded as the principal vector.

Diagnosis is made by skin biopsy deep enough to include dermal tissue. Microfilariae must be differentiated from those of *O. volvulus,* since both species occur in the skin and frequently overlap in geographic distribution.

Pathogenesis and Treatment. Streptocerciasis is regarded as innocuous, since carriers are typically symptomless. However, in some individuals there may be dermatitis characterized by pruritus, hypopigmented macules, and papules. Diethylcarbamazine is effective against both microfilariae and the adult worms. Treatment often results in an exacerbation or appearance of pruritus and the development of cutaneous papules that are at the sites of degenerating adult worms.

ZOONOTIC FILARIASIS

Certain filarial parasites of animals also occur in man. Some produce patent infections, while the majority do not. The latter are usually identified on the basis of the morphologic appearance of worms observed in the tissues.

Dirofilaria

Species of *Dirofilaria* are moderately large worms that live in the vascular system or, more commonly, in association with the subcutaneous tissues of wild and domestic animals. The microfilariae are unsheathed and circulate in the blood. Mosquitoes are the usual vectors.

Dirofilaria immitis Leidy, 1856, the heartworm of dogs and their wild relatives, is present throughout most of the temperate, tropical, and subtropical areas of the world, living typically in the chambers and connecting large vessels of the right side of the heart. In the United States, heartworm in dogs is most prevalent in the south and southeastern states, but its range extends as far north as Minnesota, Michigan, and Massachu-

Fig. 12–25. *Dirofilaria immitis.* Coin lesion *(arrow)* seen on roentgenogram in periphery of right lung. The radiographic appearance simulates that of metastatic carcinoma, but in the surgical specimen a mature *D. immitis* worm similiar to that seen in Fig. 12–26 was found in a pulmonary artery. (Courtesy of D.M. Bradburn.)

setts; except for parts of California, it is uncommon or absent west of the Mississippi River. Numerous cases of lung or heart infection with *D. immitis* in man have been reported in the United States. Infections also have been reported from other parts of the world, including Colombia, Brazil, Japan, and Australia. The great majority of these presented as a "coin lesion" in the lungs (Figs. 12–25 and 12–26).

Dirofilaria presumed to be *D. repens, D. tenuis,* or *D. ursi* have been found in subcutaneous tissues or abscesses in various anatomic locations in man, including particularly the palpebral conjunctivae, the orbit, and the subcutaneous tissues of the face (Fig. 12–27). *D. tenuis,* a parasite of raccoons *(Procyon lotor),* apparently is responsible for most such cases seen in the United States, although *D. ursi* of bears in the northern states and Canada and *D. striata* of wild cats in the southeastern coastal states are believed to occasionally infect man as well. *Dirofilaria repens,* a subcutaneous parasite of the dog, has been identified in human infections in France, Italy, and other Mediterranean countries of Europe, in the U.S.S.R., and in Sri Lanka. Although these and other species of *Dirofilaria* usually reach sexual maturity in man, they rarely produce microfilariae.

Onchocerca

Species of *Onchocerca* are common in ungulates throughout the world, including the United States. Best known among them are *O. gutturosa, O. lienalis,* and *O. stilesi* in cattle and *O. cervicalis* and *O. reticulata* in horses. They live typically in or on the ligaments and tendons. Biting midges *(Culicoides)* and black flies *(Simulium)* are natural vectors. Human infections

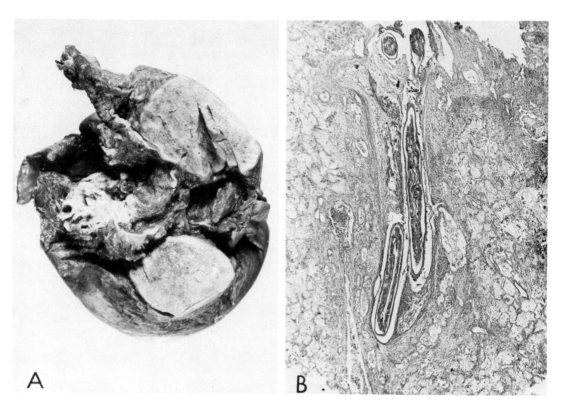

Fig. 12–26. *Dirofilaria immitis. A,* Right lower lobe of lung containing a sharply circumscribed infarct-like lesion, bisected and with tissue blocks removed from upper half. The lesion was discovered on a roentgenogram and the affected lobe was removed on suspicion of carcinoma. *B,* Tissue section showing longitudinal and transverse *(at top)* sections of a mature female in a pulmonary artery. (× 20.) (From Beaver, P.C., and Orihel, T.C. 1965. Human infection with filariae of animals in the United States. Am. J. Trop. Med. Hyg., *14*:1010–1029.)

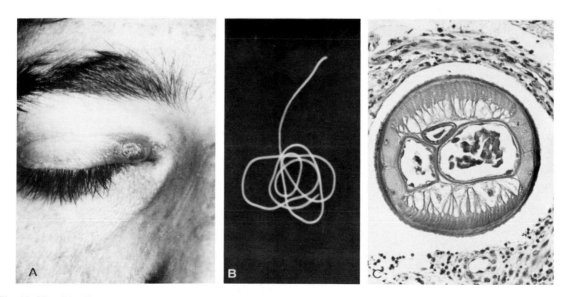

Fig. 12–27. *Dirofilaria "conjunctivae." A,* Nodule in upper lid of right eye of man in Texas. *B,* Sexually mature female worm released by incision of nodule shown in A and identified as *Dirofilaria tenuis. C,* Transverse section of worm with longitudinally ridged cuticle and other features characteristic of *D. tenuis* removed in a nodule from the thigh of a woman in Florida. (× 100.) (*A* and *B* courtesy of Dr. Whitman Rowland. *C* from Beaver, P.C., and Orihel, T.C. 1965. Human infection with filariae of animals in the United States. Am. J. Trop. Med. Hyg., *14*:1010–1029.)

have been reported from Illinois (U.S.A.), Switzerland, the U.S.S.R., and Canada.

Brugia

Filariae identified as *Brugia* have been found in lymph nodes removed from people who could not have acquired the infection outside the northern or northeastern regions of the United States, where *B. malayi* and *B. timori* do not occur. In most cases, the worms were sexually mature, all were in lymph nodes, and none was identifiable to species. In one case microfilariae were found in blood of an immunodeficient infant (Simmons *et al.*, 1984). Two species of *Brugia* are found in animals in the U.S.— *B. beaveri* in raccoons and *B. lepori* in rabbits.

Two cases of *Brugia* infection have been reported from Colombia, where no *Brugia* species has been recorded in animals, although a species was described from nearby Guiana (see page 178).

Other Zoonotic Filariae

Human infections with filariae belonging to the genus *Dipetalonema* have been reported in three or more cases in the United States. In one, a parasite was removed from the eye of a man in Oregon and was identified as possibly *Dipetalonema arbuta* from the porcupine or *D. sprenti* from the beaver. Two others found in subcutaneous nodules of the arm and abdominal wall in patients from Louisiana and Mississippi might possibly have been *D. reconditum*, a subcutaneous parasite of the dog in the United States. In a fourth case, a single microfilaria was seen in a 12-year-old girl from rural Alabama, and it, too, was identified as *Dipetalonema*, possibly *D. reconditum*.

Microfilariae named *Dipetalonema semiclarum* have been reported in the blood of people in northwestern Zaire. The adult worms have not been found.

Microfilaria rodhaini, a dipetalonematid species, was reported in the skin of natives in Gabon, West Africa. This worm is a natural parasite of anthropoid apes.

Godoy *et al.* (1980) found a microfilaria in the blood of Amerinds in the interior of Venezuela, which they named *Microfilaria bolivarensis*. The adult worms are unknown.

The microfilaria of *Meningonema peruzzi*, a filaria normally found in the subarachnoid space of monkeys in Central Africa, has been found at least twice in man (Orihel, 1973). It is probable that this parasite is responsible for a significant amount of central nervous system disease attributed to other filariae across much of Africa.

SUMMARY

1. Filarial worms have a microfilarial stage that distinguishes them from other nematodes. Deposited by the female as sheathed or unsheathed, the microfilariae migrate to the bloodstream, lymphatics, or cutaneous tissues. When picked up by an arthropod host, they transform into rhabditoid larvae, then into infective filariform larvae. When the arthropod next feeds on the definitive host, the larvae enter the skin and migrate to the site where they develop into mature worms.

2. Eight species of filariae are important natural parasites of man: *Wuchereria bancrofti*, *Brugia malayi*, and *Brugia timori*, *Onchocerca volvulus*, *Loa loa*, *Mansonella ozzardi*, *Mansonella perstans*, and *Mansonella streptocerca*.

3. *Wuchereria bancrofti*, a tropical species, is most frequently found in lymphatic vessels of the groin and pelvic regions. The sheathed microfilariae circulate in the blood and in most geographic areas circulate more abundantly at night. Mosquitoes serve as intermediate hosts. Lymphangitis and lymphadenitis develop around

and retrograde to the sites where the worms are located, resulting in elephantiasis, most frequently of the genitalia and lower extremities. Diethylcarbamazine clears the blood of microfilariae and more slowly kills the worms. Control consists of administering diethylcarbamazine to carriers and use of insecticides to control the mosquitoes.

4. *Brugia malayi*, in most respects comparable to *W. bancrofti*, is widely distributed in countries bordering on the China Sea, in Indonesia, and in southwestern India. The urban type is transmitted by anopheline mosquitoes, the rural type by *Mansonia* species whose larvae obtain oxygen from the roots of certain aquatic plants.

5. *Onchocerca volvulus* lives in fibrous subcutaneous tumors. Unsheathed microfilariae migrate through tissue of the skin. Black flies *(Simulium)*, the intermediate hosts, breed in rapidly flowing streams. Onchocerciasis is endemic in tropical Africa, on the Pacific slopes of Guatemala and adjacent states of Mexico, and in Venezuela, Brazil, Colombia, and Ecuador. Microfilariae migrate into the tissues of the eye and are responsible for failing vision and eventual blindness. Specific diagnosis is made by recovering microfilariae from superficial skin snips. Treatment consists of surgical removal of nodules and administration of diethylcarbamazine to kill the microfilariae and suramin to kill the adults. Control of the vector is by application of insecticides to the breeding sites.

6. *Loa loa*, a filaria of West and Central Africa, migrates through subcutaneous tissues periodically causing subcutaneous swellings and is occasionally seen under the conjunctiva. Microfilariae are sheathed and diurnal in periodicity. A tabanid fly, *Chrysops*, which breeds in flowing streams, is the vector. Treatment with diethylcarbamazine usually is effective.

7. *Mansonella perstans*, which has extensive distribution in tropical Africa, Atlantic coastal areas of South America, and some of the West Indies, lives in the peritoneal cavity and *Mansonella ozzardi*, which is indigenous to tropical America, lives in the subcutaneous tissues. Their unsheathed microfilariae circulate aperiodically in peripheral blood. *Mansonella streptocerca*, which inhabits cutaneous connective tissues, is endemic in parts of Central Africa. Its unsheathed microfilariae are found in the skin. These three species are transmitted by biting gnats, *Culicoides* spp. and, in the case of *M. ozzardi*, by simuliid flies as well.

8. *Dirofilaria immitis*, the dog heartworm, occasionally is a human parasite affecting the heart and lungs.

9. *Dirofilaria conjunctivae* is the name applied to certain zoonotic filariae found in subcutaneous nodules or abscesses in people of the United States, Europe, and elsewhere. The lesions often involve the conjunctivae and other tissues around the eye, as well as superficial tissues elsewhere.

REFERENCES

Beaver, P.C. 1970. Filariasis without microfilaremia. Am. J. Trop. Med. Hyg., *19*:181–189.

Bosworth, W., Ewert, A., and Bray, J. 1973. The interaction of *Brugia malayi* and *Streptococcus* in an animal model. Am. J. Trop. Med. Hyg., 22:714–719.

Danaraj, T.J., Pacheco, G., Shanmugaratnam, K., and Beaver, P.C. 1966. The etiology and pathology of eosinophilic lung (Tropical eosinophilia). Am. J. Trop. Med. Hyg., *15*:183–189.

Duke, B.O.L. 1977. Onchocerciasis. Br. Med. Bull., *28*:66–71.

Eberhard, M.L., and Orihel, T.C. 1984. The genus *Mansonella* (Syn: *Tetrapetalonema*): A new classification. Ann. Parasitol., *59*:483–496.

Godoy, G.A., Orihel, T.C., and Volcan, G.S. 1980. *Microfilaria bolivarensis:* A new species of filaria from man in Venezuela. Am. J. Trop. Med. Hyg., *29*:545–547.

Neva, F.A., and Ottesen, E.A. 1978. Current concepts in parasitology, tropical (filarial) eosinophilia. N. Engl. J. Med., *298*:1129–1131.

Orihel, T.C. 1973. Cerebral filariasis in Rhodesia—a zoonotic infection? Am. J. Trop. Med. Hyg., *22*:596–599.

———, and Eberhard, M.L. 1982. *Mansonella ozzardi:* A redescription with comments on its taxonomic relationships. Am. J. Trop. Med. Hyg., *31*:1142–1147.

———, and Lowrie, R.C., Jr. 1975. *Loa loa:* Development to the infective stage in an American deerfly, *Chrysops atlanticus*. Am. J. Trop. Med. Hyg., *24*:606–609.

Partono, F., Purnomo, A., Dennis, D.T., Atmosoedjono, S., Oemijati, S., and Cross, J.H. 1977. *Brugia timori* sp.n. (Nematoda: Filarioidea) from Flores Island, Indonesia. J. Parasitol., *63*:540–546.

Rougemont, A., Thylefors, B., Ducam, M., Prost, A., Ranque, Ph., and Delmont, J. 1980. Traitement de l'onchocercose par la suramine à faibles doses progressives dans les collectivités hyperendémiques d'Afrique occidentale. 1. Résultats parasitologiques et surveillance ophthalmologique en zone de transmission non interrompue. Bull. W.H.O., *58*:917–922.

Sasa, M. 1976. *Human Filariasis. A Global Survey of Epidemiology and Control.* Baltimore, University Park Press.

Simmons, C.F., Winter, H.S., Berde, C., *et al.* 1984. Zoonotic filariasis with lymphedema in an immunodeficient infant. N. Engl. J. Med., *310*:1243–1245.

Chapter 13

Acanthocephala and Gordiacea

T. C. Orihel

ACANTHOCEPHALA
(Thorny-headed worms)

The thorny-headed worms compose the phylum Acanthocephala, with affinities to both the Aschelminthes and the Platyhelminthes. All acanthocephalans are parasitic throughout their life cycle, except for the interval required for completion of embryonation of the eggs passed in the feces on the ground or in water. They infect the digestive tract of a variety of vertebrates, mainly fish, birds, and mammals, and are found in fresh water, marine, and terrestrial hosts. Occasionally species of three genera infect man.

Adult acanthocephalans are elongate, somewhat flattened and saclike, and at the anterior end have a spinous, eversible proboscis that serves for attachment to the intestinal wall of the host (Fig. 13–1). They vary in size from a few millimeters to several centimeters in length; males are considerably smaller than females. The living worms are milky-white to pink in color; they lack segmentation but may have superficial, transverse constrictions *(Macracanthorhynchus hirudinaceus)* or beadlike annulations *(Moniliformis moniliformis)*. Acanthocephalans have no mouth, digestive tube, or anus; nutrients are absorbed through the body surface. Excretory organs, when they exist, are of a protonephridial type and open into a terminal portion of the reproductive system. An extensive lacunar system, present within the body wall, may serve for nutrient distribution. Both sexes have complex reproductive systems.

Acanthocephalans are parasites of the intestine of their definitive hosts. Eggs (Fig. 13–2) evacuated in the feces, contain a partially developed larva called the *acanthor*, which continues its development after the egg is ingested by the invertebrate intermediate host (insects, crustaceans). It has a rudimentary proboscis with hooklets that are used by the hatched larva to bore through the gut wall and into the hemocoel of the vector. The acanthor develops within the hemocoel into a more advanced *acanthella* stage with an armed proboscis. It, in turn, matures into a juvenile stage referred to as the *cystacanth*, which contains the rudiments of structures found in the adult (Fig. 13–4). Development requires 6 to 12 weeks in the invertebrate host. When the invertebrate host is ingested by an appropriate vertebrate, the cystacanth develops into a sexually mature adult and mates; egg-laying begins thereafter.

Four different acanthocephalans have been reported as incidental parasites of man. *Macracanthorhynchus hirudinaceus*, normally found in domestic and wild pigs, has been recorded on several occasions from man in most parts of the world. A large number of cases have been reported in children in several provinces of China (Zhong *et al.*, 1983). Infections were typically nonpatent and often resulted in intestinal perforation.

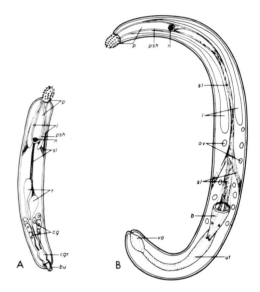

Fig. 13–1. Acanthocephala, male *(A)* and female *(B)*. Diagrams to illustrate the principal reproductive and attachment organs. *b,* Uterine bell. *bu,* Bursa. *cg,* Cement glands. *cgr,* Cement gland receptacle. *l,* Lemnisci. *n,* Nerve mass. *ov,* Floating ovaries. *p,* Proboscis. *psh,* Proboscis sheath. *sl,* Suspensory ligament. t, *Testes.* *ut,* Uterus. *va,* Vagina. (Adapted by T.C. Orihel from drawing by E.C. Faust in Faust, E.C. 1949. *Human Helminthology,* 3rd ed. Philadelphia, Lea & Febiger, p. 334.)

Infection was attributed to ingestion of infected beetles. Human infections with *Moniliformis moniliformis*, a natural parasite of rats transmitted by insect intermediate hosts, have been reported on several occasions from various parts of the world. Human infections with a species of *Bolbosoma* normally found in marine mammals and acquired by eating raw fish have been reported in Japan (Beaver *et al.*, 1983). *Macracanthorhynchus ingens*, a large species commonly found in the American raccoon, has been reported once as a human parasite in a child in Texas (Dingley and Beaver, 1985).

GORDIACEA OR HAIRWORMS

The gordiids belong to the phylum Nematomorpha. They are long, slender, wiry worms, creamy-white to dark brown in color, intensely opaque, and measure 10 to 50 cm in length

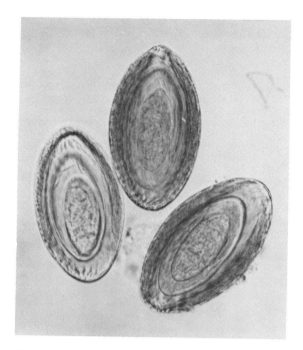

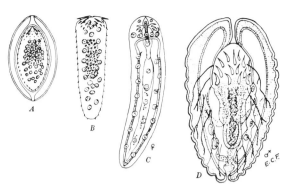

Fig. 13–4. *Macracanthorhynchus hirudinaceus*. Chief developmental stages, enlarged but not drawn to scale. *A*, Egg, fully embryonated. *B*, Acanthor, with rostellar hooks in relaxed position. *C*, Acanthella, female. *D*, Cystacanth, male. (Adapted by E.C. Faust from Van Cleave, H.J. 1947. A critical review of terminology for immature stages in acanthocephalan life histories. J. Parasitol., *33*:118–225.)

Fig. 13–2. *Macracanthorhynchus hirudinaceus*. Eggs containing fully developed, infective acanthor. (× 340.) (By P.C. Beaver.) (From Beaver, P.C., Jung, R.C., Cupp, E.W. 1984. *Clinical Parasitology*, 9th ed. Philadelphia, Lea & Febiger, p. 545.)

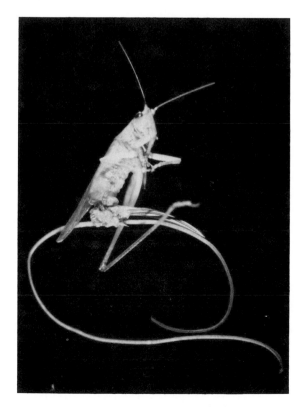

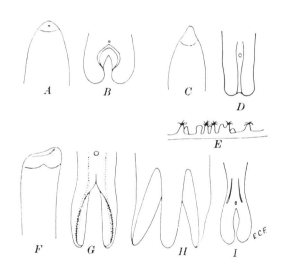

Fig. 13–5. Gordiacea, characteristic features. *A* and *B*, Anterior and posterior extremities, respectively, of male *Gordius villoti*, enlarged. *C* and *D*, Anterior and posterior extremities, respectively, of male *Chordodes*, enlarged. *E*, Section through papillae and cuticular hairs of *Chordodes*, greatly enlarged. *F* and *G*, Anterior and posterior extremities, respectively, of male *Paragordius varius*, enlarged. *H*, Posterior extremity of female *Paragordius varius*, enlarged. *I*, Posterior extremity of male *Parachordodes*, enlarged. (*A* through *D* and *I*, Adapted from Camerano, L. 1897. Monografia dei Gordii. Mem. R. Accad. Sc. Torino, *47*:339–419. *E*, From Römer, F. 1896. Beitrag zur Systematik der Gordiiden. Abhandl. Senckenb. Naturf. Gesellsch., *23*:247–295. *F* through *H*, Adapted from Stiles, C.W. 1907. Three new American cases of infection of man with horsehair worms (species *Paragordius varius*), with summary of all cases reported to date. U.S. Hyg. Lab. Bull., no. *34*:53–68, and from May, H.G. 1919. Contributions to the life histories of *Gordius robustus* Leidy and *Paragordius varius* (Leidy). Illinois Biol. Monogr., *5*, no. 2, Fig. 133.)

Fig. 13–3. *Gordius* sp. Adult ruptured free from body cavity of katydid. (× ca. 2) (By M.L. Eberhard.)

(Fig. 13–5). The sexes are separate but both have a cloaca. The posterior end of the male is bifurcated or grooved and that of the female either entire or trilobed. The digestive tract is usually degenerate. Adults are free-living, whereas the developmental stages are parasites of insects, mainly grasshoppers and other orthopterans.

Mature worms live in fresh water, where they mate; the female discharges strings of eggs into the water. Following embryonation, a larva hatches and penetrates the tissues of an insect such as a grasshopper, cricket, or cockroach and develops in the hemocoel. As it approaches maturity, the worm ruptures the body wall of the insect (Fig. 13–3) and begins its free-living aquatic existence. Recognized genera include *Gordius, Chordodes, Paragordius, Neochordodes,* and *Pseudogordius.*

There are numerous accounts of gordiid worms parasitic in man, including instances of passage of the living organisms in vomitus or feces (Ali-Khan and Ali-Khan, 1977) and, in some cases, discharged from the urethra. Some of the accounts possibly are fanciful, others erroneous. Gordiids retrieved from the toilet bowl are submitted for identification on the mistaken presumption that they migrated or were passed from the body. In no instance has pathogenicity of a gordiid been demonstrated.

REFERENCES

Ali-Khan, F.E.A., and Ali-Khan, Z. 1977. *Paragordius varius* (Leidy) (Nematomorpha) infection in man: A case report from Quebec (Canada). J. Parasitol., *63*:174–176.

Beaver, P.C., Otsuji, T., Otsuji, A., Yoshimura, H., Uchikawa, R., and Sato, A. 1983. Acanthocephalan, probably *Bolbosoma,* from the peritoneal cavity of man in Japan. Am. J. Trop. Med. Hyg., *32*:1016–1018.

Dingley, D., and Beaver, P. 1985. *Macracanthorhynchus ingens* from a child in Texas. Am. J. Trop. Med. Hyg., 34: In press.

Zhong, H-L., Feng, L-B., Wang, C-X., Kang, B., Wang, Z-Z., Zhou, G-H., Zhao, Y., and Zhang, Y-Z. 1983. Human infection with *Macracanthorhynchus hirudinaceus* causing serious complications in China. Chinese Med. J., *96:*661–668.

Chapter 14

Leeches

Leeches, class Hirudinea, phylum Annelida, have true segmentation, but they lack appendages. They have an elongated muscular body with two suckers—one surrounding the mouth and one at the posterior end (Fig. 14–1)—by which they move like "measuring worms." They are also good swimmers. Leeches take vertebrate blood as food, and most species are avidly sanguinivorous. Like ticks, leeches ingest a large quantity of blood, which they store in greatly distended ceca and digest slowly over periods of weeks or months. Some leeches are aquatic, others are terrestrial in rain forest areas, and still others are amphibious.

Morphology and Life Cycle

Morphology. Leeches vary in size up to about 12 cm in length and in shape from elongated cylindroid to broadly pyriform. They are dorsoventrally compressed, but frequently they have a convex dorsum and a concave ventral side (Fig. 14–1). There is a maximum of 34 true segments in the body, with a similar number of median ventral paired nerve ganglia and of rows of sensory papillae. Each segment has three to many external annulations.

A tough cuticula covers the body. Seventeen paired nephridiopores are located in the median annulus of segments 7 to 23. On the dorsal surface of each of the first five segments in most leeches, there are minute pairs of eyespots or light-sensitive end organs. Depending on the species, the surface of the leech may be essentially plain, may be striped longitudinally, or symmetrically patterned in colors.

The *digestive system* is provided anteriorly with a protrusile proboscis in the order Rhynchobdellida or three very muscular jaws with marginal denticles in the order Gnathobdellida. Leeches of medical importance belong to the order Gnathobdellida. Their three cutting jaws produce a characteristic triradiate (Y-shaped) laceration in the victim's skin. The small mouth leads into a muscular pharynx, which is surrounded by many secretory glands that provide anticoagulin *(hirudin)* when the leech is taking a blood meal (Fig. 14–2). Behind the pharynx there is a long, thin-walled median crop, with 11 pairs of distensible diverticula or ceca. The distal end of the crop joins the midgut, where digestion of the stored blood takes place. However, leeches apparently have no digestive gland. Behind the midgut is a short intestine followed by a short rectum and anus.

The *blood vascular system* is composed of blood vessels with muscular walls and two blood sinuses (one dorsal and one ventral) that represent the greatly reduced body cavity. Branches and capillaries extend to all parts of the body.

The *nervous system* consists of a pair of median ventral, partially fused ganglia for each segment, with connecting longitudinal twinned nerve cords, and at the anterior end a large cephalic ganglion.

The *reproductive organs* of both sexes in the same worm

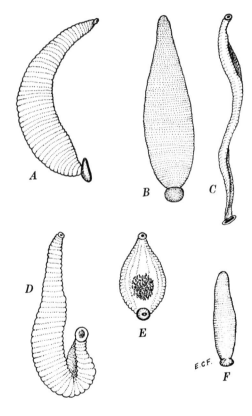

Fig. 14–1. Habit sketches of leeches, about natural size. *A, Limnatis nilotica.* B and C, *Hirudo medicinalis.* D, *Haemopis sanguisuga.* E, *Planobdella parasitica,* with brood of young attached to ventral side. F, *Haemadipsa zeylanica.* (By E.C. Faust.)

consist of 1 to 10 (or more) pairs of small spherical *testes,* each with a *vas efferens;* paired *vasa deferentia, seminal vesicles, prostate glands, ejaculatory ducts* and muscular *penial organs;* and one pair of *ovaries* with *oviducts* that unite and join a muscular *uterus* that opens through a short *vagina* one segment behind the male genital pore.

Life Cycle. Insemination is characteristically accomplished by cross-fertilization, either by reciprocal copulation or by implantation of a horny spermatophore containing the spermatozoa of one onto the cuticula of another. In some groups the eggs

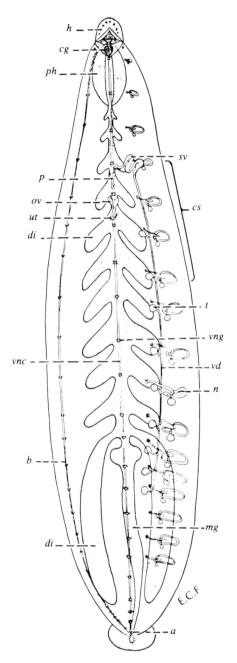

Fig. 14–2. *Hirudo medicinalis,* the medicinal leech. Only one of each pair of nephridia and male structures is shown. *a,* Anus. *b,* Lateral blood vessel. *cg,* Cephalic ganglion. *cs,* Clitellar somites. *di,* Diverticulum of crop. *h,* Head, with eyespots. *mg,* Midgut. *n,* Nephridium. *ov,* Ovary. *p,* Penis. *ph,* Pharynx. *sv,* Seminal vesicle. *t,* Testis. *ut,* Uterus. *vd,* Vas deferens. *vnc,* Ventral nerve cord. *vng,* Ventral nerve ganglion. (× ca. 2.) (From Faust, E.C. 1949. *Human Helminthology,* 3rd ed. Philadelphia, Lea & Febiger, p. 561.)

are deposited soon after fertilization; in other groups the hatched young are carried for some time in a cocoon.

Medical Importance of Leeches (Hirudiniasis)

Since the days of early Greek medicine the "medicinal leech" *(Hirudo medicinalis)* has been employed by physicians to extract blood from patients. It is still dispensed in some pharmacies of Europe and Latin America. Leeches injurious to man include aquatic forms that are responsible for internal and, at times, external hirudiniasis, and terrestrial species that cause external hirudiniasis only.

Internal Hirudiniasis. Small leeches that get into the mouth when people drink from natural streams or bodies of water may reach the pharynx, larynx, epiglottis, and esophagus or may wander into the nasopharynx, become attached, and suck blood. They increase greatly in size and cause congestion and inflammatory swelling of the area, at times producing occlusion of the respective passages. When engorged, they produce pain and tenderness of the affected region. A leech attached to the trachea or a bronchus may produce blockage of the air passage and at times suffocation.

Internal hirudiniasis involving the pharynx and upper respiratory tract has been widely reported from southern Europe, northern Africa, and Asian countries extending from the Mediterranean coast to India and China. In many of these regions the leech is *Limnatis nilotica* (Fig. 14–1A), which is so small as to be hardly noticed in clear water of quiet brooks, pools, ponds, or lakes; but after attachment to mucous membranes and engorgement it may grow and enlarge to reach a length of 8 to 12 cm and a width of 1 to 1.5 cm near the posterior end. Other species of *Limnatis* have similar habits. *Dinobdella ferox* is a common culprit in India, Sri Lanka, Burma, southern China, Thailand, and Formosa. Nasal infestation with *D. ferox* was reported in military personnel in Vietnam and with *Limnatis maculosa* in people in Malaysia and Singapore (Hii et al., 1978).

Internal hirudiniasis may also occur as a result of bathing, swimming, or wading in leech-infested fresh water, with involvement of the vagina, labium majus, or male urethra. Leeches attached to the vaginal mucosa cause severe and prolonged bleeding (Lepage et al., 1981). Following 8 days of vaginal bleeding, a 6-cm engorged leech was removed from the uterus of a 16-year-old victim in India (Prasad and Sinha, 1983).

When a leech is located in the nares or elsewhere internally, the area may be injected with procaine and the intruder removed with a probe. Irrigation with strong saline solution also may assist in removal of the worm.

External Hirudiniasis. Leech infestation of the skin is a relatively common occurrence among people who travel through tropical rain forests. Moreover, it has been reported from the Chilean Andes, Australia, and Micronesia. A considerable number of terrestrial leeches have been incriminated, including the notorious *Haemadipsa zeylanica* of India, Sri Lanka, and Burma. Travelers through leech-infested tropical rain forests are frequently plagued by these worms, which are able to get inside closely woven pants or insinuate themselves into tightly laced, stout, knee-length leather boots.

Although the leech's puncture of the skin is essentially painless, there may be a serous discharge from the wound for some time because of the remaining presence of hirudin at the puncture site. Healing is slow and frequently complicated by invasion of pyogenic organisms. Leeches found attached to the skin should not be pulled off without first applying a few drops of brine or procaine to the worm or touching it with a match flame, after which it can be removed by gentle traction. The wound should then be staunched and covered with an aseptic dressing.

Dimethyl phthalate, and probably other insect repellents, can be used to ward off leeches.

Medicinal leeches have been used to decongest skin flaps after plastic surgery (Henderson *et al.*, 1983). However, a bacterium, *Aeromonas hydrophila,* constantly present in the gut of *H. medicinalis* and thought to be involved in the slow digestion of the leech's blood meal, possibly could be a source of infection (Whitlock *et al.*, 1983). In view of the long and extensive use of leeches without reported complications, the risk of transmitting *Aeromonas* infection from leech to man seems remote (Ross, 1983).

SUMMARY

1. Leeches (class Hirudinea, phylum Annelida) are aquatic or terrestrial, vary in size from a few millimeters to several centimeters in length, are dorsoventrally compressed, and have a sucker at each end of the body. The species of medical importance have three muscular jaws with marginal denticles that produce Y-shaped lacerations for sucking blood. They inject anesthetic and anticoagulant secretions into the lacerated skin.

2. Leeches have a digestive tract capable of storing large amounts of blood that is digested slowly over periods of several months.

3. Aquatic species entering the mouth become attached to the lining of the pharynx or upper respiratory passages and enlarge as they engorge with blood, producing swellings and at times blockage of the respiratory passages; those entering the urethra or vagina cause bleed-ing and discomfort. Terrestrial species resting on vegetation in tropical rain forests attach themselves to the skin of people passing along paths, frequently getting under clothing, where they suck blood and produce relatively painless lacerations. Fully engorged leeches detach themselves spontaneously; burning heat, strong salt solution, or procaine can be used to force detachment.

4. Impregnation of clothing with dimethyl phthalate is usually effective as a repellent of terrestrial leeches.

REFERENCES

Henderson, H.P., Matti, B., Laing, A.G., Morelli, S., and Sully, L. 1983. Avulsion of the scalp treated by microvascular repair: The use of leeches for post-operative decongestion. Br. J. Plastic Surg., *36*:235–239.

Hii, J.L.K., Kan, S.K.P., and Au Yong, K.S. 1978. A record of *Limnatis maculosa* (Blanchard) (Hirudinea: Arynchobdellida) taken from the nasal cavity of man in Sabah, Malaysia. Med. J. Malaysia, *3*:247–248.

Lepage, P., Serufilira, A., and Bossuyt, M. 1981. Severe anaemia due to leech in the vagina. Ann. Trop. Pediatr., 1:189–190.

Prasad, S.B., and Sinha, M.R. 1983. Vaginal bleeding due to leech. Postgraduate Med. J., *59*:272.

Ross, M.R. 1983. The leech: Of dermatologic interest? Arch. Dermatol., *119*:276–277.

Whitlock, M.R., O'Hare, P.M., Sanders, R., and Morrow, N.C. 1983. The medicinal leech and its use in plastic surgery: A possible cause for infection. Br. J. Plastic Surg., *36*:240–244.

Section IV

Arthropods as Agents and Vectors

Chapter 15

Arthropods and Human Disease

J. H. Esslinger

The discipline of medical entomology is of central concern in tropical medicine and parasitology; many arthropods directly affect the health of man through transmission of pathogens or by serving as disease agents themselves. It is with these aspects that the present chapter is concerned. Entomology in a broader sense, of course, is a vast area and includes economic and veterinary entomology, both of which also have a vital impact on man's well-being indirectly through the effects of arthropods on his sources of food and shelter.

The history of medical entomology is colorful and ancient; however, as an identifiable discipline it is only about a century old, with most of the major "breakthrough" discoveries (*e.g.,* understanding of the transmission of malaria and yellow fever) occurring around the turn of the century. A succinct and fascinating account of the development of medical entomology and its landmarks has been published by Service (1978).

Consideration of the arthropods of medical importance in the present text is necessarily brief. For additional information, readers may wish to consult other sources for general medical entomology, such as Harwood and James (1979), Smith (1973), and Beaver *et al.* (1984); for arthropods of dermatologic interest, Parish *et al.* (1983); and for details on venomous arthropods and their effects on man, Bucherl and Buckley (1971) and Bettini (1978).

ARTHROPODS IN GENERAL

Arthropods (phylum Arthropoda) constitute the largest group of related organisms in the Animal Kingdom. They are segmented invertebrates that are bilaterally symmetrical, have an anteroposterior axis, are provided with an exoskeleton, and have paired jointed appendages. In the ancestral arthropod all of the segments (metameres) were distinctly marked off from one another, with a twinned nerve ganglion and a pair of jointed appendages of similar type for each body segment. As evolutionary changes developed, the six anteriormost segments became consolidated into a head portion, and the head appendages became modified into sense organs (antennae) and feeding organs (chelicerae, mandibles, maxillae), while the appendages of other regions were transformed into walking legs, swimming or genital appendages, or completely suppressed on some segments. The general anatomy of an arthropod, represented by an insect, is shown in Fig. 15–1.

Morphology. All arthropods have a *digestive tract* divided into three portions, *viz.* (1) a foregut lined with chitin, divided successively into a mouth cavity, a muscular pharynx, an esophagus, and a proventriculus, for the ingestion and trituration of food; (2) a nonchitinized midgut or "stomach," in which nutriment is digested and from which it is absorbed; and (3) a chitin-lined posterior region or hindgut, including a rectum for the accumulation and elimination of excreta.

The *excretory organs,* present in all but a few arthropods, consist of the malpighian tubules, usually two or more in number, which lie freely in the hemocoel ("body cavity") and open into the hindgut near its junction with the midgut. They serve to collect liquid wastes, which are then discharged into the hindgut.

There is an open *circulatory system* consisting of a dorsally situated pumping organ (heart), aorta, and sometimes paired blood vessels that open into the hemal cavity (hemocoel) which extends into all parts of the body and communicates with the heart. The blood (hemolymph) consists of plasma and

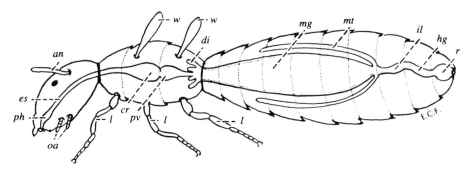

Fig. 15–1. Primitive winged insect, schematic representation, lateral view. *an*, Antenna. *cr*, Crop. *di*, Food diverticulum. *es*, Esophagus. *hg*, Hindgut. *il*, Ileum. *l*, Legs. *mg*, Midgut. *mt*, Malpighian tubule. *oa*, Oral appendages. *ph*, Pharynx. *pr*, Proventriclus. *r*, Rectum. *w*, Wings. (From Beaver, P.C., Jung, R.C., and Cupp, E.W. 1984. *Clinical Parasitology*, 9th ed. Philadelphia, Lea & Febiger, p. 609.)

ameboid white cells; respiratory pigment when present (gill- and book lung-breathing forms) is hemocyanin in the plasma rather than hemoglobin.

The *respiratory system* has been developed into gills for aquatic species and a tracheal system for terrestrial forms. The "book lungs" of scorpions and spiders constitute a special adaptation of gills to a nonaquatic environment.

The *central nervous system* consists of an anterior "brain" composed of dorsal and ventral fused cephalic ganglia connected by circumesophageal commissures to the median ventral paired nerve trunks and to twinned ganglia of each postcephalic body segment. Nerve fibers extend from the central nervous system to all important organs and tissues. In many groups there are light-sensitive organs in the head, either individual eyespots (ocelli) or compound eyes composed of ommatidia.

Arthropods have no trace of a ciliated tegument. The musculature, which is mostly striated, is highly developed in many species, particularly in the organs of locomotion.

Life Cycle. Growth is accompanied by periodic *molting* (shedding) of the entire exoskeleton and the chitinous lining of foregut, hindgut, and tracheae, in the course of which these are replaced by secretion of new and larger components. Molting divides the life cycle, after hatching from the *egg*, into *stages* or *instars*. The young are called *nymphs* when they resemble the adults in appearance and *larvae* when they are markedly different from the adult. The simplest type of cycle (*"without metamorphosis"*) consists of the egg, several nymphal instars resembling the adult except for smaller size and lack of sex organs, and the wingless adult stage (*e.g.*, spiders, lice). Some groups have wingless nymphs and winged adults (*"grad-*

ual metamorphosis," *e.g.*, true bugs), while others undergo a more complex development with several wormlike larval instars, a transitional nonfeeding *pupal stage* in which external and internal reorganization occurs, and the adult, which may or may not have wings (*"complete metamorphosis,"* *e.g.*, flies, fleas). Usually no further growth occurs in the adult stage, which has a narrowly restricted range of size for each species.

Biology of Arthropods. Arthropods were originally aquatic. Groups like the copepods and larger crustaceans have continued to inhabit water and to respire through gills. Many species have become terrestrial, and as a result have developed tracheal respiration. Others, which are aquatic during larval and pupal stages and aerial during adult life, have tracheae for respiration during both immature and sexually mature stages.

Classification of Arthropods. Most species of medical importance belong to one or the other of the following broad groups.

CRUSTACEA. Examples: copepods (*Cyclops* and *Diaptomus*); decapods (crabs and crayfish); pentastomids ("tongue worms"). [Intermediate hosts, parasitic.]

CHILOPODA. Example: centipedes. [Venomous.]

DIPLOPODA. Example: millipedes. [Vesicating.]

ARACHNIDA. Examples: scorpions, spiders, ticks and mites. [Venomous, biologic vectors, parasitic.]

INSECTA. Examples: sucking lice, true bugs, beetles, bees, wasps and ants, moths, flies and gnats, fleas. [Venomous, urticating, biologic and mechanical vectors, intermediate hosts, parasitic.]

ARTHROPODS AND DISEASE

Arthropods may be responsible for disease in man by a number of means. These are briefly categorized here.

Vesication. Discharge of body fluids that cause blisters on the skin or mucous membranes. An example of an arthropod causing vesication is a blister beetle.

Urtication. Nettling from poison "hairs" that come into contact with the skin or mucous membranes, such as may be caused by Io and saddleback caterpillars, among others.

Envenomation. Injection of poisonous fluid into the skin by a specific stinging apparatus or other structure of the arthropod. Examples of such arthropods are scorpions, bees and ants.

Sensitization. Introduction of salivary secretions or other substances into the body that evoke an immunologic response. Examples of causes of sensitization reactions are bites of bloodsucking arthropods (ticks, mosquitoes), allergens from mites inhaled in dust and stings of bees, wasps, or ants. Sensitization may, of course, accompany or follow envenomation.

Tissue Invasion. Invasion of the skin or other organs may be natural or accidental and may be by the adult or one of the immature stages of an arthropod. Examples are penetration of or burrowing in the skin by myiasis-producing flies, the chigoe flea, and the itch mite.

Psychological Disturbance. Inordinate fear of certain arthropods (arachniphobia, entomophobia), or delusional parasitosis. Included here also should be the irritation and restlessness resulting from the persistent crawling, biting, and buzzing of arthropods about or upon one's person.

Transmission of Disease Agents. Arthropods are involved as vectors in the dissemination of etiologic agents from man to man or animal to man.

ARTHROPODS AS VECTORS

The role of arthropods in the transmission of disease agents is generally placed in one of two broad categories: *mechanical transmission* and *biologic transmission*. The former may be considered as merely contaminative or even accidental, whereas the latter is far more complex and represents a great degree of coevolution and interorganismal adaptation on the part of the etiologic agent, the arthropod vector, and the vertebrate host.

Mechanical Transmission. Characteristically, the arthropod as a mechanical vector obtains the pathogen from human (or animal) feces, blood, superficial ulcers, or exudates. The contamination may be solely on the surface of the legs, body, or exposed mouthparts of the arthropod. In many instances, however, the infective substances are ingested and are then voided in vomit drops or in the excreta of the arthropod. In either, the disease agent does not undergo any development or appreciable multiplication within the arthropod, and the process of transmission is simply the transport of organisms from one place to another.

The most common example of such mechanical transmission is seen with the house fly *(Musca domestica)* and similar "filth flies." These insects often feed and sometimes breed in human excreta and are known to transmit some of the enteric pathogens such as *Salmonella typhosa* (and other species of *Salmonella), Shigella dysenteriae, Escherichia coli,* and the cholera organism to human food and drink. This subject is dealt with in detail by Greenberg (1971, 1973). Other flies such as the tiny eye gnats *(Hippelates)* have been involved in epidemics of acute conjunctivitis in the United States. Cockroaches may also serve as mechanical disseminators of enteric organisms, including the cysts of intestinal protozoa such as *Entamoeba histolytica* from human excreta to food.

The role of the many hematophagous (bloodsucking) arthropods in the mechanical transmission of organisms found in the blood is minor. Occasional mention will be made of such instances under discussions of particular groups of arthropods.

Biologic Transmission. In a situation involving biologic transmission, the disease agent must spend a predetermined amount of time (the *"extrinsic incubation period"*) within the vector, during which it either undergoes a series of developmental stages or reproduces, or does both. Only at the end of this obligatory phase of the life cycle within the vector is the disease agent infective to the vertebrate host. The most important arthropod-borne diseases involve biologic transmission; hence, special attention is directed toward this subject. Three types of development within the vector are recognized: propagative, cyclopropagative and cyclodevelopmental. These are readily correlated with the type of etiologic agent.

PROPAGATIVE. Propagative development is an increase in numbers only. This usually implies that a certain minimal number of organisms within the vector must be attained before an infective dose can be introduced into the definitive host. It may also be that subtle biochemical or physiologic changes in the microorganisms must occur before they are infective. Examples: all bacteria, rickettsiae, and viruses.

CYCLOPROPAGATIVE. The cyclopropagative process is both an increase in number and the fulfillment of certain developmental sequences in the life cycle of the agent. Examples: the arthropod-transmitted protozoa such as those causing malaria or trypanosomiasis.

CYCLODEVELOPMENTAL. This refers to passage through essential life-cycle stages, but with no increase in number. Example: the filarial nematodes.

Dynamics of Arthropod-Borne Disease. As implied previously, a successful arthropod-borne disease has a history of an intimate and long-standing association among its three components: the agent, the vector, and the vertebrate host. This interaction has often developed under conditions of relative geographic isolation. Because of this, an arthropod-borne disease of man in a given location in the world may involve particular species, subspecies, or even geographic or biologic strains of the etiologic agent and vector, and their genetic peculiarities are often manifested in ways that directly influence the epidemiology, prevention, and control of the disease. Moreover, several of these diseases are zoonotic, with animals other than man serving as the principal reservoirs, thus adding another parameter to this integrated complex. Although generalizations suffice for the "big picture" of the different arthropod-transmitted diseases, when an actual situation is confronted, the unique nature of each disease "system" must be understood before appropriate and effective measures can be taken against it.

The reasons why a particular arthropod serves as a vector for a given pathogen are manifold and are usually considered from the aspects of (1) *vector competency,* and (2) *vector potential.* The first encompasses those innate or internal conditions and processes of the arthropod that enable it to support the "needs" of the pathogen to the stage where the agent is infective to the vertebrate host. These include the many anatomic and physiologic characteristics that determine susceptibility; examples of such are type of mouthparts, rate of digestion, longevity (the vector must obviously live long enough for the disease agent to complete its development), and size of blood meal. Also included are the largely unknown biochemical and genetic qualities that result in the essential "compatibility" between vector and agent. The second aspect, vector potential (or *vector efficacy*), is concerned with

those factors involved in determining how well a competent vector will serve to transmit the disease. Included here are primarily behavioral characteristics of a given arthropod, such as reproductive rate (usually the more abundant the vectors, the greater the efficacy), host preferences (a vector of a zoonotic disease must feed on both man and the reservoir host), closeness to human habitations, time and frequency of biting, and flight range. Many of these factors can be exploited in devising preventive and control tactics. This subject is discussed further in the context of mosquito-borne diseases in Chapter 16.

SUMMARY

1. Medical entomology as a distinct scientific discipline came into being at the turn of the century, when the role of arthropods in the transmission of certain major diseases (*e.g.,* malaria, yellow fever, filariasis) was elucidated.

2. Arthropods are characterized by bilateral symmetry, true segmentation, an exoskeleton, and paired jointed appendages.

3. Arthropods have a complete digestive tract, an excretory system, an open circulatory system with a hemocoel, a respiratory system consisting of gills, book lungs or tracheae, and a central nervous system; the adults are dioecious.

4. The life cycle of arthropods involves a stepwise growth pattern determined by periodic molting. Metamorphosis in varying degrees accompanies molting. When metamorphosis is absent or gradual, the cycle consists of eggs, nymph and adult; when complete, the cycle consists of egg, larva, pupa, and adult. The larval and nymphal stages may be divided into instars by successive molts.

5. Species of arthropods may be completely aquatic, completely terrestrial, or have sequential aquatic, terrestrial, and aerial phases during the life cycle.

6. Arthropods are responsible for disease in man through vesication, urtication, envenomation, sensitization, tissue invasion, psychologic disturbances, and transmission of disease agents.

7. Disease transmission by arthropod vectors may be mechanical or biologic. In biologic transmission, the most common and significant type, an obligatory "extrinsic incubation period" occurs in the vector before the agent becomes infective. This may involve propagative (bacteria), cyclopropagative (protozoa), or cyclodevelopmental (filarial nematodes) processes.

8. The determination of whether a certain arthropod will serve as a vector for a specific disease agent in a particular geographic area depends upon a complex set of dynamic parameters that are categorized as vector competence (ability of the arthropod to support development of an agent to the infective stage) and vector potential or efficacy (behavioral aspects of a competent arthropod fostering actual transmission of the agent from host to host).

REFERENCES

Beaver, P.C., Jung, R.C., and Cupp, E.W. 1984. *Clinical Parasitology.* 9th ed. Philadelphia, Lea & Febiger.

Bettini, S., ed. 1978. *Arthropod Venoms. (Handbook of Experimental Pharmacology,* n.s., vol. 48). New York, Springer-Verlag.

Bucherl, W., and Buckley, E.E. (eds.). 1971. *Venomous Animals and Their Venoms.* 3. *Venomous Invertebrates.* New York, Academic Press.

Greenberg, B. 1971. *Flies and Disease.* Vol. I. *Ecology, Classification and Biotic Associations.* Princeton, N.J., Princeton University Press.

———— 1973. *Flies and Disease.* Vol. II. *Biology and Disease Transmission.* Princeton, N.J., Princeton University Press.

Harwood, R.F., and James, M.T. 1979. *Entomology in Human and Animal Health.* 7th ed. New York, Macmillan.

Parish, L.C., Nutting, W.B., and Schwartzman, R.M. 1983. *Cutaneous Infestations of Man and Animal.* New York, Praeger.

Service, M.W. 1978. A short history of early medical entomology. J. Med. Entomol., *14*:603–626.

Smith, K.G.V. 1973. *Insects and Other Arthropods of Medical Importance.* London, British Museum (Natural History).

Chapter 16

Insects

J. H. Esslinger

Insects (class Insecta) are the most numerous class of arthropods and constitute about 70% of all known animal species. Both economically and medically, the insects rank as perhaps the most important group in the Animal Kingdom.

General Aspects

Adult Morphology. All adult insects have three pairs of thoracic legs; hence the frequent reference to this class as *"hexapods."* There are three distinct portions of the body, *i.e.,* head, thorax, and abdomen (see Fig. 15–1, p. 202).

The head is developed from six fused segments. The paired appendages are all highly modified from the jointed legs of the primitive arthropod. The anteriormost pair are the *antennae.* The mouthparts consist of an unpaired anterior lip or *labrum,* a pair of *mandibles,* a pair of *maxillae,* and an unpaired posterior lip or *labium.* The maxillae and labium commonly bear sensory *palps.* In the grasshopper, cockroach, and beetle, these mouthparts are adapted for chewing (*mandibulate* mouthparts); in sucking lice, bugs, butterflies, flies, and fleas, they have been transformed in various ways into piercing or nonpiercing structures and form a sucking tube for liquid food (*haustellate* mouthparts).

The thorax contains three segments *(prothorax, mesothorax,* and *metathorax),* each with a pair of walking legs. Most insects also have wings. The full number of wings consists of two pairs, one pair each on the mesothoracic and metathoracic segments, although many of the insects adapted to an ectoparasitic mode of life are secondarily wingless. Flies have retained only the mesothoracic pair.

The abdomen consists of 12 original segments, most of which can be seen on external examination.

Life Cycle. In the ancestral insect the stage

hatched from the egg was essentially adult in character. Some present-day groups, such as the sucking lice, have only an inconspicuous metamorphosis between larva and adult. Others, like the true bugs, have wingless nymphal stages before transformation into the winged adult. In still other groups, *i.e.,* beetles, ants, butterflies, and fleas, the larva is wormlike and has mandibulate mouthparts. In these insects, following the last larval instar there is a pupal period during which a profound reorganization of internal and external structures takes place before the insect emerges as an adult. The pupa does not feed and may be enclosed in a cocoon constructed by the larva. In some of the flies the pupa is retained within the hardened last instar cuticle of the larva; this type of protective case is termed a *puparium.*

The sections that follow consider the various orders of insects of medical importance.

Beetles (Coleoptera)

Adult beetles have chewing mouthparts and two pairs of wings, the first of which is thickened to form a protective covering *(elytra)* over the membranous second when both pairs are at rest over the abdomen.

Small grain beetles serve as intermediate hosts for the tapeworms *Hymenolepis nana* and *H. diminuta* of rodents and man.

Certain beetles are medically important because they are vesicating agents. The most notorious group of the vesicating beetles belongs to the family Meloidae, whose adults produce cantharidin, a substance present in all body tissues but most concentrated in the genitalia. The effective principle is a volatile fluid of pungent odor and weakly acid taste. The most widely known cantharidin-produc-

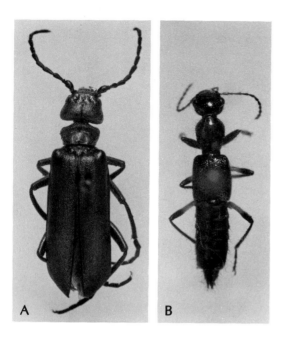

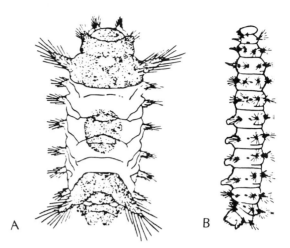

Fig. 16–1. Vesicating beetles. *A, Lytta vesicatoria* ("Spanish fly"). *B, Paederus* sp. (rove beetle). (Photographs by Howard Lyon, Cornell University.) (From Beaver, P.C., Jung, R.C., and Cupp, E.W. 1984. *Clinical Parasitology,* 9th ed. Philadelphia, Lea & Febiger, p. 710.)

Fig. 16–2. Urticating caterpillars. *A,* Saddleback caterpillar *(Sibine stimulea).* (× 3.) *B,* Io moth caterpillar, *Automeris io.* (× 2.) (Adapted from Scott, H.G., and Stojanovich, C.J. 1969. Stinging caterpillars: Pictorial key to some important United States species. In CDC, *Pictorial Keys to Arthropods, Reptiles, Birds and Mammals of Public Health Significance.* Atlanta, Ga., Publ. Health Serv. Publ. No. 1955, p. 96.)

ing species is *Lytta* (syn. *Cantharis*) *vesicatoria* ("Spanish fly"). When this beetle (Fig. 16–1*A*) is accidentally crushed on the skin, an epidermal blister develops in which histaminelike substances can be demonstrated.

A more potent vesicating fluid (not containing cantharidin) is elaborated by adults of certain rove beetles (family Staphylinidae), including species of the cosmopolitan genus *Paederus* (Fig. 16–1*B*). Both types of fluid cause intensely painful blisters on contact with the skin or conjunctiva.

If a vesicating beetle alights on the skin, it is much safer to blow it off than to crush it. Calamine lotion or topical anesthetics applied to the site of the blister partly alleviate the burning pain caused by the vesicating fluid.

Moths and Butterflies (Lepidoptera)

Moths and butterflies are characterized in the adult stage by having two well-developed pairs of wings that, like the body, are covered with minute, flat, often brightly colored scales. The medical significance of these insects lies in the urticating prop-

erties of the larval stages (caterpillars) of some members.

The specialized mechanism for urtication consists of hair- or spinelike cuticular projections formed by the hypodermis and filled with poisonous fluid that is released when the thin tip is broken.

Many species of moths and butterflies throughout the world have larvae capable of urtication. In the United States, the most commonly encountered are the saddleback and Io moth caterpillars (Figs. 16–2*A*, 16–2*B*) and the asp or puss caterpillars (Fig. 16–3*B*).

All larval instars of poisonous species have urticating hairs. Accidental contact with the living caterpillar is the usual manner of exposure, although the poisonous hairs may become incorporated into the cocoon. The sharp poison setae readily penetrate tender skin or in the instance of wind-blown hairs from cocoons, may lodge in the conjunctivae or the nasal or buccal mucosa. Although little is known of the chemical composition of the toxic substances, histamine and several kinds of enzymes, including proteases and hyaluronidases, have been identified (Schmidt, 1982).

Pathogenesis and Symptomatology. The amount of injury and the severity of symptoms in caterpillar urtication depend on the species of caterpillar and its type of poison, the number of hairs that have pierced the body surface, and the age and sensitivity of the victim.

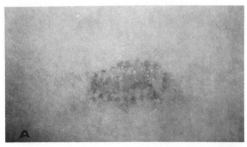

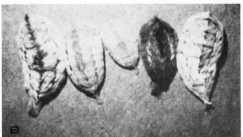

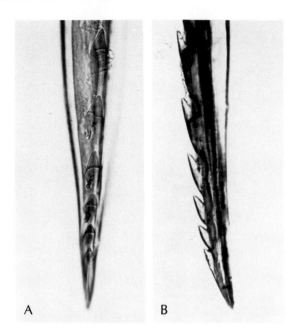

Fig. 16–3. *Megalopyge* sp. (asp or puss caterpillars). *A*, Lesion on thigh of child 48 hours after contact with a puss caterpillar. (× 1.) *B*, Specimens collected in southern Texas, showing variation in size and pigmentation. (× 1.) (Courtesy of Adam Ewert.) (From Beaver, P.C., Jung, R.C., and Cupp, E.W. 1984. *Clinical Parasitology*, 9th ed. Philadelphia, Lea & Febiger, p. 714.)

Fig. 16–4. Sting shaft of a worker honeybee. Six distalmost barbs of left shaft, viewed from lateral *(A)* and dorsal *(B)* sides. (× 300.) (By P.C. Beaver.)

At the time the poison is introduced, there is a local burning, stinging sensation. The affected area becomes erythematous and then elevated and whitish, with a reddish border extending radially as much as 2.5 cm and a peripheral reddish macular zone 2.0 cm beyond. Occasionally, urticarial wheals may develop over the entire body, accompanied by systemic manifestations suggesting a neurotoxic syndrome. A typical reaction to the puss caterpillar is seen in Fig. 16–3*A*.

Treatment. There is no satisfactory treatment other than topical application of calamine lotion or corticosteroid ointments. Usually there is no ulceration, and the reaction subsides in a few hours. Occasionally the lesion may heal slowly, like a chemical burn.

Bees, Wasps, and Ants (Hymenoptera)

The hymenopteran insects have two pairs of membranous wings, a distinct constriction (pedicel) between the thorax and abdomen, and mouthparts adapted to sucking or lapping (bees) or for lancing and chewing (ants). Metamorphosis in this group is complete. These insects are known for the trauma caused to man through envenomation. Less often mentioned are the deaths and injuries resulting from drivers who panic when a bee or wasp flies into a moving vehicle.

Sting Apparatus. In the worker honeybee (a modified female), the ovipositor at the caudal extremity is transformed into a sting apparatus (Fig. 16–4). The envenomating mechanism consists of a pair of tubular acid glands, the contents of which are conducted through a long duct to a venom receptacle (a single alkaline gland that opens at the base of the sting cavity), a strong chitinous bulb below the venom receptacle, and the chitinized sting apparatus. The puncture is made by the sting shaft, and then the poison secretion is injected into the wound. All species of hornets and wasps, most bees, and some ants have an efficient sting mechanism and potent venom.

Envenomation. The workers of the honeybee and of some wasps leave the posterior tip of their abdomen, including the entire sting mechanism, at the site of penetration in the victim's skin. Muscle attachments continue to contract for some time, forcing the sting shaft more deeply into the wound and releasing additional venom. These individuals are unable to sting again, having eviscerated themselves in the process. Bumblebees and many wasps retain their sting and may inflict repeated wounds.

The active venom fraction in general resembles viperine snake venom; it is present in the acid gland secretion. These venomous substances are complex mixtures of enzymes, polypeptides, and various smaller molecules (histamine, 5-hydroxytryptamine) that may be pharmacologically active or neurotoxic (O'Connor and Peck, 1978; Edery *et al.,* 1978). Hyaluronidase is also commonly present.

Pathogenesis and Symptomatology. In some people the sting of bees or wasps produces only a temporary local swelling with moderate pain that disappears in a few hours. In others, the entire member becomes swollen and systemic reactions of a considerable or even profound nature develop. Such individuals may require desensitization, since subsequent envenomation can have a rapid, fatal outcome owing to an *anaphylactic* reaction.

Ants. Many of the common ants are capable of inflicting painful bites; the secretions introduced into the skin by the sharp, strong mandibles contain formic acid. The reaction is usually transient, and the topical application of baking soda or anesthetics is sufficient to bring relief. Other ants, however, may additionally have a stinging mechanism. Ants that produce particularly painful wounds are the large aggressive species found in the tropics, such as the tucandeira *(Paraponera clavata)* of South America, which at times literally sting their victims to death. The harvester ants *(Pogonomyrmex* spp.) found in the United States and other parts of the Western Hemisphere are likewise capable of a vicious sting. The small "fire ants" *(Solenopsis invicta* and *Solenopsis richteri),* introduced into the United States from South America early in this century, have become an increasingly serious problem in the Southeast. These ants are aggressive stingers; because their nests (mounds) contain many thousands of individuals, multiple stings are common and infants who fall on the mounds are at particular risk. The venom is strongly hemolytic and produces a vesicle or pustule at the site of the skin puncture. In some people envenomation may result in a systemic reaction of an allergic type and desensitization may be necessary.

Treatment. The honeybee sting is extracted by use of a sharp needle or knife blade. Local injection of an antihistaminic drug will ease the pain resulting from the accumulation of histaminelike substances at the wound site. In cases of anaphylactic reaction, epinephrine, or preferably ethylnorepinephrine, should be administered hypodermically as promptly as possible. Application of 10% household ammonia to the injured site will often ease the throbbing pain. Ice packs and palliative lotions applied topically to sites of bumblebee, wasp, and hornet envenomation may be helpful in reducing the swelling and relieving the pain.

Control. Accidental sting by bees, wasps, and hornets is sometimes unavoidable. However, sensitized persons should reduce exposure by wearing protective clothing, gloves, and nets for the face and neck when they approach swarms or active hives. Hypersensitized individuals should receive desensitizing treatment carried out with specific venom extract. Domestic wasps and fire ants may be controlled through the use of a variety of insecticides (malathion and dichlorvos for wasps; diazinon for fire ants).

Sucking Lice (Anoplura)

Morphology. Lice are small but macroscopic, wingless, dorsoventrally flattened insects that have 3- to 5-jointed short antennae and three pairs of conspicuous legs, each ending in a sharp, curved claw used for clinging to hairs or fibers. The lice, restricted to an ectoparasitic life on mammals, are hematophagous and have mouthparts adapted for piercing and sucking. A bundle of stylets *(haustellum* or *fascicle)* lies within the head and is extruded only during the act of feeding.

The three types of lice that infest man are the *head louse (Pediculus humanus capitis),* the *body louse (P. h. humanus),* and the *pubic louse (Phthirus pubis).* Although the head and body lice are morphologically identical (Fig. 16–5), the pubic louse (Fig. 16–6) is readily distinguishable from these two, and its broad, robust body with the enlarged claws on the posterior two pairs of legs have led to its common name of the "crab" louse.

Life Cycle and Bionomics. The female begins to oviposit in a day or two after she has matured and been inseminated. Head lice characteristically cement their eggs to the hair of the head or back of the neck; body lice to fibers of body clothing; and pubic lice to hairs of the pubic region, chest, axilla, eyebrows, and eyelashes. These eggs (Fig. 16–7), the so-called "nits," hatch in 4 to 14 days at body temperature, with emergence of a nymphal stage that feeds and molts three times before becoming an adult 12 to 28 days after oviposition. Adults live for about 30 days, during which time each female produces 5 to 10 eggs daily.

Lice are host-specific, and the three found on man are exclusively human parasites. Their nymphs and adults depend on man for food and

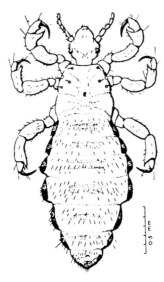

Fig. 16–5. Body louse *(Pediculus humanus)*, male, dorsal view. (Adapted from Buxton, P.A. 1939. *The Louse*. London, Edward Arnold and Co., p. 6.)

warmth but actively transfer from one person to another. Body lice engorge at frequent intervals, discharging relatively large pellets of dark red excrement as they feed.

Lice are readily transmitted from person to person, especially under circumstances leading to crowding and poor personal hygiene. Head lice are more commonly found on individuals with long hair, and outbreaks among elementary school children are now frequent in the United States. Body

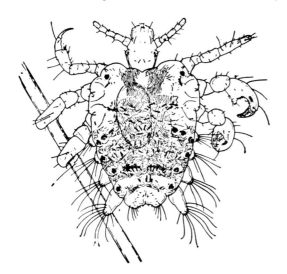

Fig. 16–6. Pubic louse *(Phthirus pubis)*. Adult female attached to hair, dorsal view. (Adapted by E.C. Faust from Martini, E. 1923. *Textbook of Medical Entomology*. Stuttgart, Gustav Fischer.) Reproduced in Beaver, P.C., Jung, R.C., and Cupp, E.W. 1984. *Clinical Parasitology*, 9th ed. Philadelphia, Lea & Febiger, p. 613.)

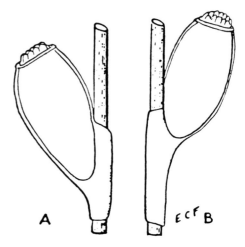

Fig. 16–7. Eggs of human lice. *A, Pediculus humanus capitus. B, Phthirus pubis*. Greatly enlarged. (Adapted by E.C. Faust. *A,* From Patton, W.S., and Evans, A.M. 1929. *Insects, Ticks, Mites and Venomous Animals*. London, H. Grubb Ltd. *B,* From Matheson, R. 1932. *Medical Entomology*. Springfield, Ill., Charles C Thomas. Reproduced in Beaver, P.C., Jung, R.C., and Cupp, E.W. 1984. *Clinical Parasitology*, 9th ed. Philadelphia, Lea & Febiger, p. 613.)

lice are usually found in temperate to cold regions where heavy clothing is worn for long periods of time. Except when feeding, these lice reside among the fibers of the clothing rather than upon the body itself. Pubic lice are more intimately associated with the host and tend to remain attached to the body hair, particularly that of the pubic area. Although pubic lice are usually acquired through sexual contact, fomites may also be involved in their dispersion.

Pediculosis. Louse infestation is known as pediculosis. The local lesion produced by lice develops at any site on the body where nymphs or adults feed. Saliva introduced by the louse into the puncture wound results in the development of a roseate elevated papule, accompanied by intense pruritus. Involuntary scratching of the lesion causes an eczematous dermatitis, striated scarring from use of the fingernails, and at times induration and bronzing of the area. Topical application of soothing lotions relieves the pruritus and allows the lesions to heal.

Disease Transmission. Only the body louse *(Pediculus h. humanus)* is involved in the transmission of diseases, and the most important of these is *epidemic (or louse-borne) typhus*.

EPIDEMIC TYPHUS. This disease has a cosmopolitan distribution, and its impact has been seen throughout history. Although its prevalence is now irregular, it still occurs in areas where crowding, poor sanitation, and malnutrition exist, including Central and South America, Africa, Asia, and Europe, and it is usually encountered during the winter when heavy clothing is worn for extended periods of time.

The etiologic agent of epidemic typhus is *Rickettsia prowazekii*. The rickettsiae, which are present in the blood of the patient, are ingested by the louse and enter the gut epithelium of the vector, where they multiply intracellularly. The organisms are shed in the *feces* of the louse and man becomes infected by *crushing* the louse on the skin or by contaminating the lesion with its dejecta. The rickettsiae are capable of surviving in dried louse feces contaminating clothing, and this may provide another source of infection for man through contact or inhalation. Lice have a narrow range of temperature that is tolerated, so when a patient is feverish or dead, the lice readily move to an optimally warm host. The transmission of epidemic typhus is strictly from man to man, since lice are extremely host-specific.

Epidemic typhus is an acute, exanthematous, febrile disease which, if not treated, may often result in the death of the patient in about 2 weeks. Treatment with antibiotics (tetracycline or chloramphenicol) is usually effective.

EPIDEMIC RELAPSING FEVER. Body lice may on occasion transmit *relapsing fever* (a spirochetal disease) from man to man in *epidemic* form. In recent years this disease has been a serious problem in some areas of Africa.

Control. For persons infested with head or pubic lice, shampoo or ointment containing 1% lindane (gamma HCH) rubbed into the parasitized area is a practical, specific measure. For body lice, dusting of the body and clothing with insecticidal powder is used. Although DDT has been effective, worldwide resistance of lice to this substance has led to the alternative use of dusts containing 1% malathion, lindane, or permethrin. Infested clothing or bedding can be fumigated with ethyl formate (Busvine, 1980).

True Bugs (Hemiptera)

Adult Morphology. Members of this order of insects typically have two pairs of wings, the anterior pair of which are thickened basally and membranous distally, while the posterior ones are entirely membranous. Bedbugs have only wing pads that never develop into functional organs. The most conspicuous external feature of true bugs is the

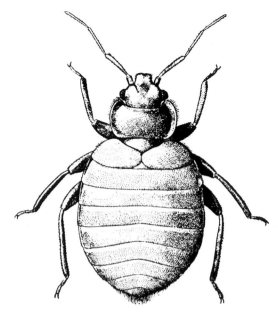

Fig. 16–8. Bedbug, *Cimex lectularius*. Adult female, dorsal view. (× 10.) (Adapted from M.E. MacGregor. In Byam, W., and Archibald, R.G. 1921–1923. *Practice of Medicine in the Tropics.* New York, Oxford University Press. Reproduced in Beaver, P.C., Jung, R.C., and Cupp, E.W. 1984. *Clinical Parasitology,* 9th ed. Philadelphia, Lea & Febiger, p. 621.)

hinged proboscis, which lies under the head and thorax when at rest but is directed ventrally at right angles to the body when engaged in piercing and sucking.

Life Cycle and Bionomics. Metamorphosis is gradual. Following hatching of the eggs there are five nymphal instars, followed by the sexually mature male or female, which typically has wings that develop from external buds visible on the later nymphs.

In *bedbugs* (family Cimicidae), the adults and immature stages hide in the dark cracks and crevices in human habitations during the daytime and come out to suck blood from their victims at night. Each female lays about 100 to 500 glutinous eggs in batches over a period of several weeks. The female requires 4 to 12 minutes to become engorged. The two bedbugs that commonly attack man are *Cimex lectularius* (temperate zone) and *C. hemipterus* (tropical). The former is more urban, the latter more rural. Both species are shiny, mahogany brown in color, and have a body about 5 mm long and 3 mm broad, flattened dorsoventrally; they lack wings, are covered with many hairlike spines, and have conspicuous compound eyes (Fig. 16–8).

The *kissing-bugs* or *cone-nosed bugs* (family Re-

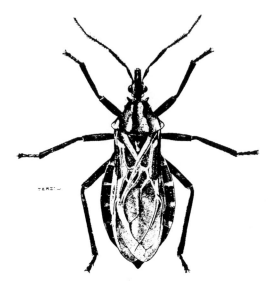

Fig. 16–9. Kissing-bug, *Panstrongylus megistus*. Female, dorsal view. (× 2.) (From Castellani, A., and Chalmers, A.J. 1919. Manual of Tropical Medicine. London, Ballière, Tindall, and Cox, p. 769.)

duviidae; subfamily Triatominae) are more elongated, considerably larger than the bedbugs (Fig. 16–9A) and have conspicuous, well-developed wings. Seen from the lateral view, the head is more or less conical and is provided with a prominent 3-segmented proboscis (Fig. 16–9). Kissing-bugs that are medically important reside in warm regions. Some species, such as *Triatoma infestans, Panstrongylus megistus,* and *Rhodnius prolixus* of South America, are primarily domestic in their habits and lay their nonglutinous eggs in cracks and crevices of poorly constructed adobe and thatched houses, from which the active stages emerge to feed on sleeping victims. *Triatoma* spp. are associated with the nests or dens of wild mammals and are found in some areas of the United States.

Bedbug and Kissing-Bug Bite. All these species are avid blood suckers. Bedbugs are usually more annoying than injurious, but in some persons their bites are responsible for a swollen, inflamed, cutaneous lesion with an indurated area at the site of each puncture, occasionally accompanied by systemic sensitization. Many of the kissing-bugs expertly puncture the skin and almost painlessly withdraw blood from the victim. The common location of their bites is the face, particularly on the lips and outer angle of the eyes. Topical application of soothing lotions, ointments, or antihistaminic drugs relieves the dermatitis. Anaphylactic reactions to triatomine bites have been reported (Edwards and Lynch, 1984).

Disease Transmission. In spite of their ubiquity and intimate association with man, bedbugs are not known to transmit any diseases. The triatomine bugs serve as the vectors of *Trypanosoma cruzi;* this is discussed in Chapter 3, page 31.

Control. Once bedbugs have invaded and established themselves in a domicile, eradication is difficult. Fumigation with aerosols of pyrethroids or dichlorvos may be useful, but the application of residual insecticides such as malathion, propoxur, or the organochlorines is probably necessary (Busvine, 1980). In areas where kissing-bugs are present, the application of appropriate insecticides within the dwelling will aid in preventing the residents from being bitten. The complete control or elimination of these insects is rarely practicable, however, since it is the type of housing (adobe, thatched huts) that promotes the establishment of the kissing-bugs in the first place.

Flies (Diptera)

Morphology and Taxonomy. The flies constitute a large and diverse group of insects that includes several families with species of medical importance. Adult flies typically have a single pair of wings that arise from the 2nd thoracic segment; a pair of club-shaped "balancing organs" *(halteres)* on the 3rd thoracic segment replaces the second pair of wings. Adult dipterans have *haustellate* mouthparts; some are adapted for piercing (as with the hematophagous mosquitoes) and others for lapping (as with house flies). Hematophagous diptera are of two basic types: the *capillary feeders (solenophages)* such as mosquitoes, in which the mouthparts are inserted into the skin and blood is withdrawn directly from the lumen of a small vessel; and the *"pool" feeders (telmophages)* such as the black flies, in which the mouthparts are much shorter and are used to lacerate the skin, forming a superficial lesion into which blood and tissue fluids flow and are then ingested by the fly. Flies undergo complete metamorphosis. Most are oviparous but some deposit larvae. There are three or more larval instars followed by a pupal stage, with the eventual emergence of the adult. The larvae are *mandibulate* and the pupal stage is a nonfeeding transitional stage, which may be motile (mosquitoes) or not (house fly).

Taxonomically the Diptera consist of three suborders: the Nematocera, which includes the mosquitoes, "sand" flies, "punkies," and black flies; the Brachycera, containing the horse flies and

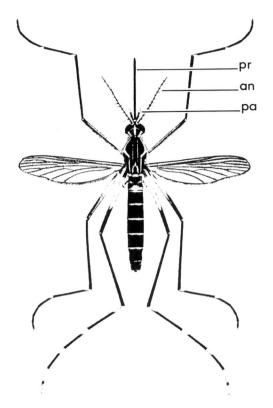

Fig. 16–10. *Aedes (Stegomyia) aegypti.* Adult female. *an,* Antenna. *pa,* Palp. *pr,* Proboscis. (Adapted from Carpenter, S.J., and LaCasse, W.J. 1955. *Mosquitoes of North America.* Berkeley, University of California Press, plate 98.)

deer flies; and the Cyclorrhapha, to which belong the house flies and their relatives, the tsetses, and a number of families that are involved in myiasis.

Flies As Sensitizing Agents. All flies that puncture human skin to suck blood introduce droplets of salivary secretions containing a mixture of digestive enzymes, anticoagulants, and other substances, and the longer the fly probes or feeds, the more secretions enter the skin. This usually produces a local reaction (pruritus, erythema) that lasts from a few hours to a few days. The severity of the reaction varies with the species of the fly as well as the degree of hypersensitivity of the host. In some people an intense allergic response more generalized in nature may result. The treatment of local reactions is symptomatic, and a number of effective proprietary ointments and lotions are available.

Mosquitoes (Culicidae)

Morphology and Taxonomy. Mosquitoes are slender, long-legged, delicate flies that have a cosmopolitan distribution and number several thou-

sand species. Several major subgroups of mosquitoes are known, but those of medical concern are, for the greater part, the anophelines (with the genus *Anopheles*) and the culicines, to which the genera *Culex, Aedes, Mansonia,* and *Culiseta* belong. Excellent sources for the identification of the mosquitoes of the continental United States and Canada are the works by Darsie and Ward (1981) and Carpenter and LaCasse (1955). All mosquitoes are characterized by the presence of minute scales on the body and appendages; the colors and distribution of these scales provide useful features for the identification of species. Morphologic features of mosquitoes are shown in Figs. 16–10 to 16–13. The antennae are long, multisegmented, and have whorls of hairs at the nodes; males appear to have very bushy antennae, while the antennal hairs of females are sparse. The mouthparts are assembled into a long proboscis in both sexes, but only the females are capable of piercing the skin; males are not hematophagous but rather feed on plant juices. The maxillary palps are much shorter than the proboscis on female culicine mosquitoes; these structures are long in anopheline females and in all males, but there are conspicuous distal swellings on the palps of anopheline males. The different resting positions of anophelines and culicines, as shown in Fig. 16–12, are characteristic. Mosquito larvae *("wigglers")* are readily separated into the two subgroups by their appearance in water (Fig. 16–13A,B). Anopheline larvae lie parallel to the surface, being suspended by *palmate hairs* (Fig. 16–13C) on the dorsal part of the abdomen; culicine larvae hang downward, with a specialized air tube *(siphon)* at the posterior end providing support at the water surface.

Life Cycle and Bionomics. Egg production and egg-laying are typically dependent on a previous blood meal. Females oviposit on the water surface or on moist areas adjacent to water that are subject to inundation when it rains. Although most mosquitoes breed in fresh water, some are adapted to brackish habitats. The larvae feed on plankton and organic matter, and after 10 to 14 days the 4th instar larvae pupate. Mosquito pupae *("tumblers,"* Fig. 16–13D) are active in the water, although they do not feed. In a few days they become quiescent at the surface, and the adult emerges. The longevity of the adult mosquito is variable but is usually measurable in terms of only a few weeks.

Certain behavioral tendencies of the adult females, characteristic of a given species, are of ut-

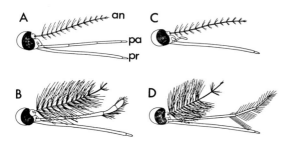

Fig. 16–11. Head and appendages of mosquitoes. *A*, Female *Anopheles*. *B*, Male *Anopheles*. *C*, Female culicine. *D*, Male culicine. *an*, Antenna. *pa*, Palp. *pr*, Proboscis. (Adapted from Carpenter, S.J., and LaCasse, W.J. 1955. *Mosquitoes of North America*. Berkeley, University of California Press, p. 9.)

most importance with respect to their potential as vectors of specific diseases. In general terms, these include the following: (1) host preference (narrow or broad) and whether they readily feed on man *(anthropophilic)* or animals *(zoophilic)*; (2) whether they are closely associated with man *(domestic)*; (3) whether they enter dwellings to feed *(endophilic)* or will bite only outdoors *(exophilic)*; and (4) whether they feed at night *(nocturnal)*, during the day *(diurnal)*, or at dawn and dusk only *(crepuscular)*.

Mosquito Bite and Sensitization. The notoriety achieved by the mosquitoes as pests is well deserved. The economic impact of their biting habits alone may be considerable in areas where outdoor activity or tourism is significant. The general aspects of mosquito bites are covered earlier in the section on flies as sensitizing agents.

Disease Transmission. As a group, mosquitoes are responsible for the transmission of a number of diseases of global significance. *Malaria* is indisputably the most important of these. The role of *Anopheles* spp. as the vectors of *Plasmodium* is discussed in Chapter 6, page 60. Certain types of *filariasis* are transmitted to man by mosquitoes. Although a number of genera and species are involved in different areas, the most commonly encountered vector of *Wuchereria bancrofti* is the cosmopolitan, highly domesticated, nocturnal-feeding *Culex quinquefasciatus*. *Brugia malayi*, which is restricted to southeast Asia and certain areas of the Pacific, is often transmitted by species of *Mansonia*.

The remaining major diseases transmitted by mosquitoes are *viral* in etiology and consist of *yellow fever, dengue,* and certain types of *encephalitis*. The classification and nomenclature of arboviruses have recently been reviewed by Matthews (1982).

Fig. 16–12. Resting positions of mosquitoes. *A* and *B*, *Anopheles*. *C*, Culicine. (Adapted from King, W.V., Bradley, G.H., Smith, C.N., and McDuffie, W.C. 1960. *A Handbook of the Mosquitoes of the Southeastern United States*, Agriculture Handbook No. 173. Washington, D.C., Agricultural Research Service, U.S.D.A., p. 86.)

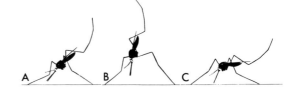

Fig. 16–13. Immature stages of mosquitoes. *A, Anopheles* larva in characteristic position parallel to surface of water. *B,* Culicine larva suspended from surface of water by siphon. *C,* Palmate hair on dorsal surface of *Anopheles* larva (greatly magnified). *D,* Generalized pupa of mosquito. (*A* and *B,* Adapted from King, W.V., Bradley, G.H., Smith, C.N., and McDuffie, W.C. 1960. *A Handbook of the Mosquitoes of the Southeastern United States,* Agriculture Handbook No. 173. Washington, D.C. Agricultural Research Service, U.S.D.A., p. 58. *C,* Adapted from Darsie, R.F., Jr., and Ward, R.A. 1981. *Identification and Geographic Distribution of the Mosquitoes of North America North of Mexico.* Fresno, California, American Mosquito Control Association p. 122. *D,* Adapted from Carpenter, S.J., and LaCasse, W.J. 1955. *Mosquitoes of North America.* Berkeley, University of California Press, p. 16.)

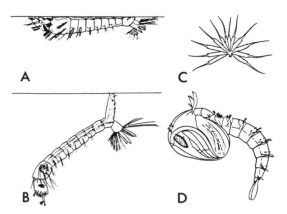

YELLOW FEVER

The yellow fever virus (YF virus) belongs to the genus *Flavivirus* in the family Togaviridae and is viscerotropic, producing an acute, febrile, and often fatal disease. Yellow fever is a disease of moist tropical climates and is found primarily in Africa and in Central and South America (Fig. 16–14). Epidemiologically, yellow fever is considered to exist in two states: *urban* yellow fever, which may be epidemic in form and is centered in concentrations of human habitations, and *sylvan* (or "jungle") yellow fever, which is maintained in areas of forest in an enzootic form, with monkeys serving as the primary vertebrate hosts.

Sylvan yellow fever involves several mosquito hosts, but most commonly the canopy (tree-top) dwelling *Haemagogus* spp. in the Western Hemisphere and comparable species of zoophilic *Aedes* in Africa. In the Americas when man, through his activities, encroaches upon the enzootic areas, he may become infected by *Haemagogus* and will take the virus back home with him. A similar pattern may occur in Africa as well, but more important is the practice of bands of monkeys moving into or adjacent to villages to feed on crops. Under these circumstances, the principal vector is considered to be *Aedes simpsoni,* which is semidomesticated and feeds on both man and monkeys.

Urban yellow fever in both hemispheres is transmitted from man to man by the very common, highly domesticated *Aedes (Stegomyia) aegypti* (Fig. 16–10), assisted in Africa by A. *simpsoni.* This mosquito has a nearly worldwide distribution and lives in very close association with man. *Aedes aegypti* is extremely well adapted to urban conditions and readily breeds in man's artifacts and refuse—notably his discarded containers such as cartons, cooking pots, tin cans, old tires, and others that collect rain water. Catch basins, water barrels, and flower vases likewise provide breeding sites for this species.

Thus, yellow fever may exist quietly in the forest, but when man or monkey brings it to human habitations, the more epidemic type of man-*Aedes aegypti*-man cycle is initiated. The common occurrence of *Aedes aegypti* in many parts of the world (including the United States) where yellow fever does not currently exist presents a very real threat that the virus may be introduced.

Although it has been thought that yellow fever was entirely dependent upon monkeys or man serving as the reservoirs, recent evidence suggests that

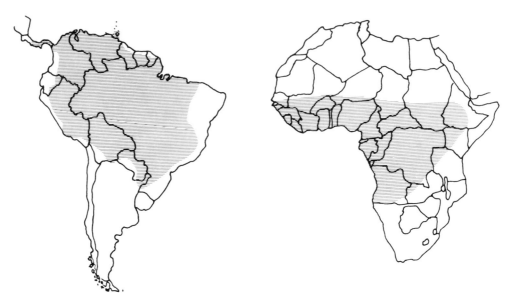

Fig. 16–14. Yellow fever endemic zones in America and Africa, based on cases reported to the World Health Organization, 1965–1980. (Adapted from CDC, 1984 Yellow fever vaccine, Morbidity and Mortality Weekly Reports, *32*:679–682, 687–688.)

the mosquitoes *(Haemagogus, Aedes aegypti)* themselves, which become infected for life, may maintain the virus through *transovarial transmission* (Beaty *et al.*, 1980; Dutary and LeDuc, 1981). This is a process in which the viruses (or other agent) infect the ovaries of the female vector, become incorporated into the eggs, and are thus passed on to the next generation. Although transovarial transmission does not proceed *ad infinitum,* it greatly enhances the efficacy of the vector when the usual vertebrate reservoirs are present in low numbers or even absent.

For people living in or particularly traveling to areas in which yellow fever is endemic, immunization with chick embryo live attenuated 17 DYF virus vaccine is recommended (CDC, 1984).

DENGUE

Another *Flavivirus* of considerable significance is that which produces dengue in man. The disease is characterized by fever and debilitating pain, particularly of the muscles, joints, and behind the eyeballs. The term "break-bone fever" is aptly used in describing this disease. Although the mortality rate from classic dengue is quite low, the manifestation of *dengue hemorrhagic fever* (DHF) and its frequently associated shock syndrome has a death rate of 10% to 50%. Dengue is cosmopolitan in the tropics; DHF is more common in Asia than in the Western Hemisphere.

Epidemiologically, dengue shows many simi-

larities to yellow fever, but the role of vertebrate reservoir hosts (monkeys) appears to be relatively unimportant. Most transmission is from man to man, with *Aedes aegypti* being the principal vector. As with yellow fever, the dengue virus has been shown to be transovarially transmitted in *A. aegypti* (Tesh, 1980). Since dengue at present is hyperendemic in the Caribbean and along the northern coast of South America, its potential for establishment within the United States is high.

ENCEPHALITIS

A growing number of mosquito-borne viral encephalitides have been described in recent decades throughout the world. These are zoonoses in nature, usually maintained enzootically in birds, and occasionally transmitted to man and other mammals. Most of these viruses are neurotropic and produce a mild febrile disease. In some instances, however, there may be serious central nervous system involvement with disabling sequelae. Strain differences play a major role in the specific manifestations and degree of pathogenicity in these infections.

Some of the more important mosquito-borne viral encephalitis types, their distribution, and principal vectors are

1. Western equine encephalomyelitis (WEE): Western Hemisphere (including U.S.); *Culex tarsalis* and others.
2. Eastern equine encephalomyelitis (EEE):

Western Hemisphere (including U.S.); *Culiseta melanura* and others.

3. Venezuelan equine encephalomyelitis (VEE): Western Hemisphere (including U.S.); *Culex* spp., *Aedes* spp., and others.

4. St. Louis encephalitis (SLE): Western Hemisphere (including U.S.); *Culex quinquefasciatus* and others.

5. Japanese encephalitis (JE): Asia and Indian subcontinent; *Culex* spp. and others.

Mosquito Control. A broad spectrum of methods for controlling mosquitoes exists, and those selected for use in a given instance depend upon a number of requirements and restraints, not the least of which is economic feasibility. The goal of any attempt at control (*e.g.,* reduce annoyance vs. eliminate disease) must be clearly defined.

Occasional mosquitoes entering houses may be dealt with successfully by using screens on windows and doors and applying a common aerosol space spray. The topical application of one of the many available insect repellents is useful to the individual undertaking outdoor activities. Temporary invasion of urban or suburban neighborhoods by large populations of pest mosquitoes (such as *Aedes sollicitans,* the salt marsh mosquito) can be alleviated through the application of insecticidal fogs or mists.

If, however, the goal is the eradication or more realistically the control or reduction of an endemic mosquito-transmitted disease such as malaria, yellow fever, or filariasis, the means employed must be more selective and thorough. To this end the cycle of transmission must be broken and the responsible vector significantly reduced in numbers, if not eliminated. The objective in the use of *residual insecticides* (DDT and others) is to break the transmission cycle. Insecticides with persisting activity are applied to the interior walls of a dwelling. Those mosquitoes that feed on an infected person usually rest on the nearby walls, and hence they are selectively killed before they become infective.

The control of vectors involves measures directed toward the larval stages as well as the adults. Before effective control efforts can be initiated, the *identity* of the specific vector (or vectors) for the particular disease in the area concerned, its *behavior* (*e.g.,* feeding, resting, flight range), and its specific *breeding sites* (*i.e.,* where the larvae develop) must be known. Current programs usually employ an *integrated approach* involving such procedures as *source reduction* (destroying larval breeding sites by swamp drainage, landfills) and the application of appropriate formulations of insecticides both as larvicides and adulticides, selecting substances to which the *local strains are not resistant.*

In recent years *biologic control* has received special attention, although many of these approaches are still in the investigative stage and not yet in widespread use. These measures include the application of specific *insect pathogens* (bacteria, viruses, nematodes) to breeding sites, *genetic manipulation* of vector populations to make them unsusceptible to the disease agent, *release of sterile males* to foster population decline, the introduction of certain other nonvector species *(competitive displacement),* and the introduction of natural enemies such as *Gambusia* (mosquito fish; a long-recognized practice) and the large nonhematophagous mosquito *Toxorhynchites,* whose larvae are predacious (a relatively new approach).

Sand Flies (Psychodidae)

Morphology and Bionomics. Bloodsucking members of the Psychodidae belong to the genera *Phlebotomus* (Old World) and *Lutzomyia* (New World) and have widespread distribution in warm and temperate climates. The adults (Fig. 16–15) are small, delicate, and light in color, with conspicuous black compound eyes and a pair of long filiform antennae. These flies have long, narrowly obovate wings that form a V-shape outline above the thorax when at rest, long straggling legs, and many fine hairs on the body, wings, and legs. Sand flies progress by short hopping flights and ordinarily are not found more than 5 meters above the ground or far from their breeding sites. Only the females are hematophagous. Sand flies feed at night and hide in dark places in the daytime.

Life Cycle. Eggs are laid in batches in moist dark sites, such as under decaying leaves on the ground, in damp mossy places, in rank vegetation, or in hollow tree trunks. The four larval instars feed on organic debris in the moist soil or mud but are not strictly aquatic. After pupation the adults emerge, with the entire cycle taking a little over a month.

Sand Fly Sensitization. The bite of a female sand fly, which is telmophagous, often produces a local, frequently indurated inflammation, at times with a wheal 1 to 2 cm in diameter. This is accompanied by a needling pain, which may be followed

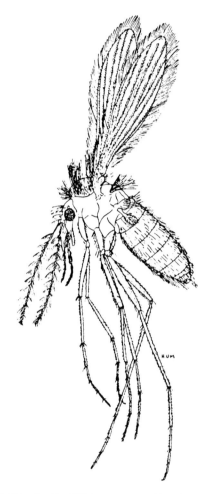

Fig. 16–15. Sandfly (*Phlebotomus* sp.). Female. (× ca. 16.) (From Monnig, H.O. 1950. *Veterinary Helminthology and Entomology*, 3rd ed. Baltimore, Williams & Wilkins, p. 301.)

by an irritating local pruritus lasting hours or weeks. Some people develop a severe allergic reaction, with swelling of the bitten member, fever, nausea, and general malaise. Topical application of phenolated camphor in mineral oil or anesthetic ointment usually alleviates the local pruritus, and residual spraying of insecticides around doors and windows kills flies entering houses.

Disease Transmission. The principal significance of the sand flies is in their transmission of the leishmaniases. This subject is discussed in Chapter 3, pages 17 to 26. Two other sand fly–transmitted diseases, sand fly fever and bartonellosis, are worthy of note.

Sand fly fever (also known as phlebotomus fever and pappataci fever) is endemic in the Mediterranean, Middle East, and portions of southern U.S.S.R. It is viral in etiology and is known only

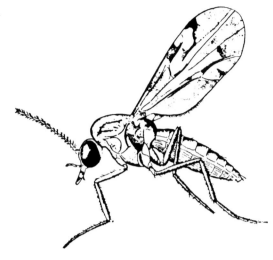

Fig. 16–16. *Culicoides* sp. Female. (From Harwood, R.F., and James, M.T. 1979. *Entomology in Human and Animal Health*, 7th ed. New York, Macmillan, p. 160.)

in man; the virus is transovarially transmitted and the flies themselves serve as reservoirs. This disease is seasonal and may occur in epidemic form following the emergence of new broods after the summer rains. The most important vector is *Phlebotomus papatasi*.

The second disease, *bartonellosis,* is also called *Carrión's disease, Oroya fever,* or *verruga peruana*. This sometimes fatal disease is characterized by a painful, acute hemolytic febrile stage followed by warty cutaneous eruptions. The etiologic agent is the pleomorphic organism *Bartonella bacilliformis*. This disease is found only in the high valleys of the Andean region in South America and is usually transmitted by *Lutzomyia verrucarum*.

Biting Midges (Ceratopogonidae)

Morphology and Bionomics. The ceratopogonid midges are tiny (about 1 mm) dark flies also known as *punkies, no-see-ums, biting gnats,* and *culicoids* (Fig. 16–16). These common pests have long delicate antennae and broadly ovate wings characteristically bearing distinct light and dark spots or mottled areas. The mouthparts are short (these midges are telmophagous), and only the females are hematophagous. Species of medical importance belong to the genus *Culicoides*. Eggs are laid in decaying vegetation in water, in tree holes, crab holes, in the scum of a wet sand bed, or even in piles of wet manure. Some species breed in brackish water. The adult females are aggressive biters and are commonly crepuscular in their feed-

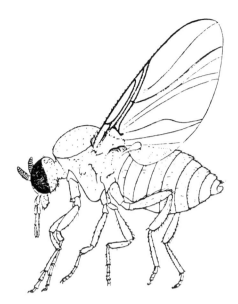

Fig. 16–17. Black fly (*Simulium* sp.). Female. (× 18.) (From Monnig, H.O. 1950. *Veterinary Helminthology and Entomology,* 3rd ed. Baltimore, Williams & Wilkins, p. 300.)

ing activity; frequently swarms of these minute flies attack man or mammals at dusk in areas where there is little or no breeze.

Bites and Sensitization. The bites of *Culicoides* are characterized by instantaneous, sharp needling pain and may occur on any exposed part of the body, including the scalp. The lesions typically appear with a minute droplet of blood surrounded by an erythematous macule 2 to 3 mm in diameter. These pruritic lesions may disappear within a few hours, although in some people they may persist for several days and may be accompanied by an appreciable systemic reaction.

Disease Transmission. The biting midges serve as vectors of some of the filarial nematodes of man (see Chapter 12, pages 186–188).

Control. Ordinary window screens and bednets are of no use in preventing *Culicoides* from entering dwellings and feeding, since they readily pass through the standard mesh. The application of residual insecticides within the house or the use of fogs outdoors is helpful, but only the elimination of larval habitats will effect any real control.

Black Flies (Simuliidae)

Morphology and Bionomics. Black flies (Fig. 16–17) are small, robust, and hump-backed, with relatively stout legs. The antennae are moderately short and moniliform (like a string of beads), and the short mouthparts are adapted to a bloodsucking

habit only in the females. The body is frequently very dark and the wings are broad and unspotted, with only the anteriormost veins being prominent. Black flies of medical importance belong to the genus *Simulium* and are known also as *buffalo gnats* and *coffee flies*. The breeding habitat of these flies is limited to rapidly flowing, well-oxygenated streams and this imposes restrictions on their geographic distribution. They usually are associated with mountainous areas. Females oviposit in running water, where the eggs are affixed to rocks or aquatic vegetation just below the water's surface, and in some instances to the carapace of freshwater crabs. The larvae (7 instars) and pupae are likewise adapted to clinging to such objects in flowing streams. The adults may have a flight range of about 10 to 20 km, but strong winds may extend this to several hundred km. Most *Simulium* species are diurnal in their feeding habits and are exophilic. Swarms of black flies attack man and domestic animals throughout the year in warm climates and during warm months in cooler areas; in the mountainous areas of the Northern United States, Alaska, and Canada such plagues are infamous.

Bites and Sensitization. The bite itself may not be particularly painful, but frequently it produces an intensely pruritic raised lesion. Typically, a little pool of extravasated blood (black flies are telmophagous) remains in the skin for days or weeks until it is resorbed. Individuals who are repeatedly bitten may develop hypersensitivity, with swelling of the arms or face, generalized urticaria, fever, and malaise.

Disease Transmission. Black flies are of considerable importance as vectors of onchocerciasis. This subject is covered in Chapter 12 (pp. 181–184).

Deer Flies and Horse Flies (Tabanidae)

Morphology and Bionomics. The tabanids (Fig. 16–18) are all large and robust, the deer flies (*Chrysops* and others) being about 1 cm in length and some of the horse flies (*Tabanus* and others) ranging up to 35 mm. Members of this group have large, often multicolored, compound eyes and strong wings that are held horizontally and toward the posterior when at rest. The mouthparts are short and massive, and only the females are hematophagous. The larval development, requiring a year or more, takes place in water or mud (river banks, lake shores, swamps).

Tabanid Bites. Many species of these rapidly

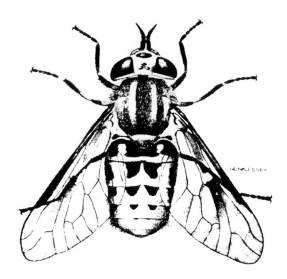

Fig. 16–18. Deer fly *(Chrysops discalis)*. Female. (Originally courtesy of Agriculture Canada. From Harwood, R.F., and James, M.T. 1979. *Entomology in Human and Animal Health,* 7th ed. New York, Macmillan, p. 237.)

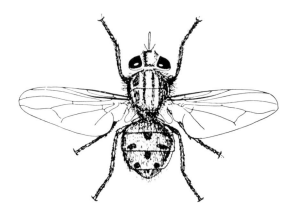

Fig. 16–19. Stable fly *(Stomoxys calcitrans)*. Adult, dorsal view. (× ca. 6.) (From Horsfall, W.R. 1962. *Medical Entomology.* New York, Ronald Press, p. 146. Reproduced in Beaver, P.C., Jung, R.C., and Cupp, E.W. 1984. *Clinical Parasitology,* 9th ed. Philadelphia, Lea & Febiger, p. 666.)

flying, diurnal feeders will take blood meals from man as well as other large mammals. All tabanids are telmophagous, and the large mouthparts lacerate the skin, producing considerable pain and a lesion that heals slowly. Sensitization occasionally develops from saliva injected into the wound, but the trauma produced is frequently more serious, and at times surgical dressing of the puncture site is required.

Disease Transmission. Species of *Chrysops* are vectors of *Loa loa,* a filarial worm of man in tropical Africa (see Chapter 12, pp. 184–186). Although tabanid flies have been suspected or accused of the mechanical transmission of a number of pathogens to man, the only other disease in which tabanids appear to play a significant role is tularemia. This zoonosis, caused by the bacterium *Francisella tularensis,* commonly is carried by rabbits as reservoir hosts in the western United States. In locations where infected rabbits are abundant, mechanical transmission to man by tabanid bites does occur.

Stable Flies (Muscidae)

Morphology and Bionomics. Muscid flies, of which the common house fly, *Musca domestica,* is the best-known example, are medium-sized, stout, and frequently dusky-gray in color. Only a few members of this family have piercing mouthparts adapted for sucking blood. A species that commonly bites man is the cosmopolitan stable fly,

Stomoxys calcitrans. It superficially resembles the house fly, which has led to the popular belief that house flies may occasionally bite. It is readily distinguished from *Musca domestica* by the long, rigid proboscis projecting conspicuously beyond the head (Fig. 16–19). Both males and females are hematophagous. Oviposition occurs in manure, decaying straw, or rotting vegetation. The larvae (maggots) pass through three instars and pupate, the last larval cuticle being transformed into the pupal case or puparium. Adults emerge from puparia in about 1 month following oviposition.

Stable Fly Bites. *Stomoxys* readily attacks man, stabbing into exposed skin or through thin clothing, and produces sharp pain at the time of puncture. Although this fly is an aggravating and persistent nuisance, it seldom produces serious local or systemic sensitization. Its role in the transmission of pathogens is insignificant.

Control. Some protection from *Stomoxys* can be achieved through ordinary door or window screening. Since breeding usually occurs in nearby wet accumulations of manure or vegetation, the provision of drains under such piles and the application of insecticides are effective.

Tsetses (Glossinidae)

Morphology and Bionomics. Tsetses (genus *Glossina*) are limited in distribution to the tropical belt of sub-Saharan Africa. They are light tan in color and a little larger than the house fly. When the fly is at rest, the well-developed proboscis is extended in front of the head and the wings are folded over one another across the abdomen (Fig.

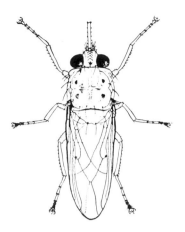

Fig. 16–20. Tsetse (*Glossina* sp.). Adult in resting position. (× 4.) (Adapted from Matheson, R. 1932. *Medical Entomology*, Springfield, Ill., Charles C Thomas. In Beaver, P.C., Jung, R.C., and Cupp, E.W. 1984. *Clinical Parasitology*, 9th ed. Philadelphia, Lea & Febiger, p. 667.)

16–20). Both sexes are voracious blood feeders and are primarily telmophagous. The adults are hardy, have exceptionally good eyesight, and are predominantly diurnal in their host-seeking. The "reproductive strategy" evolved in the tsetses is a striking departure from the usual "more-is-better" approach of most insects. Females produce one egg at a time, which hatches within the body and is nurtured through all three instars by "milk" secreted by special intrauterine glands. The larva is expelled only when it is fully grown, and it then quickly burrows into the soil and pupates. This process results in a remarkably high survival rate of the offspring. In their natural habitats, the tsetses have an abundance of wild mammals upon which to feed. Certain species, however, will readily take blood from man when he establishes settlements near their breeding sites or enters these areas to hunt, fish, or cut wood.

Disease Transmission. Tsetses are of primary importance as the vectors of trypanosomiasis in man and domestic animals (see Chapter 3, pages 26 to 31).

Control. Control of *Glossina* is difficult, and any methods used must be appropriate for the particular species involved. Clearing of the bush around native villages and boat landings, trapping of flies in game preserves, and the fumigation of vehicular transportation have been tried. The application of insecticides to infested regions by aerial spraying has met with some success (Matthews, 1979).

Fleas (Siphonaptera)

Morphology and Bionomics. Fleas are small, wingless, brown, shiny insects that are strongly compressed from side to side (Fig. 16–21). They are provided with long legs for jumping and propelling themselves through the hair of the host. Both males and females have a slender proboscis adapted for piercing and sucking. The body has numerous backwardly directed bristles, and some fleas have rows of dark stout spines (the *combs* or *ctenidia*) that are useful in species identification.

Unlike lice, fleas are not highly host-specific, although they usually are found on certain hosts. Many species are ectoparasitic on rodents, and two that commonly occur on domestic rats in many parts of the world are the Oriental rat flea *(Xenopsylla cheopis)* and the northern rat flea *(Nosopsyllus fasciatus)*. The human flea *(Pulex irritans)*, the dog flea *(Ctenocephalides canis)*, and the cat flea *(C. felis)* are cosmopolitan, the latter species being the most common on both cats and dogs in the United States.

Adult fleas spend most of their time on the host but will readily move from one individual to another. Females produce eggs that drop to the ground, usually in the resting place or nest of the host. The larvae feed on organic debris and bloody dejecta from the adults, and after three instars they pupate. The pupal period may be as short as a week or as long as a year, and the adults survive a year or more under favorable conditions.

The Chigoe Flea. The chigoe, *Tunga penetrans* (Fig. 16–22), differs from other fleas in that the female invades the skin of the host and becomes permanently buried in the cutaneous tissue and feeds on fluids within the lesion. As she begins to develop eggs, her abdomen swells to the size of a pea. Eggs are extruded through a hole in the lesion and drop to the ground, where larval development proceeds. These insects are common parasites of the feet of pigs and dogs in tropical America and Africa. People who walk barefooted on ground contaminated by infested animals are liable to become parasitized by chigoes. Sporadic cases in travelers occur in the United States (Poppiti *et al.*, 1983). The common sites of infestation are the soles of the feet and webbing between the toes, but no body surface is exempt from invasion. The lesion developed by the females may extend deeply into the dermis, causing great pain and inconvenience, and characteristically becomes secondarily

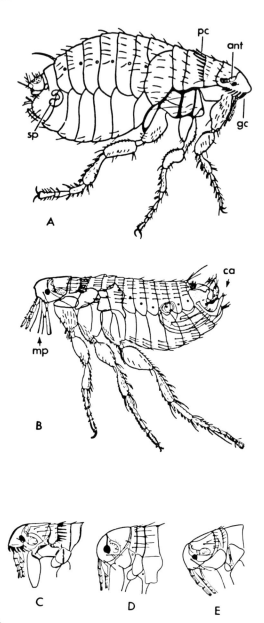

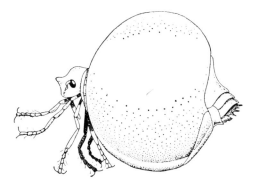

Fig. 16–22. Chigoe flea *(Tunga penetrans).* (× ca. 8.) (From Horsfall, W.R. 1962. *Medical Entomology. Arthropods and Human Disease.* New York, Ronald Press, p. 105.

Fig. 16–21. Fleas. *A,* Adult female. *ant,* Antenna. *gc,* Genal ctenidium. *pc,* Pronotal ctenidium. *sp,* Spermatheca or seminal receptacle. *B,* Adult male. *ca,* Copulatory apparatus or terminalia. *mp,* Mouthparts. *C,* Anterior of *Ctenocephalides. D,* Anterior of *Pulex irritans. E,* Anterior of *Xenopsylla cheopis.* (*A,* Adapted from CDC. 1953. Diagrammatic definitions of terms used in circular key to the flea genera of the United States, Atlanta, DHEW. *B,* Adapted from Fox, C. 1925. *Insects and Disease of Man.* Philadelphia, P. Blakiston's Son & Co., p. 113. *B* through *E,* Adapted from Beaver, P.C., Jung, P.C., and Cupp, E.W. 1984. *Clinical Parasitology,* 9th ed. Philadelphia, Lea & Febiger, pp. 697, 701.)

infected. The flea must be removed surgically or carefully teased out of the wound with a sharp needle, and then the wound is appropriately cleansed and dressed. The wearing of shoes prevents most infestations.

Flea Bites and Sensitization. Other than the acute annoyance produced by the bites, most people suffer little from fleas. In some, however, a local reaction develops at the puncture site. The lesion is roseate, raised, and frequently edematous and indurated. It is intensely pruritic and becomes inflamed and scarified as a result of scratching.

Disease Transmission. The most important diseases transmitted by fleas are *plague* and *murine typhus.* Very occasionally fleas serve as intermediate hosts for some of the tapeworms that infect man *(Hymenolepis nana, H. diminuta, Dipylidium caninum).*

PLAGUE

Plague has been known and dreaded since antiquity and bears such colorful names as "the Black Death" and "peste." This acute infectious and often fatal disease is caused by the gram-negative bacillus *Yersinia pestis.*

The clinical manifestations of plague in man are varied in both their appearance and severity. When bacteria are introduced into the skin by the bite of an infected flea, they are filtered out by lymph nodes in which they colonize. The usual findings are lymphangitis and lymphadenitis, with pronounced swelling of the lymph nodes, which become filled with caseous necrotic material. The "swollen glands," often of the inguinal or axillary regions, are called bubos, and this form of the disease is correspondingly known as *bubonic* plague. Secondarily, and commonly, bacteria enter the bloodstream, producing *septicemic* plague, and this often leads to pulmonary involvement, which is then referred to as the *pneumonic* type. With each of these progressions, the severity of the disease and the gravity of the prognosis increase. If the disease is not treated, death very likely ensues.

The means by which fleas transmit plague are varied. The flea ingests the bacteria with its blood meal when feeding on a septicemic host. Simple mechanical transfer from one host to another by contaminated mouthparts may occur when feeding is interrupted. Since the plague bacilli multiply within the gut of the insect, fecal contamination of the puncture wound (or contamination caused by crushing the flea) may effect transmission. The most important and common mode of transmission involves a process known as *blocking*. In certain fleas the bacteria become lodged in fibrinous deposits on the chitinous spines within the proventriculus. There they multiply, gradually occluding or blocking the gut. A "blocked" flea cannot feed successfully; ingested blood will pass only as far as the proventriculus before the elasticity of the anterior gut causes it to be *regurgitated*. Repeated attempts to feed on different individuals result in the "flushing" of bacteria from the blocking colony into the puncture wound at each trial. The salivary secretions are not involved in this process.

Plague is a zoonotic disease which in nature is maintained in a variety of rodents. Classic plague, the pandemic "visitations" that decimated human populations in Europe during the 14th and 17th centuries, is associated primarily with the common brown rat *(Rattus rattus)*. When an epizootic occurs and large numbers of rats die, the fleas, particularly *Xenopsylla cheopis,* turn to man as a source of blood meals. Under these conditions, an epidemic may be initiated. Once this happens, the disease may be spread from man to man by other fleas and by droplet infection from people with pneumonic manifestations. This type of plague no longer occurs as massive epidemics, but outbreaks do arise in scattered parts of the world. This disease remains a potential threat in many areas, particularly in port cities where rats abound and the introduction of infected rats and fleas is likely.

A second type of disease cycle is known as *sylvatic* or *campestral* plague. The principal hosts in this type are wild rodents such as ground squirrels, with fleas *other* than *X. cheopis* functioning as vectors (e.g., *Diamanus montanus, Hoplopsyllus anomalus*). Man acquires the infection when he enters the environs of those wild rodents and is bitten by infected fleas. Sylvatic plague in man is rural, sporadic, and often seasonal in its occurrence; most human infections occur during the summer when agricultural or recreational activities lead people into the country. Campestral plague in the United States is most common in the southwestern states. When a person having acquired sylvatic plague returns to urban areas, the introduction of *Yersinia pestis* into the domestic rat population and the initiation of the classic cycle are possible.

Plague can be treated successfully primarily with streptomycin and with the tetracycline drugs. Drug treatment has resulted in a marked lowering of the fatality rate to 5% or less in bubonic plague and to 10% in the septicemic type.

MURINE TYPHUS

Sometimes called *endemic typhus,* murine typhus is a zoonosis transmitted to man by fleas. It is an acute febrile disease of relatively mild form and is caused by *Rickettsia typhi* (syn. *R. mooseri*). Murine typhus, as its name implies, is primarily a disease of domestic rodents (*Rattus* spp.), and its principal vector is *Xenopsylla cheopis*.

Rickettsiae are ingested with the blood meal and enter the epithelial cells of the midgut, where they multiply and are later released into the lumen to pass out with the dejecta of the insect. Infection in rats, or man, is usually acquired by *contamination* of the puncture wound by *flea feces;* the rickettsiae are not injected into the wound, since they are not present in the foregut or in the salivary secretions. *R. typhi* may survive several years in dried flea feces and thus provide another means of transmission through contact with mucous membranes or inhalation.

Murine typhus is found throughout the world. Most infections in man in the United States are seen in the southeastern or Gulf Coast region, following the Mississippi river northward. The disease is sporadic in the human population and is associated with rat-infested locations (ports, grain elevators, farms).

Flea Control. The control of cat and dog fleas around the home can be accomplished by treating both the pets and their habitual resting places with appropriate insecticides. The periodic use of dips and shampoos containing rotenone (1%), malathion (4%) or pyrethrins (1%) will kill the fleas on the animals. Powders may also be used, but they are not as effective. Lindane should be avoided, particularly when cats are being treated. At the same time household insecticidal sprays or powders should be applied to the floor, carpets, pillows, and other articles associated with the animals.

The fleas associated with domestic rodents can be controlled by applying insecticides (organochlorines and others) as residual sprays or dusts along the known runways or by blowing powders into rat holes. It is essential in the control of flea-borne diseases such as plague or murine typhus that the insecticidal measures *precede* the rodenticides to prevent fleas from leaving the dying rats and moving onto human hosts.

Myiasis

Myiasis is the infestation of the body with the larvae (maggots or bots) of certain flies. This condition is often referred to in terms of the part of the body affected (*e.g., cutaneous, ocular, nasal myiasis*). Several families of cyclorrhaphid Diptera have members that may produce myiasis in man and his domestic animals (James, 1947). Myiasis is either *specific* (obligatory selection of *living tissues* for development) or *facultative* (adults are attracted to malodorous, purulent lesions, where they deposit eggs or larvae which feed only on *necrotic* matter). Accidental contamination of the skin or of the intestinal or urinary tracts may occasionally occur. Although myiasis in man is generally uncommon, certain flies causing the condition are of medical importance in particular areas of the world.

The larvae involved in myiasis have a relatively simple external morphology—a pair of sharp, curved mandibular hooks at the anterior end, a pair of spiracles (openings to the respiratory system) at the posterior end, and several body segments in between bearing bands or rows of small chitinous spines or teeth. Larvae with a narrow anterior and broader posterior extremity (Fig. 16–23A)) are called *maggots (e.g., Cochliomyia);* others, which are more robust, of more nearly uniform diameter throughout, and often with more pronounced spination on the body (Fig. 16–23B), are termed *bots (e.g., Gasterophilus).* This distinction is a matter of convenience rather than of taxonomic precision.

Screwworm. The primary screwworm, *Cochliomyia hominivorax,* is an important parasite of livestock and man in the Western Hemisphere. It occurs in tropical and subtropical areas as well as in the warmer parts of the United States, being present along the border with Mexico and in some other states. The adult flies deposit eggs in fresh wounds (*e.g.,* cuts from barbed wire) in the host's skin. First instar larvae hatch within a few hours

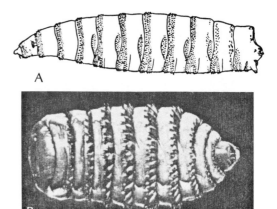

Fig. 16–23. *A,* Primary screwworm *(Cochliomyia hominivorax).* Third instar larva. (× ca 4.) Example of a maggot. *B,* Stomach bot *(Gasterophilus* sp.) of horse, third instar larva. (× ca. 4.) (*A,* Adapted from James, M.T.: *The Flies That Cause Myiasis in Man. Washington, D.C., U.S.D.A. Misc. Publ. No. 631, p. 64. B,* From Harwood, R.F., and James, M.T. 1979. *Entomology in Human and Animal Health,* 7th ed. New York, Macmillan, p. 306.)

and enter the lesion, where they feed on and destroy living tissue. They grow rapidly, reaching third instar within a week, then drop from the lesion and pupate in the soil. The adult flies emerge in a week or so. The amount of damage may be extensive, since many larvae enter the same lesion. *C. hominivorax* is responsible for most human cases of cutaneous and nasopharyngeal myiasis in the United States, and the latter type may have a fatal outcome. Control and even eradication of screwworms in southeastern United States has been successful through the release of irradiated (and hence sterile) male flies, but the reintroduction of screwworms continues to be a problem (Bushland, 1975; Steelman, 1976).

A closely related species, the secondary screwworm *(C. macellaria),* is very commonly found in the United States, but it feeds only on decaying carcasses and does not invade living tissue.

A counterpart to *C. hominivorax* found in Africa and Asia is *Chrysomyia bezziana.*

Tumbu Fly (Cordylobia). The Tumbu fly, *Cordylobia anthropophaga,* is a common parasite of man and other animals in Africa. Eggs are deposited on dirt that has been soiled by feces or urine (floors of native huts), and the larvae that hatch within a day or so penetrate the skin of people sleeping on the ground.

Dermatobia. A very important myiasis-producing fly in the neotropical area is the "human bot

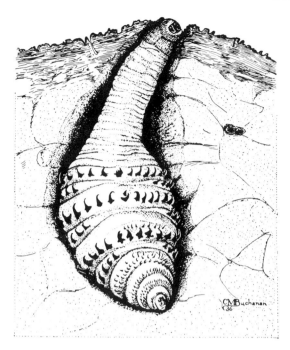

Fig. 16–24. Human bot *(Dermatobia hominis)*, maturing larva in human skin. The posterior end of the larva is at the outer end of the tunnel, so that breathing may occur through the posterior spiracles. (Drawing by C.M. Buchanan for E. C. Faust, 1936.) (From Beaver, P.C., Jung, R.C., and Cupp, E.W. 1984. *Clinical Parasitology*, 9th ed. Philadelphia, Lea & Febiger, p. 686.)

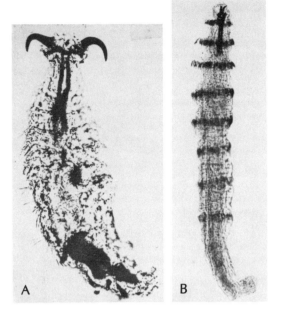

Fig. 16–26. *A, Oestrus ovis*, first instar removed from the conjunctiva at the inner canthus of the eye of a child. (× ca. 100.) *B, Cuterebra tenebrosa*, first instar (× 60.) (By P.C. Beaver. *Cuterebra* specimen courtesy of C.R. Baird.)

fly," *Dermatobia hominis*. The larva produces painful, exudative furuncular lesions in a wide variety of mammals, including man and cattle, in Central and South America (Fig. 16–24). The life cycle of this fly is curious, since it does not involve the deposition of eggs or larvae by the adult directly on the skin but rather employs a *phoretic* host; eggs are cemented to mosquitoes or other hematophagous arthropods (Fig. 16–25), and the larvae hatch

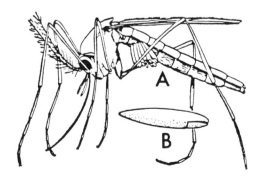

Fig. 16–25. Human bot *(Dermatobia hominis)*. *A,* Mosquito serving as phoretic host. Note *Dermatobia* eggs cemented to abdomen. *B,* Egg, greatly enlarged. (From James, M.T.: *The Flies that Cause Myiasis in Man*. Washington, D.C. U.S.D.A. Misc. Publ. No. 631, p. 103.)

and invade the skin when the mosquito feeds on man or another mammalian host.

Bots and Warbles. A number of other flies are capable of producing myiasis in man. Many of these are the *warbles* or bot flies of livestock. *Gasterophilus* (horse bots) and *Hypoderma* (cattle bots) can produce cutaneous lesions (sometimes migratory) in man. *Oestrus* (sheep bots, Fig. 16–26A), *Cuterebra* (Fig. 16–26B), and others have been reported in cases of ocular myiasis in man (Baird *et al.*, 1982).

Treatment. Simple surgical removal of the larva is the usual mode of treating cutaneous myiasis. Since these organisms leave an opening in the skin to which they periodically return for respiration, cutting off their air supply by applying petroleum jelly or bacon fat to the lesion may induce larvae to migrate to the surface, where they can be grasped with forceps. The lesion itself is treated appropriately to avoid secondary infection.

Maggot Therapy. In the 1930s and 1940s, bacteriologically sterile maggots of such flies as *Phormia* and *Phaenicia* were used in treating certain inaccessible infections (*e.g.*, osteomyelitis). These larvae, being facultative myiasis producers, do not invade living tissue, and their feeding activity cleans the infected tissues while their secretions are bactericidal. After removal of the larvae,

granulation tissue formation is enhanced and healing results. This practice was discarded with the
advent of antibiotics, but in recent years maggot
therapy has received renewed attention in the treatment of infections (*e.g.*, mastoiditis) that have
become intractable as a result of the development
of strains of antibiotic-resistant bacteria (Horn *et
al.*, 1976).

SUMMARY

1. Insects are morphologically distinguished from other
classes of arthropods in that they have three pairs of
thoracic legs. One or two pairs of wings are characteristic of the group, but many of the ectoparasitic forms
are secondarily wingless.

2. Certain beetles (order Coleoptera) contain vesicating
substances that cause painful blisters when the insect is
crushed on the skin.

3. The larval stages (caterpillars) of some moths and butterflies (order Lepidoptera) have poisonous hairs or
spines that produce severe urtication.

4. Bees, ants, and wasps (order Hymenoptera) commonly
produce envenomation in man by their stings. Reactions
are usually local, but hypersensitive people may manifest systemic responses.

5. The sucking lice (order Anoplura) that infest man include the head louse, the body louse *(Pediculus humanus
capitus* and *P. h. humanus*, respectively), and the crab
louse *(Phthirus pubis)*. Pediculosis is common throughout the world. Only body lice transmit disease agents,
the most important of which is epidemic typhus.

6. The true bugs (order Hemiptera) include the bedbugs
(Cimex spp.) and the kissing-bugs (triatomine bugs).
Bedbugs are wingless, flat, and are closely associated
with man worldwide; although their bites are irritating,
they do not transmit disease agents. The kissing-bugs
serve as vectors for *Trypanosoma cruzi* (Chagas' disease) in the Western Hemisphere.

7. The flies (order Diptera) are insects with complete metamorphosis characterized by a single pair of wings in the
adult stage. Several groups of flies are of medical importance.

8. Mosquitoes (family Culicidae) are flies with minute
scales on the wings, legs, and body; their larvae and
pupae are aquatic. Females are hematophagous solenophages (capillary feeders). Members of the genus
Anopheles are vectors of malaria throughout the world.
Several genera of mosquitoes transmit filariae *(Wuchereria bancrofti* and *Brugia malayi)* in the tropics. Mosquitoes also transmit several important viral diseases.
Yellow fever in its urban form is usually transmitted
from man to man by the common and highly domesticated *Aedes aegypti*. The sylvatic or jungle form of
yellow fever is zoonotic in monkeys in the tropics of
South and Central America and Africa and is transmitted
by other nondomesticated mosquitoes *(Haemagogus*
spp., *Aedes* spp.). Dengue, present in both hemispheres,
is also transmitted from person to person by *Aedes aegypti*. Several encephalitides (including, in the United
States, Western, Eastern, and Venezuelan equine encephalomyelitis and St. Louis encephalitis) are transmitted from wild animals, usually birds, to man. To
control mosquito-borne diseases, an integrated approach
(chemical, environmental management, and biologic
measures) is used. The exact methods employed must
be appropriate for the specific vector involved.

9. Sand flies (family Psychodidae) are small, hairy,
hematophagous gnats with a worldwide distribution in
tropical and temperate areas. They are the important
vectors *(Phlebotomus* spp. in the Eastern Hemisphere,
Lutzomyia spp. in the Western Hemisphere) of the leishmaniases.

10. Biting midges (family Ceratopogonidae), commonly of
the genus *Culicoides,* are tiny, aggressive blood feeders.
Although irritation from their persistent bites is cosmopolitan, their role as vectors is limited to the transmission of certain filariae of man.

11. Black flies (family Simuliidae) are small, robust gnats
that breed in rapidly flowing streams. The females are
telmophages ("pool feeders"), and their bites are irritating. In certain regions of Mexico, Central and South
America, and Africa, black flies (most commonly *Simulium* spp.) transmit onchocerciasis.

12. The deer flies and horse flies (family Tabanidae) are
large, robust flies that inflict bites, but in certain areas
of Africa tabanids *(Chrysops)* transmit a filarial worm,
Loa loa.

13. Stable flies (family Muscidae) are close relatives of the
common house fly but differ in having a rigid proboscis
that is used for taking blood meals. These flies have a
worldwide distribution. Their importance lies in their
irritating bites; they do not transmit disease to man.

14. Tsetses (family Glossinidae) are medium-sized hematophagous flies found only in Africa. Several species of
Glossina serve as vectors of the human and animal try-
panosomiases.

15. Fleas (order Siphonaptera) are small, wingless insects
with complete metamorphosis. Several common fleas
(Ctenocephalides on cats and dogs, *Pulex, Nosopsyllus,*
and *Xenopsylla* on rats) occasionally feed on man, producing irritation. The most important diseases transmitted by fleas are plague (bacterial) and murine typhus
(rickettsial), both zoonotic. Urban plague is associated
with domestic rats and *Xenopsylla cheopis* is the primary
vector. Sylvatic or campestral plague is enzootic in wild
rodents, and fleas (*e. g.,* *Diamanus*) transmit it to man.
Murine typhus is associated with domestic rodents and
is transmitted by *Xenopsylla cheopis*. The chigoe, *Tunga
penetrans*, of the American and African tropics penetrates and produces persistent lesions in the skin.

16. Myiasis is infestation by larvae (maggots or bots) of
certain flies. Cutaneous myiasis produced by the primary
screwworm *(Cochliomyia hominivorax)* occurs in cattle-
raising areas of the Western Hemisphere, including parts
of the United States. In tropical America, the human
bot, *Dermatobia hominis*, infests man and domestic animals. Larvae of other flies cause myiasis in different
parts of the world. Ocular myiasis involving the sheep
bot *(Oestrus)*, rodent bot *(Cuterebra)*, and others is occasionally reported.

REFERENCES

Baird, C.R., Podgore, J.K., and Sabrosky, C.W. 1982. *Cu-
terebra myiasis* in humans: Six new case reports from the
United States with a summary of known cases (Diptera:
Cuterebridae). J. Med. Entomol., *19*:263–267.

Beaty, B.J., Tesh, R.B., and Aitkin, T.H.G. 1980. Transovarial transmission of yellow fever virus in *Stegomyia* mosquitoes. Am. J. Trop. Med. Hyg., *29*:125–132.

Bushland, R.C. 1975. Screwworm research and eradication.
Bull. Entomol. Soc. Am., *21*:23–26.

Busvine, J.R. 1980. *Insects and Hygiene*. 3rd ed. New York,
Chapman and Hall.

Carpenter, S.J., and LaCasse, W.J. 1955. *Mosquitoes of North
America*. Berkeley, University of California Press.

CDC (Centers for Disease Control). 1984. Yellow fever vaccine. Recommendations of the Immunization Practices Advisory Committee. MMWR *32*:679–688.

Darsie, R.F., Jr., and Ward, R.A. 1981. *Identification and Geographic Distribution of the Mosquitoes of North America North of Mexico*. Salt Lake City, American Mosquito Control Association.

Dutary, B.E., and LeDuc, J.W. 1981. Transovarial transmission of yellow fever virus by a sylvatic vector, *Haemagogus equinus*. Trans. R. Soc. Trop. Med. Hyg., 75:128.

Edery, H., Ishay, J., Gitter, S., and Joshua, H. 1978. Venoms of Vespidae. In *Arthropod Venoms*. Edited by S. Bettini. New York, Springer-Verlag, pp. 691–772.

Edwards, L., and Lynch, P.J. 1984. Anaphylactic reaction to kissing bug bites. Ariz. Med., *41*:159–161.

Horn, K.L., Cobb, A.H., Jr., and Gates, G.A. 1976. Maggot therapy for subacute mastoiditis. Arch. Otolaryngol., *102*:377–379.

James, M.T. 1947. *The Flies that Cause Myiasis in Man*. Washington, D.C., U.S. Dept. Agric. Misc. Publ. No. 631.

Matthews, G.A. 1979. *Pesticide Application Methods*. London, Longman.

Matthews, R.E.F. 1982. Classification and nomenclature of viruses. Intervirology, *17*:1–199.

O'Connor, R., and Peck, M.L. 1978. Venoms of Apidae. In *Arthropod Venoms*. Edited by S. Bettini. New York, Springer Verlag, pp. 613–660.

Poppiti, R., Jr., Kambour, M., Robinson, M.J., and Rywlin, A.M. 1983. *Tunga penetrans* in South Florida. South. Med. J., *76*:1558–1560.

Schmidt, J.O. 1982. Biochemistry of insect venoms. Annu. Rev. Entomol., *27*:339–368.

Steelman, C.D. 1976. Effects of external and internal arthropod parasites on domestic livestock production. Annu. Rev. Entomol., *21*:155–178.

Tesh, R.B. 1980. Vertical transmission of arthropod-borne viruses of vertebrates. In *Vectors of Disease Agents*. Edited by J.J. McKelvey, B.F. Eldridge, and K. Maramorosch. New York, Praeger, pp. 122–137.

Chapter 17

Arthropods Other Than Insects

J. H. Esslinger

This section deals with groups of arthropods that range in their medical importance from occasional envenomation (centipedes, spiders, scorpions) to the transmission of microbial disease agents (ticks and mites). Some are themselves endoparasitic (the Pentastomida, certain mites), and others (Crustacea) serve as intermediate hosts of parasites.

CRUSTACEA

Crustacea are chiefly aquatic, gill-breathing arthropods, typically having two pairs of preoral antenniform appendages. Two groups of Crustacea—copepods and decapods—are of importance in the transmission of parasitic organisms to man.

Copepods (Copepoda). The nearly microscopic copepods (Fig. 17–1) are cosmopolitan and include the common freshwater genera *Cyclops* and *Diaptomus*. Copepods serve as intermediate hosts for certain tapeworms of man, notably *Diphyllobothrium latum* and *Spirometra* (causing sparganosis), discussed in Chapter 10, as well as some nematodes *(Dracunculus, Gnathostoma)*, discussed in Chapter 11. Infection by these helminths is enhanced by the fact that the tiny intermediate hosts are readily ingested by man without being noticed.

Crayfish and Crabs (Decapoda). The familiar crayfish and crabs typically have large, distinct movable claws as the first pair of legs. The role of certain freshwater species as intermediate hosts of the lung fluke *(Paragonimus westermani)* is discussed in Chapter 8. River crabs of the genus *Potamonautes* are involved in the epidemiology of onchocerciasis in East Africa, since the larvae and pupae of the black fly vector *(Simulium neavei)* characteristically attach themselves to these crustaceans.

''Tongue Worms'' (Pentastomida). The

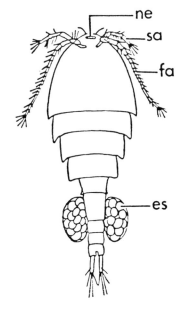

Fig. 17–1. Copepod (*Cyclops* sp.), female, dorsal view. (× ca. 50.) *es*, Egg sac. *fa*, First antenna. *ne*, Nauplius eye. *sa*, Second antenna. (Adapted from Faust, E.C. 1949. *Human Helminthology*, 3rd ed. Philadelphia, Lea & Febiger, p. 613.)

tongue worms are a small, highly modified group of endoparasitic arthropods, now thought by many workers to be most closely related to certain of the Crustacea (Riley *et al.*, 1978). The adult and most immature stages are wormlike; only the larval stage within the egg has four leglike appendages (Fig. 17–2). Human infection with this worm is sporadic and, in the United States, uncommon.

The adult forms of pentastomids infecting man are parasitic in the respiratory tract of reptiles, although one cosmopolitan species—*Linguatula serrata*—is found in the nasopharyngeal spaces of dogs. The immature stages, called nymphs, are found in the viscera of herbivorous or omnivorous

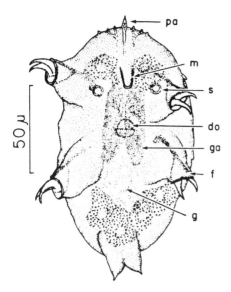

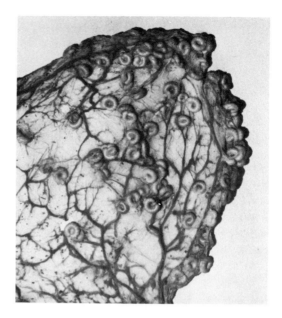

Fig. 17-2. Pentastomid larva *(Porocephalus crotali)*, ventral view. *do*, Dorsal organ. *f*, Foot. *g*, Gut. *ga*, Ganglion. *m*, Mouth ring. *pa*, Penetration apparatus. *s*, Stigma. (From Esslinger, J.H. 1962. Development of *Porocephalus crotali* [Humboldt, 1808] [Pentastomida] in experimental intermediate hosts. J. Parasitol., *48*:452–456.)

Fig. 17-3. *Armillifer* sp. Nymphs in omentum of East African vervet, *Cercopithecus aethiops*. (× ca. 1.5.) (Courtesy of R.E. Kuntz.) (From Beaver, P.C., Jung, R.C., and Cupp, E.W. 1984. *Clinical Parasitology*, 9th ed., Philadelphia, Lea & Febiger, p. 572.)

mammals that have ingested eggs passed by the definitive host. Most human infections with pentastomids involve the penetration of the viscera by the nymphs, which remain in the tissues (Fig. 17-3) and, with the exception of massive infections, cause no appreciable consequences. The pathologic course involves the development of an eosinophilic granulomatous reaction around the parasite, with the resolution of the lesion to a fibrous capsule within a few months (Esslinger, 1962). Most cases of visceral pentastomiasis in Africa are caused by *Armillifer armillatus* (Fig. 17-4) and *A. grandis,* and those in Asia by *A. moniliformis.*

Linguatula serrata (Fig. 17-5) is found in many parts of the world. In addition to the visceral involvement seen with *Armillifer,* the immature stages of *L. serrata* may establish themselves in the nasopharynx of man, a condition seen most commonly in North Africa and the Middle East. Nearly all cases of pentastomiasis in man in the United States have been caused by *L. serrata;* some of these have involved invasion of the eye. Human infections with pentastomids have been reviewed by Self *et al.* (1975) and Fain (1975).

CENTIPEDES AND MILLIPEDES

Centipedes (Chilopoda). Centipedes are elongated terrestrial arthropods ranging from 5 to 25

cm or more in length, with one pair of jointed appendages and one pair of spiracles (tracheal openings) for each body segment (Fig. 17-6). The most obvious structures at the anterior end are a pair of long, multisegmented antennae and a pair of large poison claws (maxillipeds) arising from the first body segment just ventrolateral to the short, stout mandibles. The terminal segment of each of these claws is a strong, sharply pointed, incurved piercing fang, with a subterminal pore for secretion from the poison gland in the base of the claw.

Their formidable appearance notwithstanding, the centipedes are not generally considered dan-

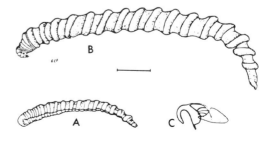

Fig. 17-4. *Armillifer armillatus. A,* Male. *B,* Female. *C,* Detail of anterior hooklet. (Scale = 1 cm.) (Adapted by E.C. Faust from Fain, A. 1961. Les pentastomides de l'Afrique Centrale, Annales de la Musée Royale de l'Afrique Centrale, ser. 8, no. 92, pp. 67, 70.)

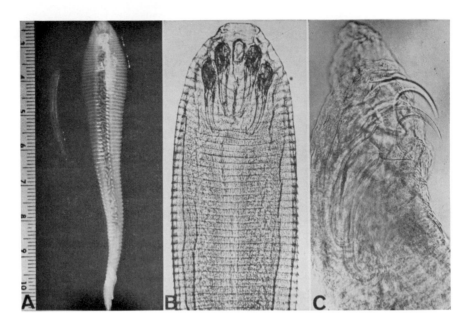

Fig. 17–5. *Linguatula serrata. A,* Adult male *(left)* and female, ventral view (centimeter scale). *B,* Nymph, anterior end, ventral view. (× ca. 20.) *C,* Head, lateral view showing two hooks at right side of mouth. (× ca. 100.) (Courtesy of J.F. Schacher.)

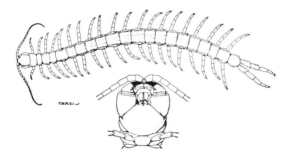

Fig. 17–6. *Scolopendra morsitans.* Dorsal view of entire centipede and ventral view of head showing poison claws (maxillipeds). (From Castellani, A., and Chalmers, A.J. 1919. *Manual of Tropical Medicine.* London, Baillière, Tindall, and Cox, p. 217.)

gerous. On the infrequent occasions when the poison claws succeed in penetrating the skin, a painful wound may result from the injection of small quantities of their acidic digestive enzymes. Only a single instance of death resulting from an uncomplicated centipede bite (a 7-year-old child) has been reported (Minelli, 1978). Treatment of a painful centipede bite is palliative, and compresses of baking soda or Epsom salts should be applied locally.

Millipedes (Diplopoda). Millipedes do not have poison claws, bear two pairs of appendages on each body segment, and generally are not dangerous. Millipedes secrete offensive substances as defense agents; in some of the giant tropical species, this

fluid may cause burning dermatitis and sloughing of the skin (Radford, 1975).

ARACHNIDA

The arachnids are arthropods in which the body is externally divided into two parts: prosoma, including cephalic structures, and opisthosoma. Antennae are lacking, and most adult forms have four pairs of legs. This large and diverse group includes a number of members of medical importance such as the scorpions, spiders, ticks, and mites.

Scorpions (Scorpiones)

Morphology and Distribution. Scorpions are widely recognized and generally feared arthropods. This group has been studied in depth by Keegan (1980). Scorpions are characterized by four pairs of spindly legs, large pedipalps terminating in stout claws, and an abdomen with a broad anterior portion and a narrow, flexible, posterior portion bearing a pyriform telson that ends in a sharp, curved spine *(aculeus)* or *stinger* (Fig. 17–7). Tiny subterminal pores in the spine serve as outlets for the venom secreted by two venom glands found within the telson.

Scorpions are found throughout the world, although they are more commonly a medical problem in arid regions. These arachnids normally prey on large insects and other arthropods at night or in

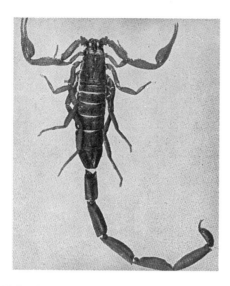

Fig. 17–7. Scorpion, *Centruroides* sp., male. (× 1.) (From Hoffman, C.C. 1936. In Brenneman, J.: *Practice of Pediatrics*, Hagerstown, Md., W.F. Prior Company.)

dark places. They usually seek shelter from direct sunlight and hide under logs and rocks and occasionally in bedrolls and boots. When disturbed, they rapidly whip the abdomen over the body, driving the terminal spine into the intruder. The more important genera of scorpions include *Buthus* and *Androctonus* in Africa and the Middle East, *Tityus* in tropical America, including some Caribbean islands, and *Centruroides* in Mexico, northern South America, and the United States. *Centruroides sculpturatus*, a relatively small species, is the only dangerously venomous scorpion in the United States, and its distribution is limited to Arizona and portions of the adjoining states.

Envenomation. The precise nature of scorpion venom varies with the species concerned, but all are complex mixtures of neurotoxic and hemotoxic substances (Bettini, 1978). Although one hesitates to classify any of the scorpions as "harmless," it is well known that some are far more dangerous than others, and often the smaller species are more deadly than their more awesome larger relatives.

The severity of a scorpion sting is related not only to the species involved but also to the age of the victim, children and infants being at much greater risk. The immediate reaction is that of intense local pain, followed in most instances by local swelling and mild systemic discomfort, which subsides within a few minutes or hours to a day. In severe cases there may be manifestations of peripheral vascular failure, respiratory paralysis, in-

coordination, and convulsions; death may occur within a few minutes or hours, or even up to a day or two.

The treatment of mild scorpion stings (the usual case) is the local application of ice to the affected part. When profound systemic reactions occur, *specific* antivenin should be administered. In the United States the antivenin for *Centruroides sculpturatus* is available only in Arizona.

The control of scorpions is feasible only in individual houses or tents. Use of many of the readily available insecticides is effective.

Spiders (Araneae)

Spiders are arachnids that have a cephalothorax and a saclike abdomen separated by a conspicuous constriction (the *pedicle*). There is no external evidence of segmentation. Spiders have four pairs of walking legs, although the long segmented *pedipalps* arising from just behind the mouth may give the impression of a fifth pair. The mouthparts include a pair of poison "fangs" (the *chelicerae*). These are comprised of a short, broad, basal segment and a clawlike terminal segment bearing a small pore through which the poison gland opens.

Bionomics and Life Cycle. The spiders constitute a diverse and ubiquitous group. Most spiders feed on insects and other invertebrates, and many are cannibalistic. They are provided with spinning organs (spinnerets), usually three pairs of glands, which open ventrally near the posterior end of the abdomen. These elaborate the material for webs that serve as nests, traps for prey, and structures for moving about. Their habitats are manifold. Fertilized eggs are laid in masses, usually within a spun cocoon. The eggs soon hatch, but the 8-legged spiderlings may remain within the cocoon for weeks or months before emerging. Molting in spiders occurs repeatedly as they grow and continues periodically throughout the life of the adult.

Envenomation. Although all spiders are venomous, relatively few are of medical importance because of the low potency or minute quantity of the venom introduced or the inability of the fangs to pierce the skin. The spiders hazardous to man belong to two groups: (1) those causing primarily systemic responses, and (2) those responsible for a local necrotizing ulcer.

SYSTEMIC ARACHNIDISM

The most commonly encountered spiders whose bite evokes a systemic response are the "widow spiders" of the genus *Latrodectus* (family Theridiidae, the comb-footed spiders), which have a worldwide distribution. In the United States *Latrodectus mactans* is often considered to be a species complex, although Gertsch (1979) holds that these are five closely related species differing in coloration and habitat. The typical female "black widow spider" (Fig. 17–8) is easily recognized by its plump, shiny, black abdomen with a red hourglass configuration on the ventral surface. These medium-sized spiders are often found in and around human habitations, where they nest in dark crevices such as woodpiles, under the flooring of houses, and beneath the seat of outdoor privies.

Latrodectus venom is neurotoxic, acting at both the adrenergic and cholinergic junctions (Bettini and Maroli, 1978). The initial result of a black widow bite is sharp pain at the site of two small red puncture marks where the chelicerae have penetrated the skin. Later the site becomes erythematous and swollen. The affected part burns and aches severely. Once the venom disseminates, general signs and symptoms develop; these include dizziness, weakness, tremor in the legs, and cramps with board-like rigidity of the abdomen. Additionally, the victim may display hypertension, profuse cold sweating, nausea, vomiting, headache, acute urinary retention, and (particularly in children) convulsions. Although numerous deaths have resulted from these bites, uncomplicated recovery usually occurs.

Treatment of latrodectism varies with its severity, and the local application of ice or anesthetics often suffices to alleviate symptoms. In more serious cases the parenteral administration of diazepam (Valium) is indicated for reducing muscle spasm and anxiety. This may be combined with intravenous injection of a 10% solution of calcium gluconate. Specific standardized antivenin (hyperimmune horse serum) given intramuscularly is usually effective.

Other spiders capable of producing systemic envenomation include some of the funnel-web spiders of Australia (*Atrax* spp.) and South America (*Trechona* spp.), the "wandering spiders" (*Phoneutria* spp.) of the neotropical region, and *Chiracanthium* in several parts of the world, including North America. The large, hairy, tropical tarantulas (family Theraphosidae), including the bird-catching spiders of South America and the "barking" spiders of Australia, contain some forms that can inflict painful and sometimes dangerous bites; these also have urticating hairs on the body. Most of the tarantulas are notably unaggressive, however, and their most common effect on man is related to their psychological impact.

NECROTIC ARACHNIDISM

Certain spiders of the genus *Loxosceles* (family Scytodidae) in the Western Hemisphere produce serious necrotic arachnidism. *Loxosceles laeta* and *L. rufipes* are responsible for most human loxoscelism in South America (Chile, Argentina, Uruguay), whereas in the United States, the important species, known as the brown recluse or fiddle-back spider, is *L. reclusa* (Fig. 17–9). This medium-sized, brownish spider is quite unspectacular in its appearance and is often not recognized as dangerous. Upon careful examination, this species can be identified by the violin-shaped area on the dorsum

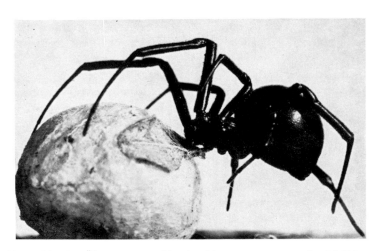

Fig. 17—8. Black-widow spider, *Latrodectus mactans*. Female with egg sac or cocoon. (× 5.) (Adapted from Needham, G.H. in Turtox News. Chicago, General Biological Supply House, 1958.)

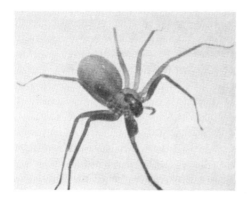

Fig. 17–9. Brown recluse or "fiddle-back" spider, *Loxosceles reclusa*, female. (× 2.) (Courtesy of C.W. Wingo.) (From Atkins, J.A., Wingo, C.W., Sodeman, W.A., and Flynn, J.E. 1958. Necrotic arachnidism. Am. J. Trop. Med. Hyg., 7:165–184.)

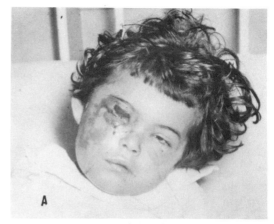

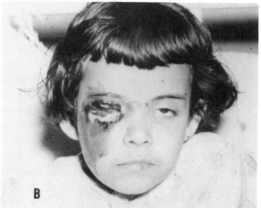

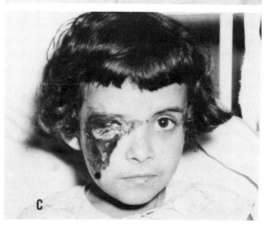

Fig. 17–10. *Loxosceles laeta*. Lesions produced on face of 7-year-old girl in Chile following envenomation. *A*, 20 hours after bite. *B*, 48 hours after bite. *C*, 21 days after bite. (Courtesy of Dr. Hugo Shenone.) (From Beaver, P.C., Jung, R.C., and Cupp, E.W. 1984. *Clinical Parasitology*, 9th ed., Philadelphia, Lea & Febiger, p. 580.)

of the cephalothorax. These spiders are often found inside human habitations, and typically are hidden away in closets, under piles of clothing or debris, in basements, under porches, or behind picture frames.

The manifestations produced by the necrotoxic venom of *Loxosceles* are reviewed in detail by Schenone and Suarez (1978) and by Foil and Norment (1979). Some sharp pain is associated with the bite, and the site becomes ischemic and edematous. Central necrosis appears and gradually spreads in the dermal tissue. The skin may become covered with vesicles and eventually slough (Fig. 17–10). Deeper tissues including muscles may also be involved. Healing is slow, requiring weeks or months, and disfiguring cicatrization commonly results.

In some instances grave systemic manifestations are seen. These may begin within about 2 days after the bite. Hemolytic anemia, hemoglobinuria, hematuria, jaundice, fever, and sensorial impairment resulting from diffuse intravascular involvement lead to a high mortality in such cases, particularly in small children (Berger, 1982).

There is no established specific treatment for loxoscelism, although dapsone in low doses (50 to 100 mg/day) has been cautiously recommended for that purpose (King and Rees, 1983). The administration of corticosteroids within a few hours of the bite may lessen the early symptoms and partially control the toxic necrosis.

Ticks and Mites (Acari)

The ticks and mites constitute a large group of arachnids in which neither the usual body divisions nor external segmentation is evident. The mouth-parts are contained in a discrete anterior structure known as the *gnathosoma* or *capitulum*.

Ticks (Parasitiformes; Ixodida)

Ticks are distinguished from mites in being generally larger, in having backwardly projecting teeth on the median component of the mouthparts (*i.e.,* an *armed hypostome,* Fig. 17–11), and in having a pair of conspicuous spiracles on the ventrolateral surface of the body.

Ticks have a relatively simple and straightforward life cycle. The female deposits eggs. From each egg a larva hatches that generally resembles the adult but has only three pairs of legs. The tick then passes through one or more nymphal stages that have four pairs of legs and finally becomes a sexually functional adult. The complete cycle usually requires from 1 to 2 years and may take longer.

Larvae, nymphs, and adults are all hematophagous. When ticks feed, the paired chelicerae (Fig. 17–11) lacerate the skin and the toothed hypostome is inserted, serving as a holdfast, and in apposition to the chelicerae it functions as a duct for the salivary secretions and the ingested blood.

There are two distinct families of ticks, the *hard ticks* (Ixodidae) and the *soft ticks* (Argasidae), which differ from one another with respect to morphology, habits, and medical importance.

HARD TICKS (IXODIDAE)

Morphology and Bionomics. The hard ticks (Fig. 17–12) are the more widely recognized of the two families. These are characterized by a dorsoventrally flattened body (when not engorged), by the placement of the capitulum, which extends anteriorly beyond the margin of the body, and by the presence of a distinct chitinous plate, the *scutum,* on the dorsum. The scutum covers the entire body in the male but only the anterior portion in the larva, nymph, and female.

The larval stages, commonly called "seed ticks," are frequently encountered in large numbers where they have hatched from a mass of several hundred eggs laid by the female. Larvae, as well as nymphs and adults, are seen on blades of grass or low vegetation, often at the margins of wooded areas, where they attach and wave their legs about while awaiting contact with a passing host. This behavior is termed *questing.* After feeding, the larva drops to the ground, molts to the nymphal stage, and seeks a new host. Nymphs and adults behave similarly; a blood meal is usually necessary for the development of eggs in the female. The feeding process is quite slow, taking several days to a week or so, and upon repletion the body is greatly distended with blood.

Hard ticks exhibit a moderate degree of host specificity and distinct preferences are seen. A few ticks feed on the same host in all stages, but most utilize at least two different vertebrate hosts during their development, with the earlier stages tending to parasitize small hosts (rodents, rabbits) and adults (or both adults and nymphs) selecting larger animals (deer, dogs, man). Those ticks whose life

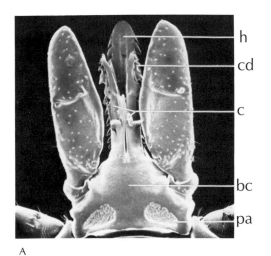

A

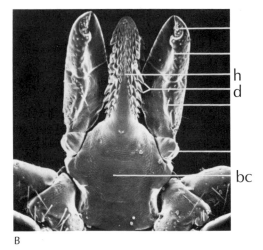

B

Fig. 17–11. *Ixodes affinis.* Gnathosoma of female. *A,* Dorsal view. *B,* Ventral view. (× ca. 90.) *bc,* Basis capitulum. *c,* Chelicerae. *cd,* Cheliceral digits. *d,* Denticles of the hypostome. *h,* Hypostome. *pa,* Porose area. *pl,* Segments 1 to 4 of palp. (From Keirans, J.E., and Clifford, C.M. 1978. The genus *Ixodes* in the United States: A scanning electron microscope study and key to the adults. J. Med. Entomol., Suppl. 2:41.)

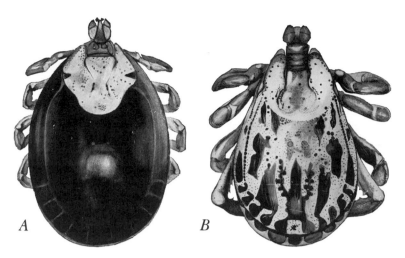

Fig. 17–12. Hard tick, *Dermacentor andersoni,* dorsal view. *A,* Female. *B,* Male. Enlarged. (From Stitt, E.D. 1929. *Diagnostics and Treatment of Tropical Diseases.* New York, The Blakiston Division, McGraw-Hill.)

cycles involve two or more hosts, the second of which is man, are instrumental in the transmission of the zoonotic diseases. Since ixodid ticks remain on the host for relatively long periods of time, dropping off randomly at the cessation of feeding, their distribution tends to be widespread and follows the range of their host.

Medical Importance. The hard ticks produce a certain amount of trauma to the skin when they feed, and the usual problems related to hypersensitivity to arthropod bites may arise in some individuals. Additionally, toxic substances in the salivary secretions of some ticks may lead to a serious disease known as *tick paralysis.* The hard ticks are also responsible for the transmission of a number of diseases of varying etiology in man or animals.

TICK BITES

The actual penetration of the skin by the chelicerae and hypostome of the feeding tick ordinarily goes unnoticed, since the procedure is usually painless. The fluid from a pair of salivary glands prevents coagulation of blood. The properties of the salivary secretions of ticks and other acarines have been reviewed by Sauer (1977). The combined mechanical and digestive action provokes an inflammatory reaction in the perivascular tissues of the corium, with local hyperemia, edema, pruritus, and hemorrhage, together with a thickening of the stratum corneum. Lesions may persist for several days to a week or more after the tick is removed, and certain individuals may exhibit a generalized hypersensitivity reaction.

When people are exposed to infestation by ticks

an end of the day tick inspection is in order, particularly with children. Care should be taken in removing ticks that are firmly anchored in the skin. The application of substances such as chloroform, lighter fluid, oil, petroleum jelly, or fingernail polish will often cause the tick to relax its hold. The anterior portion of the tick should then be grasped with forceps, and a slow but steady pull exerted straight out from the skin. This will usually remove the entire tick. If the mouthparts break off in the skin, attempts should be made to remove them because a severe and often painful foreign body reaction may result.

TICK PARALYSIS

A serious disease associated primarily with the Ixodidae is tick paralysis. This condition has been reported in man and animals (dogs, cattle, birds) throughout the world and is discussed in detail by Murnaghan and O'Rourke (1978) and Gothe *et al.* (1979). Paralysis may develop from a tick attached to any part of the body but is more serious when the tick is located in the occipital region, back of the neck, or along the spinal column.

The syndrome involves no etiologic agent other than the tick itself and is characterized by a general toxemia with elevations of temperature to 40°C (104°F), rapidly developing ascending paralysis, difficulty in swallowing and breathing, and at times is fatal. Children are more adversely affected than adults. Manifestations may develop within 24 hours to several days following attachment and progress in severity as long as the tick is still feeding. The disease appears to be caused by substances in the tick's salivary secretions that prevent impulses from traversing the terminal nerve fibers. Prompt removal of feeding ticks is instrumental in preventing tick paralysis, or if the disease has developed, the removal of the tick usually results in immediate improvement and complete remission within 1 to 3 days, even in severe cases.

The toxin is most highly concentrated in adult female ticks. The species most frequently involved in the United States are *Dermacentor andersoni* in the western and northwestern part and *D. variabilis, Amblyomma americanum,* and *A. maculatum* in the eastern and southeastern areas.

THE SPOTTED FEVERS

The spotted fevers constitute a group of zoonotic diseases in different parts of the world (North and South America, Asia, Australia, and the Mediterranean region). Although bearing different names, they are clinically similar and are produced by closely related rickettsiae. The North American form is *Rocky Mountain spotted fever* (RMSF), also known as *tick typhus.* Contrary to the implication of its name, RMSF is found predominantly in the eastern portion of the United States, with most human infections being reported from the Appalachian region.

Small wild rodents and rabbits are known to be infected in nature. Ticks acquire the etiologic agent *Rickettsia rickettsii* during feeding and these microorganisms invade the tissues of the tick, including the salivary glands and ovaries. A propagative type of development occurs within the tick and the rickettsiae are introduced into the vertebrate host (including man) through the *salivary secretions.* The invasion of the tick's ovaries and the developing eggs leads to the *transovarial transmission* to the tick's progeny. This mechanism enables the ticks themselves to serve, at least for a few generations, as reservoir hosts of the agent.

The disease in man is of an acute, febrile, exanthematous type. Onset is sudden after an incubation period of 3 to 10 days, with high fever, chills, and headaches. A maculopapular rash, usually starting on the palms and soles on about the third day, spreads rapidly to the whole body. Petechial and ecchymotic hemorrhages are common. The disease lasts 2 to 3 weeks and has a fatal outcome in about one fifth of the untreated cases. Complement fixation tests with group-specific spotted fever antigens are positive in the second week of infection. The treatment of RMSF with tetracyclines or chloramphenicol generally yields

a good prognosis. A single infection confers long-lasting immunity.

The prevention of RMSF can be achieved by immunization or through avoidance of tick bites. Persons spending extended periods of time outdoors in enzootic areas should receive the vaccine (dead rickettsiae) and maintain immunity with annual booster inoculations. Proper dress is useful in avoiding tick bites. Shirttails should be tucked in and trouser legs should be covered with long socks or stuffed inside boot tops. Since ticks quest on low vegetation and crawl upward on the body to seek a feeding site, dressing as suggested usually forces them to move to the neck, where they are more readily felt and can be brushed or picked off. Feeding ticks should be removed as soon as possible, since the probability of becoming infected with the rickettsiae increases with the length of time they remain attached to the skin. The use of tick repellents is also recommended.

The prevalence of RMSF has increased in the eastern and southeastern United States over the last two decades, with women and children accounting for a large proportion of this rise (Burgdorfer, 1977). The movement of large populations into newly developed suburban areas has apparently influenced the changes (Hoogstraal, 1981). The role of pets (dogs in particular) has been recognized. Infected ticks brought back to the environs of homes by dogs drop off and transovarially infected populations may build up locally. The use of tick repellent collars appears to aid in reducing this risk.

The most important vectors of RMSF in the United States are the Rocky Mountain wood tick *Dermacentor andersoni* in the west, the American dog tick *D. variabilis* in the east and southeast, and the Lone Star tick *Ambylomma americanum* in Texas and Oklahoma.

OTHER IXODID-TRANSMITTED DISEASES

Colorado tick fever, a self-limiting benign zoonosis of viral etiology, is encountered in the western portions of the United States and Canada. Small rodents serve as reservoir hosts and *Dermacentor andersoni* is a common vector. Most human infections occur during the warmer months of the year, coinciding with outdoor recreational and occupational activities.

In different parts of the world there are several tick-borne viral diseases, some of considerable severity. These are all zoonotic in nature, usually involving wild rodents and rabbits as reservoirs. They include such encephalitides as *Russian spring–summer encephalitis* (RSSE), *central European encephalitis* (CEE), *louping ill* (in the British Isles), and *Powassan encephalitis* (sporadic in the northwest United States and in Canada). Likewise of viral etiology and sometimes fatal are *Omsk hemorrhagic fever* in Siberia and *Crimean-Congo hemorrhagic fever* in Europe, Asia, and Africa (Simpson, 1978).

Human *babesiosis* (see Chapter 6, p. 72) caused by the protozoan *Babesia microti* has been reported in man in New England. Small rodents serve as reservoirs for this organism and the tick *Ixodes dammini*, which normally feeds on deer in its adult stage, is the presumed vector for human infections (Spielman *et al.*, 1979).

Lyme disease, a curious form of inflammatory oligoarticular arthritis with occasional resultant cardiopathy, was first observed in Old Lyme, Connecticut (Steere *et al.*, 1977). This was associated with the bite of *Ixodes dammini*, but only recently (Steere *et al.*, 1983) has a spirochetal etiology of this puzzling disease been established.

Although hard ticks have been implicated in the *mechanical transmission* of several infectious diseases, including Q fever caused by the rickettsia *Coxiella burnetti* and tularemia or "rabbit fever" caused by the bacterium *Francisella tularensis*, the actual role of these hematophagous arthropods in the epidemiology of these agents is probably marginal.

SOFT TICKS (ARGASIDAE)

Morphology and Bionomics. The soft ticks are characterized by a flexible, leathery body that lacks a chitinous dorsal scutum (Fig. 17–13). The capitulum is located on the anteroventral surface and does not project beyond the anterior margin of the body. Argasid ticks, in contrast to the ixodids, pass through up to five nymphal instars in their development. Soft ticks differ markedly from the hard ticks in their habitats and behavior, spending nearly all their time secreted away in the dwelling of the host (rodent nest, den, thatched hut). Feeding is rapid and frequent, being completed within only a few minutes, usually while the host is sleeping. Since these ticks do not remain on their hosts for any appreciable amount of time, their dispersion is limited and isolated stable focal concentrations tend to occur. Of the four genera in this family, only the genus *Ornithodoros* has species of particular medical concern.

Medical Importance. The bites of argasid ticks

may be irritating and at times painful, but reactions are usually transient. Problems encountered with the prolonged attachment by hard ticks are not seen.

ENDEMIC RELAPSING FEVER

Endemic relapsing fever, also known as *recurrent fever* or *tick-borne relapsing fever*, is of spirochetal etiology, being caused by various strains of *Borrelia duttoni* and other closely related species. This relatively mild disease is characterized by repeated episodes of fever lasting 2 to 9 days, separated by afebrile periods of 2 to 4 days. The epidemic form of relapsing fever transmitted by body lice (Chapter 16, p. 211) is usually more severe. Treatment is by administration of tetracycline antibiotics.

Transmission of the spirochetes involves multiplication of the organisms within the tissues of the tick and their subsequent injection into the skin with the *salivary secretions*. Additionally, the *coxal glands*, structures unique to the soft ticks, are invaded, and when the tick feeds, fluid elaborated from these glands spills onto the surface of the skin, supplying still more spirochetes which enter the lesion. As is common with the acari in general, *transovarial transmission* of the disease agent occurs within the *Ornithodoros* population.

Tick-borne relapsing fever exists enzootically in many parts of the world where a variety of mammals, most commonly wild rodents, function as the principal (reservoir) hosts. In most regions, including the western United States, human infections are sporadic and result from man's encroachment on the habitats of the reservoir hosts and their ticks (camping, military operations). The epidemiologic conditions in parts of Africa are different, however; there the vectors establish themselves within the thatching of the huts, and the spirochetes are transmitted from person to person.

Several species of *Ornithodoros*, each with its own serotypically distinct strain of *Borrelia*, are involved in the transmission of the relapsing fevers throughout the world (Hoogstraal, 1979). In the United States, *O. turicata*, *O. parkeri*, *O. hermsi*, and *O. talaje* are the important vectors. The principal domestic vector in Africa is *O. moubata*.

Control. The control of soft ticks and the avoidance of their bites are difficult in view of their elusive nature; however, the use of acaricidal dusts such as propoxur, lindane, malathion, and carbaryl may be effective.

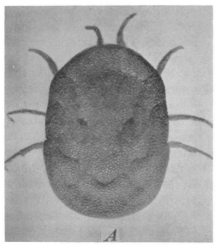
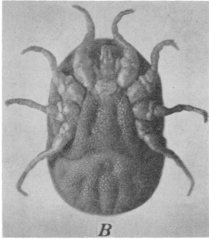

Fig. 17–13.   Soft tick, *Ornithodoros moubata*, female. *A*, Dorsal view. *B*, Ventral view. (× 7.) (From Jirovec, O.: Parasitologie pro Lékare. Prague, Melantrich, 1948.)

Mites (Acariformes)

While sharing many features with the ticks, the mites can be distinguished by their minute size (usually less than 1 mm long) and by the absence of teeth on the hypostome. The Acariformes is an enormous and for the most part confusing assemblage of highly diversified arthropods. Mites are to be found throughout the world occupying nearly every conceivable ecologic niche; most are free-living, existing as scavengers or predators of other small organisms. Some are important parasites of wild and domestic animals. Relatively few members of only three or four of the major subgroups are of direct medical concern.

The life histories of mites resemble those of the ticks. Additional stages may occur in some, but such details are not essential in the present consideration. Compared with ticks, the mites have a much shorter generation time and individual life span—days or weeks as opposed to months or years.

RODENT AND BIRD MITES: ORDER PARASITIFORMES
(Suborder Gamasida or Mesostigmata)

Members of the Parasitiformes are more ticklike in their appearance than the other mites of medical concern (Fig. 17–14). The genera most commonly affecting man are *Ornithonyssus, Dermanyssus,* and *Liponyssoides (= Allodermanyssus)*. These mites live in nests of rodents and birds closely associated with man. They periodically feed on the blood and tissue juices of their preferred host, but

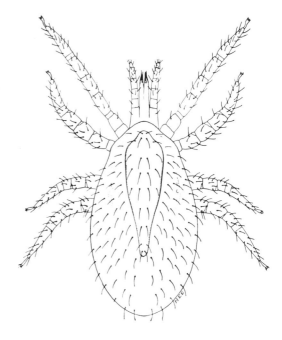

Fig. 17–14.   Tropical rat mite, *Ornithonyssus bacoti*. Greatly enlarged. (From Ewing, H.E. 1929. *External Parasites.* Springfield, Ill., Charles C Thomas, p. 15.)

when those hosts die or leave, or the nests are disturbed, the mites often seek blood meals elsewhere, and will attack man.

Ornithonyssus bacoti is the common rat mite of warm climates, including the southern United States, and frequently causes problems in any structure or habitation infested with rats. Other species of *Ornithonyssus (e.g., O. bursa)* and of the genus *Dermanyssus* are associated with sparrows and pigeons that nest under eaves or in attics of houses, and with domestic poultry. The bites of these and other related mites are somewhat painful, quite irritating, and may produce sleepless nights and disruption of domestic tranquility when they invade houses. The lesions produced are varied but ordinarily benign; urticarial wheals, papules, vesicles, and occasionally hemorrhagic necrosis may develop at the site of the puncture. Treatment is the same as that followed for insect bites.

Although most of these common mites are not known to transmit disease to man, an exception is seen with *Liponyssoides sanguineus,* an ectoparasite of mice and rats. A mild exanthematous febrile zoonosis *(rickettsialpox)* caused by *Rickettsia akari,* immunologically related to the rickettsia causing RMSF, has been reported from several cities in the northeastern United States (New York, Boston, Hartford, and Cleveland), where it occurs endemically and occasionally in epidemic form.

The control of rat and bird mites in dwellings usually requires the elimination of the hosts, accompanied by the use of acaricidal dusts or residual sprays, particularly in nesting areas and portals of access for the mites, such as windowsills and air ducts.

CHIGGERS AND RELATED MITES: OTHER ACARIFORMS
(Suborder Actinedida or Prostigmata)

Chiggers

Chiggers, also called *harvest mites* and *"red bugs,"* belong to the family Trombiculidae and are well known for their irritating bites (Fig. 17–15). Only the 6-legged larval trombiculid is parasitic; subsequent stages are free-living and are found in habitats such as leaf litter and beneath loose tree bark. Most larval trombiculids can be recognized by the presence of plumose (featherlike) hairs on the body and legs.

Chiggers (the larval stage) have a broad host range that includes birds, reptiles, and mammals. These minute acarines are not strictly hematophagous but rather feed on the contents of dermal cells. In the process of feeding, which may take several days, a conduit *stylostome* is induced within the tissue. The larval trombiculid does not burrow as is commonly thought but remains on the surface of the skin.

DERMATITIS. People throughout most of the world are familiar with the irritation of chigger bites. In tropical and subtropical regions, biting

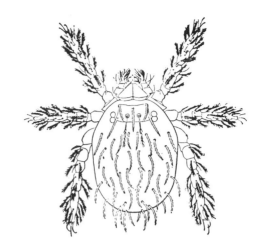

Fig. 17–15. Chigger (*Leptotrombidium akamushi,* larva). Greatly enlarged. (Adapted from Nagayo, M., et al. 1921. Five species of tsutsugamushi (the carrier of Japanese river fever) and their relation to the tsutsugamushi disease. Am. J. Hyg., *1*:569–591.)

activity may be felt all year long; in temperate areas, definite "chigger seasons" occur during the warmer months.

The cutaneous reaction to the trauma and salivary secretions begins 12 to 24 hours after attachment, appearing as a minute red elevation. This becomes pruritic and is followed by development of a wheal. As a result of unrestrained scratching, secondary infection with pustule formation is common. This may become serious when infection of adjoining bites becomes confluent. Chiggers often feed on the body in sites where the clothing is tightly appressed, such as the elastic bands on socks and underwear and at the beltline. Although various "remedies" for chiggers abound (application of nail polish or removing the mite with tape or digging it out with a sharp needle), none of these is particularly useful, since once the chigger has begun to feed the duration of the dermatitis is not appreciably affected.

Prevention of infestation by chiggers can be achieved to a great extent by simply tucking trouser legs into boot tops, since these mites are usually encountered on grass or low vegetation. Like ticks, larval trombiculids crawl upward on the body until they reach skin. The additional use of common repellents such as dibutylphthalate and dimethylphthalate is also effective.

SCRUB TYPHUS. An acute exanthematous febrile disease known as scrub typhus or *tsutsugamushi fever* is caused by *Rickettsia tsutsugamushi* and is enzootic principally in field mice, wild rats, shrews, and voles. Its geographic distribution encompasses parts of east and southeast Asia and northern Australia, and of the Pacific islands in that general area. The disease is usually mild and lasts only about 2 weeks. In some areas, however, largely dependent on the rickettsial strain, an appreciable mortality rate of up to 40% may occur. In general, an excellent prognosis is afforded by treatment with chloramphenicol or tetracycline antibiotics.

The vectors of scrub typhus (*Leptotrombidium deliense, L. akamushi,* and others) pass the rickettsiae *transovarially* from one generation to the next within the mite population. This mechanism is *essential* for the transmission of the disease to man or other vertebrate hosts, since *only* the larval stage of the mite is parasitic and each larva feeds only on *one* host. The trombiculids responsible for transmitting scrub typhus are often closely associated with a particular reservoir host. As a result, a very spotty distribution of infected vectors may occur; this corresponds to the locations of stable populations of burrowing rodents that maintain the enzooticity of the rickettsiae. These rather sharply delimited foci are known as "mite islands," and when their locations are known they can be avoided or control measures (*e.g.,* forcing acaricidal dusts into the rodent burrows) can be undertaken. These and other epidemiologic aspects of scrub typhus are reviewed by Traub and Wisseman (1974).

Other Actinedid Mites

FOLLICULAR MITES. Two species of follicular mites, *Demodex folliculorum* and *D. brevis* (family Demodicidae) very commonly infect man, being found within or associated with the sebaceous glands of the face, particularly in the areas of the nose and forehead. These mites are minute (100 to 400 μm long) and vermiform, with stumpy legs. Although related species produce devastating mange in dogs and other mammals, the *Demodex* of man are usually nonpathogenic and remain unnoticed. Occasionally there may be a mild rosaceous pruritus with a slight local fibrous tissue response. When treatment is indicated, lindane ointment and bactericidal lotions are useful.

PREDACEOUS MITES. Some species of the family Pyemotidae such as the straw itch mite (*Pyemotes tritici*) are known to bite man, producing painful lesions that occasionally lead to transient systemic manifestations (Moser, 1975). These mites feed on the larvae of insects that infest seeds, grain, and plant stems. They are sometimes encountered in large numbers in straw mattresses, granaries, or beneath old houses in the debris from tunnels produced by wood-boring beetles.

CHEYLETIELLID MITES. Certain members of the family Cheyletiellidae associated with pets (dogs, cats, rabbits) may bite man and cause a pruritic dermatitis. These mites do not burrow within the skin, however, and infestations are transient. The clinical aspects attributed to these mites are discussed by Cohen (1980) and Shelley *et al.* (1984).

ITCH OR MANGE MITES: ORDER ACARIFORMES
(Suborder Acaridida or Astigmata)

There are several genera and species of itch mites, most of which are in the family Sarcoptidae. They produce severe mange in pets and domestic animals. Fortunately, they do not establish themselves in the skin of man, and at worst human contact may result in a slight rash of short duration. However, a single species of acaridid mite, *Sarcoptes scabiei,* does infest man and commonly produces severe dermatitis. This disease is known variously as *scabies, "seven-year itch," sarcoptic mange,* and *scabetic mange.*

Sarcoptes scabiei (Fig. 17–16) is a minute (450 μm and smaller) ovoid mite with four pairs of inconspicuous stubby legs, the anterior two being widely separated from the posterior two. The first two pairs of legs of females (first three of males) bear a terminal stalk ending in a minute disclike sucker. The cuticle has transverse striations and conspicuous hairs; the dorsal surface has several stout teeth or spines.

Sarcoptes scabiei inhabits the epidermis, where the females excavate tunnels up to 3 cm long. Oviposition takes place within these tunnels, and the life span of these mites is approximately 2 months. Larvae migrate to the surface of the skin where, within about a week, development to the adult stage is completed. After mating, the males and females burrow into the skin.

Scabies

Scabies may occur on any part of the body, but those regions most commonly affected are the interdigital webs and backs of the hands, beneath the breasts, and between the belly folds of babies. The metabolic products (secretions, excretions) as well as mite substances (egg shells, dead adults) are offensive to the tissues, and intensely pruritic, short, linear, reddish lesions are produced. Sometimes scabies may appear as an indeterminant urticaria (Chapel *et al.,* 1981). Vesicles and papules are frequently present. Scratching often leads to

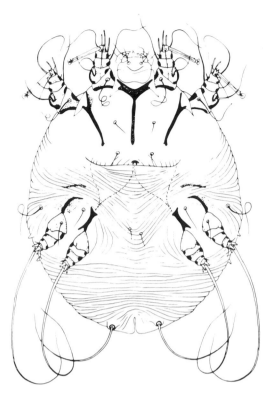

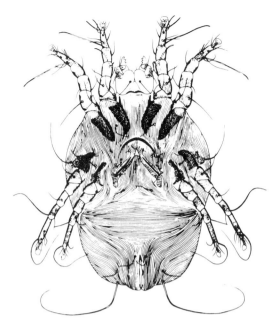

Fig. 17–17. Dust mite, *Dermatophagoides pteronyssinus*. Female, ventral view. Greatly enlarged. (From Fain, A. 1966. Nouvelle description de *Dermatophagoides pteronyssinus* [Trouessart, 1897]. Importance de cet acarien en pathologie humaine [Psoroptidae: Sarcoptiformes]. Acarologia, 8:302–327.)

Fig. 17–16. *Sarcoptes scabiei*. Female, ventral view. (From Fain, A. 1968. Étude de la variabilité de *Sarcoptes scabiei* avec une révision des Sarcoptidae. Acta Zool. Pathol. Antverp, 47:1–196.)

secondary bacterial infection with pustule formation, and in severe cases to weeping and bleeding. With time, small, rather innocuous initial lesions spread as the mite population grows and invasion of the skin progresses. An unusual type, often termed ''Norwegian scabies,'' may involve the formation of keratotic excrescences on extensive areas of the body and relatively little pruritus (Youshock and Glazer, 1981).

The diagnosis of scabies is usually made on the basis of the characteristic appearance and locations of the pruritic lesions. It is best to obtain a definitive identification by scraping the excoriated skin associated with the tunnels onto a microscope slide, adding 10% KOH as a clearing agent, and directly observing the eggs and mites.

The treatment of scabies involves the application of 10% crotamiton in a vanishing cream base or 1% lindane (gamma isomer of hexachlorocyclohexane) in a lotion or ointment base to the affected areas after the skin has been thoroughly scrubbed clean and softened by washing with soap. One to three treatments ordinarily results in a clinical cure.

Scabies is worldwide in its distribution, and although it is most commonly found in conditions of poverty, crowding, and poor sanitation, such as in institutions, its prevalence in the more affluent segments of the population is rising. *Sarcoptes scabiei* is truly contagious in its transmission from person to person by simple direct contact and by fomites.

Various aspects of *Sarcoptes* and scabies have been reviewed by Andrews and Desch (1983), Parish *et al.* (1983), Millikan (1983), and Bikowski (1983).

Food and House Dust Mites

Several genera of acaridid mites are commonly found in foodstuffs and plant materials. Contact with them may lead to temporary irritation of the skin, although they neither bite nor burrow. The benign but annoying condition known as ''grocer's itch'' is of this type and involves mites contaminating cheese and a wide variety of stored food products. These mites may also act as allergenic agents of asthmatic bronchitis (Ingram *et al.*, 1979).

Of somewhat more serious nature are the consequences of human exposure to the so-called house dust mites (Fig. 17–17). Members of the genus *Dermatophagoides* (*D. farinae* in the United States) are most commonly found in intimate association with man. They feed on organic debris such as sloughed human skin flakes, fungi, spilled food, and pollen. They, their fecal pellets, cast-off cuticula, and fragments of the dead mites are ubiquitous within the home, being found in dust and particularly on carpeted floors and in upholstered furniture. These mites not only concentrate antigens that they use for food but the mite substances themselves are allergens (Wharton, 1976).

A previously unrecognized disease, now known as Kawasaki syndrome, was first described in Japan and reported soon afterward in the United States. The etiology of the syndrome is uncertain, although it is associated with house dust and with *Dermatophagoides* in particular. Clinically, Kawasaki syndrome includes fever, bilateral conjunctival infection, inflammation of the mucous membranes of the mouth, erythema of the palms and soles, rash, and cervical lymphadenopathy. This syndrome is usually self-limiting, but rheumatic changes may occur in some children. Coronary aneurysms are seen in 15% to 20% of the patients and subsequent coronary thrombosis leads to sudden death in 1% to 2% of patients with Kawasaki syndrome (Yanigahara and Todd, 1980; Melish, 1981).

Several isolated cases and outbreaks have been reported in the United States (CDC, 1983). This syndrome is usually seen in infants and preschool children and its onset often occurs within 1 month after shampooing carpets.

SUMMARY

1. Certain crustaceans (*e.g.,* crab and crayfish) serve as intermediate hosts for the lung fluke, *Paragonimus*. Minute aquatic copepods are intermediate hosts for some nematodes (*Dracunculus*) and cestodes (*Diphyllobothrium,* sparganum).
2. Pentastomids, or tongue worms, are parasitic in the respiratory tracts of reptiles and some mammals. Immature stages of these highly modified organisms infect man, particularly in tropical Asia and Africa, although a few infections with *Linguatula* have been reported from the United States.
3. Centipedes have poison glands in specialized claws; their bites may be painful but are usually benign. Millipedes, except for certain tropical species, are harmless. They do not bite but rather secrete offensive (rarely vesicating) substances.
4. Arachnids are arthropods that are distinguished from insects in that they have four pairs of legs in the adult stage and their body is divided into two rather than three parts. Scorpions, spiders, ticks, and mites belong to this group.
5. Scorpions are characterized by large pedipalps modified

into claws and by the slender posterior part of the abdomen that terminates in a spine through which a venom gland opens. Most scorpion stings are painful but not deadly. *Centruroides sculpturatus* in the area of Arizona is the only dangerous species in the United States.
6. Only a few spiders are dangerous. The venom may be neurotoxic, producing a systemic reaction (*e.g.,* black widow or *Latrodectus mactans),* or necrotoxic, producing ulcerous cutaneous lesions (*e.g.,* brown recluse spider, *Loxosceles reclusa).*
7. Hard ticks (Ixodidae) spend prolonged periods of time on their hosts. Bites can be irritating, and some species have substances in their salivary secretions that may produce a systemic neurologic reaction—tick paralysis. The most important diseases (all zoonotic) transmitted to man by hard ticks are the spotted fevers (rickettsial), Colorado tick fever (viral), some of the European and Asian hemorrhagic fevers (viral), and Lyme disease (spirochetal).
8. Soft ticks (Argasidae) spend most of their time in burrows of their host animals. Their primary medical importance is in the transmission of endemic relapsing fever (spirochetal) worldwide (including the western United States).
9. Mites resemble ticks in structure but are much smaller. Some rodent and bird mites (*Ornithonyssus, Dermanyssus)* occasionally invade houses and produce irritating bites. Chiggers (larvae of *Trombicula* and others) cause irritation by their bites worldwide; in Southeast Asia certain chiggers transmit scrub typhus (rickettsial) from wild rodents to man. The itch mite *Sarcoptes scabiei* invades the skin and produces a severe dermatitis—scabies. Transmission is by direct contact, and the prevalence of scabies is increasing in the United States. Some mites found in stored food products may produce dermatitis or asthma. Certain house dust mites (*Dermatophagoides* spp.) have been associated with Kawasaki syndrome, a severe disease of preschool children in Japan and the United States.

REFERENCES

Andrews, J.R.H., and Desch, C.E., Jr. 1983. The morphology, life history and habitat of *Sarcoptes scabiei.* In *Cutaneous Infestations of Man and Animal.* Edited by L.C. Parish, W.B. Nutting, and R.M. Schwartzman. New York, Praeger, pp. 53–69.

Berger, R.S. 1982. Spider (brown recluse and black widow) bites and scorpion stings. In *Current Therapy 1982.* Edited by H.F. Conn. Philadelphia, W.B. Saunders Co., pp. 959–960.

Bettini, S. (ed.) 1978. *Arthropod Venoms. Handbook of Experimental Pharmacology,* n.s., vol. 48. New York, Springer-Verlag.

———, and Maroli, M. 1978. Venoms of Theridiidae, genus *Latrodectus.* A. Systematics, distribution and biology of species; chemistry, pharmacology and mode of action of venom. In *Arthropod Venoms.* Edited by S. Bettini. New York, Academic Press, pp. 149–184.

Bikowski, J.B. 1983. Institutional instructions for treatment of scabies. In *Cutaneous Infestations of Man and Animal.* Edited by L.C. Parish, W.B. Nutting, and R.M. Schwartzman. New York, Praeger, pp. 100–105.

Burgdorfer, W. 1977. Tick-borne diseases in the United States: Rocky Mountain spotted fever and Colorado tick fever. Acta Trop., *34*:103–126.

Centers for Disease Control. 1983. Epidemiologic notes and reports. Kawasaki syndrome—United States. Morbidity and Mortality Weekly Reports, *32*:98–100.

Chapel, T.A., Krugel, L., Chapel, J., and Segal, A. 1981. Scabies presenting as urticaria. J.A.M.A., 246:1440–1441.

Cohen, S.R. 1980. *Cheyletiella* dermatitis. Arch. Dermatol., 116:435–437.

Esslinger, J.H. 1962. Hepatic lesions in rats experimentally infected with *Porocephalus crotali* (Pentastomida). J. Parasitol., 48:631–638.

Fain, A. 1975. The Pentastomida parasitic in man. Ann. Soc. Belge Med. Trop., 55:59–64.

Foil, L.D., and Norment, B.R. 1979. Envenomation by *Loxosceles reclusa*. J. Med. Entomol., 16:18–25.

Gertsch, W.J. 1979. *American Spiders*. New York, Van Nostrand Reinhold Co.

Gothe, R., Kunze, K., and Hoogstraal, H. 1979. The mechanisms of pathogenicity in the tick paralyses. J. Med. Entomol., 16:357–369.

Hoogstraal, H. 1979. Ticks and spirochetes. Acta Trop., 36:133–136.

———. 1981. Changing patterns of tickborne diseases in modern society. Annu. Rev. Entomol., 26:75–99.

Ingram, C.G., Jeffrey, I.G., Symington, I.S., and Cuthbert, O.D. 1979. Bronchial provocation studies in farmers allergic to storage mites. Lancet, 2:1330–1332.

Keegan, H.L. 1980. *Scorpions of Medical Importance*. Jackson, University Press of Mississippi.

King, L.E., and Rees, R.S. 1983. Dapsone treatment of a brown recluse bite. J.A.M.A., 250:648.

Melish, M.E. 1981. Kawasaki syndrome: A new infectious disease? J. Infec. Dis., 143:317–324.

Millikan, L.E. 1983. Scabies in the compromised host. In *Cutaneous Infestations of Man and Animal*. Edited by L.C. Parish, W.B. Nutting, and R.M. Schwartzman. New York, Praeger, pp. 79–84.

Minelli, A. 1978. Secretions of centipedes. In *Arthropod Venoms*. Edited by S. Bettini. New York, Academic Press, pp. 73–86.

Moser, J.C. 1975. Biosystematics of the straw itch mite with special reference to nomenclature and dermatology. Trans. Roy. Entomol. Soc. London, 127:185–191.

Murnaghan, M.F., and O'Rourke, F.J. 1978. Tick paralysis. In *Arthropod Venoms*. Edited by S. Bettini. New York, Academic Press, pp. 419–464.

Parish, L.C., Witkowski, J.A., and Cohen, H.B. 1983. Clinical picture of scabies. In *Cutaneous Infestations of Man and Animal*. Edited by L.C. Parish, W.B. Nutting, and R.M. Schwartzman. New York, Praeger, pp. 70–78.

Radford, A.J. 1975. Millipede burns in man. Trop. Geogr. Med., 27:279–287.

Riley, J., Banaja, A.A., and James, J.L. 1978. The phylogenetic relationships of the Pentastomida: The case for their inclusion within the Crustacea. Int. J. Parasitol., 8:245–254.

Sauer, J.R. 1977. Acarine salivary glands—physiological relationships. J. Med. Entomol., 14:1–9.

Schenone, H., and Suarez, G. 1978. Venoms of Scytotidae. Genus *Loxosceles*. In *Arthropod Venoms*. Edited by S. Bettini. New York, Academic Press, pp. 247–278.

Self, J.T., Hopps, H.C., and Williams, A.O. 1975. Pentastomiasis in Africans. Trop. Geogr. Med., 27:1–13.

Shelley, E.D., Shelley, W.B., Pula, J.F., and McDonald, S.G. 1984. The diagnostic challenge of nonburrowing mite bites: *Cheyletiella yasguri*. JAMA, 251:2690–2691.

Simpson, D.I.H. 1978. Viral haemorrhagic fevers of man. Bull. W.H.O., 56:819–832.

Spielman, A., Clifford, C.M., Piesman, J., and Corwin, M.D. 1979. Human babesiosis on Nantucket Island, U.S.A.: Description of the vector, *Ixodes (Ixodes) dammini* n. sp. (Acarina: Ixodidae). J. Med. Entomol., 15:218–234.

Steere, A.C., Grodzicki, R.L., Kornblatt, A.N., Craft, J.E., Barbour, A.G., Burgdorfer, W., Schmid, G., Johnson, E., and Malawista, S.E. 1983. The spirochetal etiology of Lyme disease. N. Engl. J. Med., 308:733–740.

———, Malawista, S.E., Hardin, J.A., Ruddy, S., Askenase, P.W., and Andiman, W.A. 1977. Erythema chronicum migrans and Lyme arthritis: The enlarging clinical spectrum. Ann. Intern. Med., 86:685–698.

Traub, R., and Wisseman, C.L., Jr. 1974. The ecology of chigger-borne rickettsiosis (scrub typhus). J. Med. Entomol., 11:237–303.

Wharton, G.W. 1976. House dust mites, J. Med. Entomol., 12:577–621.

Yanagihara, R., and Todd, J.K. 1980. Acute febrile mucocutaneous lymph node syndrome. Am. J. Dis. Child., 134:603–614.

Youshock, E., and Glazer, S.D. 1981. Norwegian scabies in a renal transplant patient. J.A.M.A., 246:2608–2609.

Section V

Aids to Diagnosis and Treatment

Chapter 18

Diagnostic Materials and Methods

M. D. Little and R. G. Yaeger

In order to properly evaluate the clinical and public health implications of parasites and vectors, the organisms involved must be accurately diagnosed. Thus, adequately trained personnel and suitable laboratory facilities are indispensable, whether the focus is on the individual patient or on population groups.

EQUIPMENT AND SUPPLIES

Unless the laboratory is devoted exclusively to parasitology, provision must be made in the general laboratory, preferably in a separate room, for doing the essential coprologic, hematologic, and other parasitologic examinations.

There must be a good compound microscope for the person doing parasitologic diagnosis. For study of macroscopic specimens such as helminths, surgical biopsies, or arthropods, it is desirable to have a binocular dissecting microscope. Additional microscopic equipment should include a micrometer disc to be placed in the eyepiece and a micrometer slide to calibrate the divisions in the micrometer disc for the particular microscope and for each of the eyepieces and objectives employed. If a micrometer slide is not available, the units in a hemacytometer slide may be substituted in making the calibration. Laboratories using fluorescent antibody diagnostic methods will require a compound microscope designed for such work. There should be a good incubator, water bath, drying oven, clinical centrifuge, and steam sterilizer. Reagent bottles, Petri dishes, staining dishes, Pyrex-type beakers, flasks, centrifuge tubes, test tubes, and pipettes of graded sizes, graduate cylinders, microscope slides, and coverglasses (22 × 22 mm) must be available in good supply. A suitable type of specimen container is a 2-oz glass or plastic bottle with a screw top, which can be used for samples of feces, urine, and sputum.

Routine examination of fresh fecal films requires conveniently placed dropping bottles of physiologic salt solution and aqueous iodine solution. Concentration techniques require large supplies of the principal reagents. For fixation of fecal films, Schaudinn's fluid is most frequently employed. For fixing tissues, buffered (pH 7.2) 10% formalin is recommended. For staining of fecal films, the iron-hematoxylin technique or the trichrome technique can be used. For blood films, best results usually are obtained with the Giemsa stain.

EXAMINATION OF FECES

Collection of Specimens

The following sections describe some of the commonly used methods for collecting stool specimens and examining them for intestinal parasites. More comprehensive coverage may be found in a laboratory manual by Melvin and Brooke (1982).

A normal stool consists almost exclusively of feces, but the dysenteric stool may consist of blood and mucus and a considerable amount of cellular exudate and sloughed tissue. At times these portions of the stool provide evidence of parasitic infection when the specimen is otherwise negative. Similarly, *Ascaris, Enterobius,* and proglottids of *Taenia* and *Dipylidium* may be passed without the presence of their eggs in the fecal part of the specimen. Stools may also contain large amounts of undigested food or medication. It is therefore important that the material submitted for examination be sufficient for dependable diagnosis. Gross inspection of the specimen should always precede microscopic examination.

Collection should be made in a clean container without contamination by water or urine. The specimen must be free of oil, magnesia, aluminum salts, and barium.

Formed stools can usually be kept for one or more days, preferably under refrigeration, without loss of the diagnostic integrity of parasite objects. Unformed stools should be examined promptly. For periods of several hours and sometimes longer good preservation is obtained by refrigeration at 3° to 10°C. For reliable and lasting preservation, chemical fixation is required.

Preservation of Helminths

Most helminths do not require delicate techniques for satisfactory preservation. Tapeworms, trematodes, and nematodes usually fix well in hot (65°C) 5% formalin or AFA fixative (10 ml formalin, 50 ml 95% ethanol, 5 ml glacial acetic acid, and 45 ml distilled water). In case large tapeworms are to be used as demonstration specimens, they should be chilled and placed in the desired position before fixation.

Preservation of Fecal Samples

Formalin. Eggs and larvae of helminths found in stool specimens or obtained by centrifugation or sedimentation of feces or urine are satisfactorily fixed and preserved for later examination in 10% formalin heated to 65°C (1 part of feces to 5 to 10 parts of 10% formalin). The sample should be thoroughly mixed at the time of fixation. Formalin fixation is less satisfactory for protozoan cysts and does not fix trophozoites in recognizable form.

MIF. The MIF (merthiolate-iodine-formaldehyde) solution can be used to preserve trophozoites and cysts of protozoa as well as eggs and larvae of helminths in fecal specimens. The MIF solution is made by adding 1 part of Lugol's iodine solution (iodine crystals, 5 g, potassium iodide, 10 g, and distilled water,

100 ml) to about 15 parts of MF stock solution immediately before use. The MF stock solution consists of distilled water, 250 ml; tincture of merthiolate (No. 99 Lilly 1:1000), 200 ml; formaldehyde, U.S.P., 25 ml; and glycerol 5 ml. A portion of the fecal sample is thoroughly mixed in about 5 parts of the MIF solution. This method is particularly adapted to field collections (Dunn, 1968). All microscopic parasite objects are well preserved and adequately stained for diagnostic reliability. The preserved material keeps well in a tightly-stoppered bottle for a year or more.

Direct Smear Saline Suspension

Fecal specimens should first be examined microscopically in direct smear preparations containing 1 to 2 mg of feces evenly suspended in 1 drop of physiologic saline solution under a coverglass. These films should be free of air bubbles and macroscopic debris. An unstained film of this type is useful for observing motile trophozoites of intestinal protozoa, helminth eggs, and *Strongyloides* larvae and has considerable diagnostic value for protozoan cysts. For studying the internal diagnostic characteristics of protozoan cysts, iodine stain (1% aqueous solution potassium iodide saturated with iodine crystals) is used. The stain may be placed at the edge of the coverglass and allowed to flow into the film or added to a new preparation before the coverglass is applied. Only enough stain should be used to give the suspension a distinctly yellow hue.

Kato Thick Smear

A cellophane-covered thick smear technique of fecal examination was introduced by Kato and Miura in 1954. It was later adapted to large-scale routine annual examination of school-children and others in an intestinal parasite control program in Japan. Because it proved to be highly effective for the diagnosis of *Necator, Ancylostoma, Trichuris, Ascaris,* and some less common intestinal helminth infections including schistosomiasis mansoni, it soon was widely used elsewhere and was modified and adapted for quantitative (egg counts) as well as qualitative diagnosis (Martin and Beaver, 1968).

Materials Required
1. Glass microscope slide, 1 × 3 inches (26 × 77 mm).
2. Cellophane coverslip, wettable, of medium thickness (No. 134 PD, E.I. DuPont de Nemours, Inc., Film Department, Wilmington, Delaware), cut into 22 × 30 mm rectangles.
3. Glycerin–malachite green solution: 10 ml pure glycerin, 100 ml water, and 1 ml 3% aqueous malachite green. Allow the cellophane strips to soak in the glycerin mixture for at least 24 hours. (Although the malachite green reduces some of the glare at the microscope, it is not essential.)
4. Wooden applicator sticks.
5. For specimens containing large amounts of fiber or seeds, use 105-mesh stainless steel bolting cloth (W.S. Tyler Co., Cleveland, Ohio) or 210-mesh nylon monofilament mesh (Small Parts Inc., Miami, Florida), cut into 4-cm squares.

Procedures
1. With applicator, transfer about 50 mg of feces to a microscope slide. (A 4-mm cube of feces weighs about 65 mg.) When required for fibrous specimens, put 1 or 2 g of feces on a disposable paper sheet, place over it a square of the wire cloth or nylon mesh, and then remove a sample of screened feces with an applicator stick by pushing the cloth into the feces and scraping the applicator stick across the surface of the cloth. If the fecal sample is hard, add drops of water and mix until it is soft enough to process.
2. Cover the fecal sample with a cellophane coverslip,

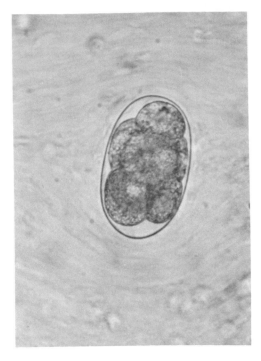

Fig. 18–1. Egg of *Necator americanus* after clearing of feces in a Kato thick smear. (× 540.) (By P.C. Beaver.)

invert the preparation, and press it down against a flat, absorbent surface (such as a sheet of thick, soft paper on a table top) until the fecal mass covers an area 20 to 25 mm in diameter.
3. Allow the smear to stand for about 1 hour at room temperature or for 20 to 30 minutes at 34 to 40°C (in a dry incubator or under an electric lamp). This clears the feces but leaves helminth eggs uncleared (Fig. 18–1). Since overclearing may cause collapse and disappearance of hookworm eggs and sometimes causes schistosome eggs to become indistinct, the preparation is best examined immediately upon clearing. To temporarily stop the clearing-drying process at any desired time, the slide can be inverted and left face-down on a flat, smooth surface.
4. Examine the entire film under low magnification; experienced microscopists can detect and identify eggs under scanning-lens magnification (35 to 45 ×). When overcleared, schistosome eggs must be verified under low power (about 100 ×).

As the film dries, the feces clear more rapidly than the eggs do, but eggs, too, become clear eventually. Thus the optimal time for drying under different conditions must be determined. In overdried films, gas pockets form and delicate eggs (*e.g.,* hookworm) disappear from view.

Permanent Fecal Film

To make a permanent, stained film of fresh feces for study of intestinal protozoa, a representative fleck of the material is smeared as evenly as possible in a thin film on a clean slide and immediately immersed in Schaudinn's solution (saturated solution of mercuric chloride in distilled water, 200 ml, and 95% ethyl alcohol, 100 ml; glacial acetic acid, 15 ml, is added just before the fixative is to be used).

Different stains may be used, but iron-hematoxylin or trichrome usually is employed. In following the steps described below, the film must not be permitted to dry and the time schedule must be adhered to except where smears are in 70% alcohol; then overnight or longer delay is allowable.

Iron-Hematoxylin Stain

1. Fix smears in Schaudinn's solution for at least 5 minutes at 50°C or 15 minutes at room temperature.
2. Immerse in 50% alcohol for 5 minutes.
3. Immerse in alcohol iodine (70% alcohol with enough iodine to give a pale amber color) for 5 minutes; if solution becomes decolorized, repeat this step with fresh solution.
4. Wash in 50% alcohol for 3 to 5 minutes.
5. Run under tap water for 3 to 5 minutes.
6. Mordant with 2% aqueous iron-alum for 5 minutes at 40 to 50°C or at least 10 minutes at room temperature.
7. Wash in 2 changes of distilled water, 3 minutes total.
8. Stain in 0.5% aqueous hematoxylin for 5 minutes at 40 to 50°C or at least 10 minutes at room temperature.

Note: The times in the mordant and stain should be about the same. A longer time produces a better, more lasting stain.
9. Wash in running tap water at least 2 minutes.
10. Differentiate in saturated picric acid solution for 10 to 15 minutes.
11. Wash in running tap water for at least 5 minutes and preferably for 30 minutes.
12. Rinse in distilled water.
13. Wash in 70% alcohol for 3 to 5 minutes.
14. Wash in 95% alcohol for 3 to 5 minutes.
15. Immerse in two changes of absolute alcohol for 3 to 5 minutes each.
16. Clear the stained smears in xylene or toluene for 3 to 5 minutes each.
17. Add coverglass with Canada balsam or one of the faster drying mounting media.

Trichrome Stain

1. Fix smears in Schaudinn's solution at least 5 minutes at 50°C or 15 minutes at room temperature.
2. Wash in 70% alcohol plus sufficient iodine to give a pale amber color for 1 minute; if solution becomes decolorized, repeat this step with fresh solution.
3. Wash in 70% alcohol for 1 minute.
4. Wash again in 70% alcohol for 1 minute.
5. Trichrome stain, 2 to 8 minutes. Preparation: Chromotrope 2R, 0.6 g; light-green SF, 0.15 g; fast-green FCF, 0.15 g; phosphotungstic acid, 0.7 g. Combine the dry ingredients and add 1.0 ml of glacial acetic acid; allow to "ripen" for 15 to 30 minutes. Add 100 ml distilled water. Stain can be used repeatedly but should be periodically filtered, depending upon usage.
6. Rinse in acid alcohol (90% alcohol plus 1 drop glacial acetic acid per 10 ml alcohol).

Note: This is a critical step. The slide should be dipped 2 or more seconds repeatedly until there is very little stain running from the smear, which is then quickly passed through the next 2 steps.
7. Wash in 95% alcohol (2 changes) for a few seconds.
8. Wash in 100% alcohol (2 changes) for 1 minute.
9. Immerse in xylene or toluene (2 changes) for 2 minutes.
10. Add coverglass with Canada balsam or one of the faster drying mounting media.

Acid-Fast Stain for *Cryptosporidium*

Reagents
1. Kinyoun's carbolfuchsin:

Basic fuchsin	4 g
Phenol	8 g
95% ethanol	20 ml
Distilled water	100 ml

Dissolve basic fuchsin in the alcohol, add phenol and water, and mix well.
2. Acid alcohol: 3 ml of concentrated hydrochloric acid is added to 97 ml of 95% ethanol.
3. Methylene blue: Dissolve 1.0 g of methylene blue in 100 ml of absolute ethanol.

Procedures
1. Prepare thin film of fresh feces on a glass slide and allow to dry; gentle heat can be used to hasten drying.
2. Fix in absolute alcohol for 5 minutes.
3. Cover fecal film with Kinyoun's carbolfuchsin for 3 minutes.
4. Wash briefly with tap water.
5. Decolorize with acid alcohol until no more stain comes out (about 2 minutes).
6. Wash briefly with tap water.
7. Cover film with methylene blue for 2 minutes.
8. Rinse with tap water, drain, and dry; gentle heat can be used to hasten drying.
9. When smear is completely dry, it can be examined under oil or a coverglass with mounting medium can be added. The oocysts of *Cryptosporidium* will be stained pink to deep red (Fig. 18–2).

Note: Fecal films fixed in Schaudinn's solution or dried films of PVA-fixed feces can be stained as above to demonstrate *Cryptosporidium*. Such films must first be treated with iodine alcohol as described for the iron-hematoxylin stain (p. 249), rinsed in 70% alcohol, and dried before adding the carbolfuchsin. Oocysts recovered by one of the centrifugal flotation techniques can be mixed with albumin before making a smear on a slide; after drying, the film should be fixed and stained as described above.

PVA-Fixed Fecal Film

The polyvinyl alcohol (PVA)–fixative solution consists of Schaudinn's solution, 93.5 ml; glycerol, 1.5 ml; glacial acetic acid, 5.0 ml; and powdered polyvinyl alcohol, 5 g. The polyvinyl alcohol is added slowly with constant stirring when the other ingredients have been heated to 75°C. For use, 1 drop of well-comminuted fecal suspension and 3 drops of the fixative are spread over the middle third of the slide, which is then dried overnight at 37°C. At a convenient time, the dry film is then placed in 70% alcohol containing iodine to remove excess mercuric chloride, as in step 2 of the trichrome staining procedure, and then stained by the iron-hematoxylin or trichrome technique.

Concentration Methods

Microscopic parasite objects may be concentrated and separated from other objects in the feces by sedimentation, flotation, or a combination of the two.

Gravity Sedimentation. Sedimentation is accomplished by suspending the fecal specimen in tap water and allowing natural settling to take place or by accelerating the process mechanically through centrifugation. For the intestinal protozoa gravity sedimentation is tedious and provides little if any concentration over the direct fecal film. On the other hand, for helminth eggs gravity sedimentation has several advantages over other meth-

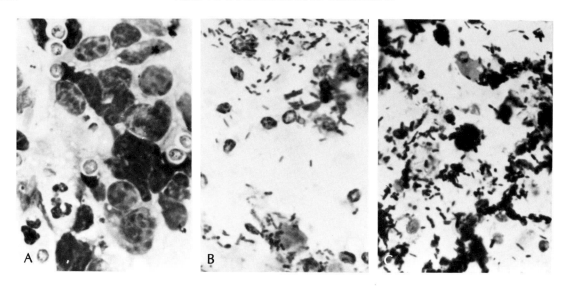

Fig. 18–2. *Cryptosporidium* oocysts. *A.* Impression smear from mucosa of ileum taken at autopsy, stained by the Giemsa technique (p. 253). Seven oocysts are evident among larger cells of exudate. *B.* Fecal smear stained by the Giemsa technique. Nine oocysts are shown. *C.* Fecal smear stained by the acid-fast technique. Only four oocysts (near bottom) are evident in this black and white photo but numerous others, all made conspicuous by bright red color, were evident in the microscope field. (×1000.) (By P.C. Beaver.)

ods of concentration, since the eggs of all species settle to the bottom of the container in a viable, undistorted condition. It is especially recommended for eggs of *Schistosoma, Clonorchis, Opisthorchis,* and heterophyid flukes.

A 10 g portion of the fecal specimen is thoroughly mixed in 10 to 20 times its volume of tap water, poured into a sedimentation glass, and the sediment is allowed to settle out. After an hour, the top two thirds with the floating debris is carefully either poured off or siphoned off, water is added to near the top of the container, and the fecal material is thoroughly resuspended in it. This procedure is repeated until the supernatant fluid is relatively clear. After final removal of the water, a small portion of bottom sediment is removed with a long pipet to a broad slide (37 × 75 mm) and examined for eggs.

For eggs of *Schistosoma* spp., 0.5% glycerol added to tap water causes increased "wetting" and more rapid sedimentation, minimizes the number of eggs decanted, and provides a yield up to about 25-fold that of the unprocessed stool. It is desirable to strain out the larger detritus in the stool through surgical gauze with about 22 meshes to the linear inch, using 2 to 4 thicknesses that have been previously soaked in water and the excess water squeezed out. The gauze is then stretched loosely over a funnel of appropriate size and the emulsified feces poured through into the sedimentation glass. Few eggs are trapped in the gauze unless there is considerable mucus in the stool. After 1 hour, the first decantation is made, 45 minutes later a second, and 30 minutes later a third and last one. Measured amounts of the sediment in the bottom are then removed to a slide and mounted with a 40 × 22 mm coverglass. Eggs of all types can be found in the sediment. It is probably the most practical method for obtaining immature, fully mature, and degenerate eggs for diagnosis in the same proportion in which they occur in the stool.

Formalin-Ether (F–E) Centrifugal Sedimentation. The formalin-ether technique is moderately effective in concentrating protozoan cysts and helminth eggs in feces. It uses formalin to fix and preserve the fecal specimen and ether to decrease the specific gravity of small fecal particles, causing them to float in the suspension while the coarser, nonabsorbent elements are left at the bottom, including eggs and cysts of parasites.

In this procedure, the fecal sample is first comminuted in sufficient water to provide 10 to 12 ml of suspension, which is strained through 2 layers of surgical gauze into a 15-ml centrifuge tube. The suspension is then centrifuged, the supernatant decanted, and the particulate matter resuspended repeatedly until the supernatant is clear. After an additional decantation the sediment is mixed with 10 ml of 10% formalin and allowed to stand for 5 minutes, after which 3 ml of ether is added and the suspension is shaken vigorously for at least 2 minutes. Following centrifugation at about 600 g for 2 minutes, the entire supernatant is poured off. A thin film of the sediment is placed on a slide, a drop of iodine stain is mixed with it, and the preparation is mounted with a coverglass for examination. Feces preserved in 10% formalin can be processed with this technique. However, the specific gravity of eggs and cysts fixed in formalin for an extended period is apparently altered, and yields eventually become unsatisfactory.

Gravity Flotation. In contrast to sedimentation, flotation utilizes a liquid suspending medium heavier than the parasite objects so that they rise to the surface and can be skimmed out of the surface film. For diagnostic usefulness, the suspending medium not only must be heavier than the object to be floated but also must not produce shrinkage sufficient to render the object undiagnosable.

The floating medium generally employed is brine, *i.e.*, saturated aqueous solution of NaCl, having a specific gravity of approximately 1.20. Eggs of common intestinal helminths, such as hookworms, *Ascaris,* and *Trichuris,* are not damaged by this process, but *Schistosoma* eggs, hookworm and *Strongyloides* larvae, and protozoan cysts become badly shrunken; furthermore, eggs of *Clonorchis, Opisthorchis,* and heterophyid species float only briefly in brine.

The procedure is simple. A sample of feces is thoroughly mixed with 10 times its volume of brine, strained through gauze to remove coarse elements, transferred to a test tube, and allowed to stand undisturbed for 20 to 30 minutes. The tube may be filled to near the brim and the eggs removed by means of a wire loop (about 4 mm. diameter) for examination under a microscope (usually without a coverglass).

A sugar solution consisting of 500 g sucrose and 6.5 ml

melted phenol in 360 ml distilled water can be used instead of brine for flotation by either gravity or centrifugation. The method has been recommended for the isolation of oocysts of *Cryptosporidium* from feces.

Zinc Sulfate Centrifugal Flotation. Concentration by centrifugal flotation is based on essentially the same principles as gravitation and flotation. A sample of feces is suspended in approximately 10 times its volume of water, strained through gauze to remove the larger objects, placed in a centrifuge tube, and by means of 2 or 3 successive centrifugations, decantations of the supernatant and resuspensions, is cleared of the fine particulate material. After the last centrifugation the entire supernatant is drained off; the sediment is then resuspended in the floating medium, recentrifuged, and after the centrifuge tube has been at rest for 10 to 20 seconds, the surface film is removed with a wire loop. The floating medium generally employed is zinc sulfate solution having a specific gravity of 1.18; however, sugar solution has also been used.

The zinc sulfate flotation technique is effective for concentration of protozoan cysts, helminth eggs, and larvae in a readily diagnosable condition. All of these parasite objects, except for operculate eggs, those of blood flukes, and eggs heavier than the floating medium, are recovered in good concentration and in a viable condition.

The steps in the original technique are as follows:

1. A fecal suspension is prepared by comminuting 1 part of feces in about 10 parts of tap water.
2. The suspension is strained through gauze, and a Wassermann tube 12 × 100 mm is filled with the strained suspension.
3. The preparation in the tube is then centrifuged for 45 to 60 seconds at 500 to 700 g. The supernatant fluid is poured off, 2 or 3 ml of water are added, the sediment is broken up by shaking or tapping, and additional water is added to fill the tube.
4. Step 3 is repeated once or twice until the supernatant fluid is clear.
5. The last supernatant fluid is poured off completely and 1 or 2 ml of zinc sulfate solution is added. The packed sediment is broken up, and enough zinc sulfate solution is added to fill the tube to 3 or 4 mm below the rim.
6. The tube is centrifuged for 45 to 60 seconds at 500 to 700 g and is allowed to stop without interference.
7. After 15 to 20 seconds and without removing the tube from the centrifuge, several loopfuls of the surface film are removed by means of a wire loop (4 mm diameter) onto the clean side, 1 drop of iodine stain (saturated iodine in 1% KI) is added, and the preparation is agitated manually to ensure uniform staining.
8. The preparation is mounted with a coverglass and is now ready for examination.

Less time-consuming and more effective modifications and simplifications of the zinc sulfate centrifugal flotation technique have been introduced (Beaver, 1952).

Baermann Larval Extraction. The most efficient technique available for the laboratory diagnosis of *Strongyloide stercoralis* infections utilizes the Baermann apparatus. Various modifications of the technique are also used for the recovery of nematode larvae or in some cases of adults from tissues, characoal cultures, or soil (see page 255). A glass or plastic funnel (10 to 15 cm in diameter) is placed vertically in a support frame. A short length of rubber tubing with a pinch clamp attached to one end is fitted to the stem of the funnel. A wire screen of hardware cloth about 25 mm smaller in diameter than the top of the funnel is placed in the funnel. A circular pad of several layers of surgical gauze is placed on the wire screen and enough warm water, at 38 to 40°C, is added to the funnel to cover the gauze pad. Using a wooden tongue depressor, the fecal sample

is smeared over the surface of an appropriate-size circle of filter paper (Whatman No. 2 or equivalent) to a depth of 3 to 4 mm. Then the filter paper is inverted and placed over the gauze in the funnel. The apparatus is allowed to stand for 30 minutes to 1 hour to permit the *Strongyloides* rhabditoid larvae to migrate into the water and settle to the bottom. Water from the bottom of the funnel is then drawn off through the tubing into one or more 15-ml centrifuge tubes, each tube receiving 10 to 12 ml. The tubes are centrifuged for 2 minutes at 500 g and then the sediment in each is transferred to a microscope slide with a pipet. The motile rhabditoid larvae can be detected under low magnification, but their characteristic features must be observed under higher magnification (100 × or more) to confirm their identification (see page 149).

Egg Counts

While the several techniques described above provide opportunity for efficient recovery and accurate identification of most parasite objects in the feces, an estimate of the parasite burden is often useful. Methods have been developed for relatively accurate calculation of hookworm, *Ascaris*, and *Trichuris* worm burden by estimating the number of eggs present in the stool.

Direct Smear Egg Count. The method of making egg counts by direct smear is based on the observation that eggs of hookworms and those of other species that inhabit the small intestine or upper colon have random distribution in the feces and that any series of direct smears of equal density taken from the same stool will contain equal quantities of fecal solids and statistically equal numbers of eggs (Martin, 1965). A method of making uniform smears has been devised, and the factor for converting eggs per slide to eggs per g or per mg of formed stool has been determined for the type of smear that is regarded as being of ideal density (Beaver, 1950). Ordinary direct fecal smears made by experienced technicians for routine diagnosis of parasitic infections almost invariably contain the equivalent of about 2 mg (1/500 g) of formed feces. For routine estimation of worm burden, counts of "eggs per smear" are therefore as useful as the more complicated time-consuming methods.

Dilution Egg Count. The technique of Stoll and Hausheer (1926) is as follows: Add 56 ml of N/10 (0.4%) sodium hydroxide to a small Erlenmeyer flask or bottle that has marks indicating 56- and 60-ml levels. Add feces until the solution reaches the 60-ml level (*i.e.*, 4 ml or approximately 4 g feces added). Add several glass beads, close the container with a rubber stopper, and shake the contents until the fecal sample is thoroughly mixed. Allow to stand 12 to 24 hours with occasional shaking. The mixture is then thoroughly shaken and 0.075 ml of the suspension is drawn into a calibrated pipet, discharged onto a clean slide, and covered with a 22 × 30 mm coverglass. The number of eggs of the particular species of helminth under observation is then counted, and this number is multiplied by 200 to obtain the number of eggs per g of feces. The estimate obtained depends on the consistency of the feces. Correction factors must therefore be used to convert the estimate to the formed stool basis (fsb). Failure to take this variable into accout will result in wide variation in the estimates. Counts on mushy-formed feces are multiplied by 1.5, mushy by 2, mushy-diarrheal by 3, flowing-diarrheal by 4, and watery by 5 or more. Thus an egg count of 5,000 per g of mushy feces is equivalent to 10,000 per g of formed feces from the same individual. *Note:* These conversion factors are not needed for counts made by direct smear.

Thick Smear Egg Count. The Kato cellophane-covered thick fecal smear can also be used for making egg counts. The procedure described by Martin and Beaver (1968), page 248, can be made quantitative by accurately estimating the amount of feces placed on the slide. A modification described by Katz

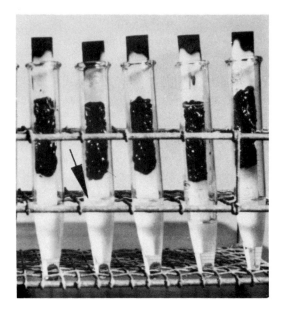

Fig. 18–3. Harada-Mori test-tube fecal culture for the diagnosis of hookworm and other intestinal nematode larvae. The cultures shown here are 3 days old, and by the upward flow and evaporation of water, the fecal film has been leached and the soluble elements deposited in the dark zone at the top of the filter-paper strip. The water level (shown by an *arrow*) is maintained by periodic replacement. After about 24 hours of leaching, the odor of feces disappears and is replaced by the aroma of damp soil. (From Beaver, P.C., Malek, E.A., and Little, M.D. 1964. Development of *Spirometra* and *Paragonimus* eggs in Harada-Mori cultures. J. Parasitol., *50*:664–666.)

et al. (1972) uses a template constructed of cardboard or plastic of such thickness that a 6 mm punched-out circular hole contains approximately 50 mg of feces. In this procedure the template is placed on a slide, the hole is filled with the screened fecal sample, the template is removed and discarded, the sample is spread under a cellophane coverslip, and the eggs are counted after the appropriate period of clearing. A kit of disposable materials to use with this procedure is commercially available. Peters *et al.* (1980) introduced a stainless steel template that delivers 20 mg feces for use in making quantitative thick smears.

Fecal Culture for Diagnosis of Hookworm Larvae

Specific identification of hookworm and hookwormlike eggs appearing in feces is often difficult or impossible, whereas the infective-stage larvae developing from the eggs are readily distinguishable. A common practical problem is the differentiation of *Necator* from *Ancylostoma* infections. For the culturing of larvae from eggs, a clean and simple test-tube method requiring only readily available materials was devised by Harada and Mori (1955) and variously modified by others (Hsieh, 1962). The method is adaptable to other purposes (Beaver *et al.*, 1964) (Fig. 18–3). For obtaining large quantities of larvae, charcoal cultures are preferred.

Test Tube Culture. Test-tube cultures are made by spreading a film of feces 1 to 2 mm thick on the middle third (one side only) of a 13 by 120 mm strip of filter paper (Whatman No. 3 MM, or similar). This is then placed in a 15-ml conical-tip centrifuge tube or a 16 by 125 mm culture tube containing about 3 ml distilled water, forcing the paper to near the bottom of the

tube. The culture is held at room temperature (24° to 28°C) in the dark for 7 to 10 days, and water is added as needed to hold the water level well above the bottom end of the paper. The capillary flow of water upward through the paper and fecal film keeps the feces moist and carries soluble elements of the feces to the top of the paper, where they either volatilize or accumulate in a dark deposit (Fig. 18–2). After 48 hours, the portion of the filter paper extending from the tube may be cut off and the tube stoppered or capped. On reaching the infective stage, the larvae migrate to the water pool, where they can be seen with a hand lens and taken up with a pipette for microscopic examination. Minor variations in the tube or filter-paper strip are not critical.

Charcoal Culture. Charcoal cultures are made by thoroughly mixing 1 part of soft or softened (with water) feces with 5 to 10 parts of fine, granular (not powdered), hardwood charcoal, which is made damp throughout and packed into a covered but not air-tight container. Excess water must be avoided or removed. After 7 to 10 days, on reaching the infective stage of development, the larvae migrate to the surface, where they can be removed conveniently by a method first described for recovering hookworm larvae from soil (Beaver, 1953). A thick, 12- to 15-ply pad of soft cotton cloth (cheesecloth or absorbent gauze) of appropriate size to fit the culture-container is dampened with warm water, pressed onto the culture surface; and the cover replaced. A majority of the larvae migrate into the pad within 30 minutes, after which the pad is picked up at the center with forceps and transferred upside down to a sedimentation flask filled to near the brim with warm water when the pad is immersed. The larvae promptly fall to the bottom of the flask, while the adherent charcoal (or soil) is held on the upper surface of the pad. Most of the larvae can be removed with a pipette after 20 minutes.

WORMS MIGRATING FROM THE ANUS

In the case of *Enterobius* infection, it is unusual for gravid worms to oviposit within the bowel. Adult females habitually migrate out of the anus and their eggs are shed onto perianal and perineal skin. Worms may be passed in the feces but more commonly crawl out of the anus at night. Mature and immature *Ascaris* are at times passed spontaneously in the feces. Such worms should be preserved in formalin and properly identified. Tapeworm proglottids (species of *Taenia* or *Dipylidium caninum*), singly or in chains, are usually discharged periodically in stools of infected patients. Specific identification of these worms can most readily be made from moist proglottids. Patients should be warned not to wrap them in toilet paper, which dries them out and usually renders identification difficult or impossible.

ANAL SCRAPINGS AND SWABS

Amebiasis cutis of the perianal area may be diagnosed by scraping material from lesions, removing it to a slide in a drop or two of tepid physiologic salt solution, mounting with a coverglass, and demonstrating typical *E. histolytica* motility.

The *Scotch tape technique* is used for obtaining eggs of *Enterobius* from the anal and perianal areas. A length of clear adhesive tape is held adhesive side out on the end of a wooden tongue depressor by the thumb and index finger and after "swabbing" is placed adhesive side down on a microscope slide. Before examination, the tape is lifted except at one end, a drop of toluene is added, and the tape is smoothed out on the side.

Perianal swabbing will often recover eggs of *Schistosoma mansoni* and other helminths; it is an excellent method for recovery of eggs of *Taenia solium* and *Taenia saginata*.

ENTERO-TEST

Duodenal contents may be obtained by use of this technique described by Beal *et al.* (1970). It consists of a weighted gelatin capsule containing a coiled nylon line, one size for adults and a smaller pediatric size. A portion of the nylon line is withdrawn and attached to the patient's face, and the capsule with the remaining line is swallowed with water. After 3 to 4 hours the string is withdrawn and the absorbed material from the distal end is squeezed onto a microscope slide for examination. *Giardia lamblia* and *Strongyloides stercoralis* are the parasites usually sought with this method, but occasionally others may be encountered. The Entero-Test capsules are available from Hedeco Health Development Corporation, 2411 Pulgas Avenue, Palo Alto, California.

PURGED AND ENEMA SPECIMENS

The purpose of examining purged and enema material is to obtain diagnostic evidence of infection with *Entamoeba histolytica,* usually in the cecal area of the intestine, when routine examination of the stools has been consistently negative and yet there is strong clinical suspicion of intestinal amebiasis. For diagnostic purposes, the purgative agent is sodium sulfate (Glauber salts) or Phospho-soda, which is preferred for delivering the amebic trophozoites in an undamaged, motile condition. For reliable diagnosis the examination must be made while the specimen is fresh. The material to be examined is the mucus and tissue detritus in the liquid portion following the evacuation of the fecal material. With a pipette, small amounts of the mucus or other sediment are transferred to a slide with as little liquid as possible, mounted under a coverglass, and examined in the unstained condition. Typical pseudopodial activity and locomotion must be demonstrated in order to make a specific diagnosis of *E. histolytica,* and care must be taken not to confuse host cells or trophozoites of nonpathogenic amebae with those of *E. histolytica.* Smears that are preserved and stained as previously described are useful to confirm identification and provide a permanent record.

Enema specimens should be obtained by high instillations of tepid physiologic salt solution to irrigate the cecal area. As in purged material, the mucous settlings in the liquid portion of the evacuation will provide the greatest likelihood of obtaining trophozoites of *E. histolytica.*

POSTANTHELMINTIC TREATMENT SPECIMENS

The most common post-treatment examinations are made in helminthic infections of the intestinal tract, particularly for hookworms, *Ascaris, Trichuris,* tapeworms, and intestinal trematodes. Depending on the type of anthelmintic, the worms may be evacuated in an undamaged, living condition or may be badly damaged. Large worms are most easily recovered by dilution, sedimentation, and decantation of the stools; smaller species are more readily found and their numbers counted by straining the diluted feces through wire gauze with the appropriate-sized mesh (Beaver, 1952).

EXAMINATION OF URINE

Trichomonas vaginalis is frequently recovered from urine sediment in both female and male patients. Rarely, trophozoites of *Entamoeba histolytica* may be present in urine of persons who have amebic ulceration of the genitalia.

Urine to be examined for eggs of *Schistosoma haematobium* is collected in a sedimentation glass and the eggs are allowed to sink to the bottom, together with erythrocytes and pus cells. The bottom sediment is then pipetted onto a slide and examined microscopically. In Bancroft's filarial infection with chyluria and in other filarial infections, notably onchocerciasis, microfilariae are discharged in the urine. They may readily be recovered in sediment from centrifuged specimens.

EXAMINATION OF SPUTUM AND GASTRIC WASHINGS

In pleuropulmonary amebiasis, rupture of the amebic abscess into a bronchus characteristically results in coughing up the contents containing trophozoites of *Entamoeba histolytica.* Similarly, rupture of a pulmonary hydatid cyst is followed by discharge of its contents, in which there will be fragments of the laminated membrane and germinal layer of the cyst wall and usually free scolices of *Echinococcus granulosus.* In the pulmonary phase of infection with *Ascaris, Necator, Ancylostoma,* and *Strongyloides,* the migrating larvae, along with eosinophils and Charcot-Leyden crystals, may be demonstrated in the sputum or, more frequently, in the washed sediment from gastric washings (Proffitt and Walton, 1962; Gelpi and Mustafa, 1967). Sputum is the most common medium of discharge from which eggs of *Paragonimus westermani* are recovered. Rarely, eggs of blood flukes are coughed up.

DETECTION OF PARASITES IN BLOOD

Next to feces, blood provides the most common medium for recovery of various stages of animal parasites. From this source, diagnosis is routinely made of malaria, African trypanosomiasis, and most types of filariasis, less frequently of Chagas' disease, and rarely of kala-azar and toxoplasmosis. It is necessary to remember that in a particular infection the etiologic agents are not consistently present.

Protozoa

Throughout the world, the standard procedure for obtaining material for diagnosis of protozoa in circulating blood is to make microscope slide preparations.

Preparation of Blood Films. The older method consisted of obtaining only thin blood films, but for rapid examination thick films are needed. Preferably, a combined thin- and thick-film should be made on the outer thirds of the same slide. (The slide should be smooth and free of all blemishes, oil, lint, and finger marks.) In making the thin film, a small drop of blood from a finger, toe (of children), or ear lobe is brought in contact with one end of the slide and is immediately drawn out into a smooth film one cell thick, with the smooth straight edge of another slide. In making the thick film, a somewhat larger drop of blood is deposited near the other end of the slide and is spread out evenly to the size of about 15 mm in diameter. Both films must be allowed to dry thoroughly without heating and without opportunity for contamination from dust or deposits of flies or roaches. Unless the slide is meticulously clean, the thick film is likely to flake off. Films that are freshly prepared and dried always stain best.

Giemsa's Stain. The most valuable single stain for blood films that are to be examined for protozoa or microfilariae was developed by Giemsa, prepared from azure blue and eosin. The thin-film end of the slide must first be fixed in absolute ethyl alcohol or absolute methyl alcohol for 30 seconds to avoid dehemoglobinization. The thick film requires no fixation, since dehemoglobinization is necessary to see through the several layers of cells. When ready for staining, the slide should be immersed for a period of 10 to 30 minutes in a mixture of 2 to 3 drops of the concentrated stain to each ml of buffered distilled water (pH 7.4), then washed off, and thoroughly dried in the air. It is now ready for examination with oil-immersion objective, but if it is to be preserved, each portion should be covered with mounting medium and a No. 1 coverglass.

Microfilariae

Giemsa's Stain. In most instances microfilariae in blood (or from skin snips, viz., those of *Onchocerca volvulus*) are satisfactorily stained by the Giemsa technique. The thick film is recommended. After the material has been spread over a circular area about 20 mm in diameter on an absolutely clean microscope slide and has been thoroughly dried, the slide is placed vertically in diluted Giemsa stain (see above). In approximately 30 minutes staining is complete, and the slide is removed, washed gently in tap water, and dried. Overstaining is not likely to occur.

Hematoxylin Staining. For microfilariae, some workers prefer hematoxylin staining. The dried thick film is dehemoglobinized in 0.5% HCl, washed in 1% lithium carbonate solution, and then stained with Bullard's, Harris', or Delafield's hematoxylin obtained commercially.

Concentration of Microfilariae. Defibrinated and dehemoglobinized blood, lymph, or chylous urine is concentrated by centrifuging for about 1 minute at about 100 g, the supernatant fluid decanted, and the sediment examined for microfilariae. These may be vitally stained or the film air-dried, fixed, and permanently stained with Giemsa or hematoxylin.

Knott (1939) modified this technique as follows: 1 ml of blood is thoroughly shaken with 10 ml of a 2% solution of formalin, centrifuged for 2 minutes, the supernatant fluid decanted, and the sediment examined microscopically for microfilariae. The sediment can be spread, dried, fixed, and stained with Giemsa, as for thick-blood films.

When they are exceptionally scanty microfilariae can be recovered from blood by filtration through modern microfilters (Chularerk and Desowitz, 1970). One ml of blood is drawn into a heparinized syringe. Nine ml of a 10% solution of Teepol (Shell Chemicals) in physiologic saline is then taken into the syringe and mixed with the blood by gentle rotation until hemolysis is complete. The needle is removed and replaced by a Swinney or similar filter holder containing a 25 mm microporous filter membrane with a 5 μm pore size. Cellulosic membranes may be used, but polycarbonate membranes have the advantage of remaining flat during dehydration and clearing. Nathan *et al.* (1982) recommended Nuclepore (Nucleopore Corp.) membranes with a 3 μm pore size. The lysed blood is forced through the filter membrane, after which physiologic saline is forced through for rinsing. After removal from the filter holder, the membrane is placed on a microscope slide, dried, and then stained by the thick blood smear technique. During field collecting, one ml blood is added to 9 ml of the Teepol-saline mixture, and after lysis is complete 1 ml of formalin is added. The filtration and staining can be carried out later.

EXAMINATION OF ASPIRATES AND BIOPSY MATERIAL

Aspirates

Recovery of protozoa and helminths from aspirated material is always a successful procedure.

Colon and Rectum. Proctoscopic aspirates and scrapings are valuable in confirming suspicion of amebic ulcers in the lower sigmoid colon and rectum, but diagnosis of the cellular content of the aspirate is frequently a difficult problem, since host tissue cells are often confused with nonmotile trophozoites or cysts of *Entamoeba histolytica*.

Duodenum. Duodenal aspiration in employed in the demonstration of infections with *Giardia lamblia*, *Strongyloides stercoralis*, *Fasciolopsis buski* (eggs), and parasites located in the gallbladder or biliary tract.

Liver and Lung. Obtaining aspirates from lesions in the liver and lungs is particularly helpful for diagnosis of amebic liver abscess as well as of hydatid cyst. In the hepatic abscess, trophozoites of *Entamoeba histolytica* are more likely to be demonstrated in aspirates obtained from the wall of the enlarging lesion than from the completely necrotic center of the abscess. Enzymatic liquefaction of viscous aspirates greatly facilitates the search for amebae. Streptodornase in sterile physiologic saline solution, 50 U/ml, is added to the fresh aspirate 1 to 5 parts. The mixture is incubated for 30 minutes at 37°C, stirring 2 or 3 times. The liquefied material is then transferred to tubes and centrifuged. Amebae in the sediment are motile and can be cultured in a preconditioned medium.

Lymph Nodes and Other Organs. Aspirates from lymph nodes, spleen, liver, bone marrow, and spinal fluid frequently provide diagnostic evidence of African trypanosomiasis, visceral leishmaniasis (kala-azar), Chagas' disease, primary amebic meningoencephalitis and toxoplasmosis. The material obtained should be used in part for direct, unstained, coverglass preparations to demonstrate motile organism (trypanosomes, amebae), in part for impression smears that are processed by the Giemsa technique, and in part for culturing the organisms that may be present.

Biopsy Material

Biopsy has become increasingly useful and common in the diagnosis of parasitic infections. It may be the most convenient and at times the only method of confirming clinical suspicion of infection.

Skin. Biopsies of skin can be used to demonstrate amebiasis cutis, cutaneous leishmaniasis, and microfilariae of *Onchocerca volvulus*. In the first two infections a representative portion of the lesion should be removed; this should be fixed and processed for serial sections to be stained by the hematoxylin-eosin technique. For microfilariae of *O. volvulus* only small, superficial specimens are required. These thin snips of skin are each placed in a drop of tepid physiologic salt solution, mounted with a coverglass, and examined for microfilariae emerging from the tissue fragment. Occasionally in areas where other types of filariasis are endemic other microfilariae may be present, particularly if the biopsy incision has been deep enough to rupture cutaneous blood vessels.

Lymph Node. Biopsy of a superficial lymph node may demonstrate organisms of African trypanosomiasis, kala-azar, Chagas' disease, and toxoplasmosis. While impression smears should be made for staining with the Giemsa technique, a representative portion should be fixed, sectioned, and stained with hematoxylin-eosin.

Muscle. A muscle biopsy may demonstrate *Trichinella* larvae and at times the cysticercus of *Taenia solium*. Some of the former material may be compressed between glass slides and examined directly for *Trichinella* cysts, but a portion should be digested in artificial gastric juice at 37°C and the excysted larvae concentrated by centrifugation. If the specimen is adequate, a portion can be fed to a laboratory rat for evidence of the viability of the larvae that may be present. Usually muscle biopsy for demonstration of trichinosis is less common than the use of immunologic techniques (see Chapter 20, pages 260–261). If a cysticercus is present in the specimen, it should be carefully dissected out of its capsule, deflated with a needle, and compressed between a slide and coverglass to demonstrate the characteristic scolex with 4 suckers and an anterior circlet of hooks.

Rectal Mucosa. Examination of a rectal biopsy specimen may confirm suspicion of amebic colitis, but biopsy is less commonly performed than aspiration. On the other hand, proctoscopic biopsy is a most valuable procedure for demonstrating eggs of *Schistosoma mansoni*, *S japonicum*, and *S haematobium*.

Rectal biopsy material taken from the level of the first valve of Houston, rendered transparent by KOH, and examined microscopically under compression provides a simple, safe procedure and is particularly valuable in chronic cases of intestinal schistosomiasis and as a follow-up of treatment when stools are negative for eggs of the parasite. It may be helpful as a check on immunologic tests. A similar technique, using the cystoscope to obtain a biopsy specimen of the bladder, may be useful in diagnosing *S. haematobium* infection.

Liver. Visceral biopsy, particularly from the liver, is the only practical clinical diagnostic procedure for demonstration of visceral larva migrans produced by larvae of *Toxocara*.

Lung. Examination of material from the lung is the usual procedure for detecting infection with *Pneumocystis carinii*. An open lung biopsy allows the surgeon to select an area most likely to contain parasites, but the patient's condition may not permit the added risk of the procedure. Transbronchoscopic lung biopsy has been used with success. Impression smears should be made from the biopsy specimen before it is preserved for sectioning. Such smears should be stained with Giemsa's stain to detect the free uninucleate forms as well as those within the cysts. The cyst walls may be stained with Gomori's silver-methenamine or by the toluidine blue method in either the tissue smears or sections. Tracheal aspirates should be concentrated by centrifugation, and smears of the sediment may be stained by the above methods.

ENVIRONMENTAL MATERIAL

Material obtained from the environment may be useful in providing evidence of a specific causal relationship of an animal agent or vector to the disease in a particular patient, as, for example, recovery of an arthropod or vertebrate animal in connection with host envenomation.

Fomites

The recognizable cysts of protozoan parasites are rarely recovered from fomites. Gross fecal pollution of underclothing and furniture may furnish evidence of *Entamoeba histolytica* or *Giardia lamblia* cysts or *Cryptosporidium* oocysts following immersion of these objects in water and concentration of the sediment by centrifugation.

In contrast to protozoan parasites, eggs of intestinal helminths are not uncommonly obtained from underclothing, household furniture, green vegetables and topsoil of potted house plants. The most common of these eggs in the immediate environment are those of *Enterobius vermicularis*. Likewise, it is frequently possible to obtain eggs of *Ascaris, Trichuris,* hookworms, *Hymenolepis,* and *Taenia* on the floors and in other locations within the homes of infected individuals.

Water

There is circumstantial evidence that infections with *Entamoeba histolytica* and other intestinal protozoa may be acquired from drinking water contaminated with human feces. Direct proof by isolation of cysts from water is difficult but may be accomplished by filtration of large volumes of water through filter membranes with appropriate pore size using a suction pump. The recovery of helminth eggs from sewage and sewage sludge has been accomplished by a variety of filtration, sedimentation, and concentration procedures.

Soil

While it is possible that under certain conditions cysts of intestinal protozoa deposited on the soil in human feces may survive and later get into the human digestive tract on contaminated objects, no practical method has been developed for recovery of these organisms from the soil. Long survival of *Toxoplasma* organisms in soil can be demonstrated by feeding soil contaminated by cats to experimental animals. Cysts may be recovered from soil by homogenizing a sample in water and then using a centrifugation-flotation procedure on the washed sediment.

In epidemiologic investigations of intestinal helminthic infections, it is frequently necessary to obtain direct evidence of soil pollution by demonstration of the eggs or larvae. When first deposited cysts, eggs, and larvae may be present in the fecal mass on top of the ground, but rain, coprophagous insects, and other agents soon cause disintegration, with dissemination of the eggs and cysts, and the larvae tend to migrate in the topsoil.

Eggs can be recovered from soil by brine or zinc sulfate flotation after initial treatment of the sample with sodium hypochloride solution (1 part soil to 2 parts 30% bleaching fluid) for 30 minutes with frequent stirring. The treated mixture is diluted with 10 parts water, strained through gauze to remove coarse elements, centrifuged, then washed twice by centrifugation in water, and separated by centrifugal brine flotation. The top film is poured off, diluted and concentrated by centrifugation, and then examined microscopically on a slide.

Larvae of hookworms can be recovered by the technique of Baermann or by the damp pad method already described (p. 252). A necessary adaptation of the latter when used on soil is to add water to the soil if it is not damp at the surface and to cover the pad with plastic to reduce evaporation (Beaver, 1953).

The *Baermann* technique requires a simple apparatus, as described on page 251. The soil sample to be tested is placed on the wire screen lined with cloth. Lukewarm water is placed in the funnel and its height is adjusted so that the soil will be immersed in the water. Within 10 to 15 minutes, nematode larvae in positive soils may be observed falling down the stem of the funnel. The maximum yield takes place within the first hour, after which the pinch-cock should be opened, 10 to 15 ml of water and sediment drawn off into a test tube, the suspension centrifuged, the supernatant fluid pipetted off immediately, and the sediment transferred to a slide for examination. The examiner needs training to differentiate hookworm and *Strongyloides* larvae from free-living soil nematodes.

PRESERVATION OF ANIMAL SPECIMENS

It is usually not sufficient merely to identify an arthropod as a tick, mite, fly, or mosquito. Similarly, adequate identification of a mollusc or vertebrate animal that has a connection with disease may be needed. When expert identification service is not available locally in such cases, specimens should be properly preserved and shipped to a specialist.

Arthropods

Centipedes, scorpions, ticks, spiders, and assassin bugs can be kept in a dry container or preserved in 70 to 80% alcohol. Trombiculid mites, sarcoptid mites, fleas, and lice can be preserved in small vials containing alcohol. Fleas can be removed from dogs and cats by touching them with a camel's hair brush moistened with xylol or chloroform. Rats caught in traps may be placed in an air-tight chloroform chamber for removal of their fleas, mites, and lice. Flea larvae can be obtained by sieving the sweepings from the floors of dwellings occupied by infested people, dogs, or cats. Eggs, larvae or pupae of mosquitoes, sand flies, or *Culicoides* can be preserved in alcohol. Soft-bodied animals should be killed in hot water (65°C) and preserved in 70% alcohol. Ticks, mites, lice, fleas, and other arthropods with hard exoskeletons may be placed directly in alcohol. Arthropods should not be stored in formaldehyde solution because this causes excessive shrinkage and hardening.

Winged adult insects are best preserved as dry specimens mounted on insect pins. Killing jars of any desired size are prepared by placing granular potassium or sodium cyanide in a wide-mouth bottle and covering it with a layer of sawdust held in place by a disc or cardboard or plaster of Paris. A chloroform tube, generally used for mosquitoes, consists of a corked test tube containing rubber bands that have been soaked in chloroform and covered with a layer of cotton and a tightly fitted disc of blotting paper. Larger specimens can be mounted on pins thrust through the thorax, while mosquitoes and other small species are placed on a minute pin carried on a small block of cork or balsa wood on the larger pin. Small specimens may also be glued to the side of a pin or to the point of a slender triangle of paper borne on a pin. Pinned specimens are not treated with a preservative but are simply allowed to dry. To protect them from dust, air currents, and museum pests, they must be stored in tight boxes lined with a pinning surface of sheet cork, balsa wood, or two layers of corrugated carton paper. Individual specimens may be pinned on a cork inserted in a vial. For transportation to specialists, unmounted flies and mosquitoes should be placed between layers of soft paper (never cotton) in a well-buffered pillbox. Dry specimens may be pinned after softening them in a moist chamber containing phenol to inhibit molds.

Molluscs

While the clinical laboratory has no special need for preserving snails or other molluscs, the laboratory may be called on to identify the specimens. This is a task for specialists, who are frequently at a distance from the laboratory, and molluscs do not ordinarily survive shipment. Snails should be relaxed by slowly adding menthol crystals or pentabarbital solution to the water in which they are placed, then killed in hot water (60 to 65°C) and preserved in 70% alcohol.

Vertebrate Animals

Fishes, reptiles, and small birds and mammals can be preserved either in 10% formalin (4% formaldehyde) or 70% alcohol and will keep well, provided that slits have been made in the animal's body cavities so that the viscera can be adequately fixed. It is not usual to preserve larger birds or mammals. Most frequently only the dried "skins" of birds and the dried pelts and skulls of mammals are kept.

REFERENCES

Beal, C.B., Viens, P., Grant, R.G.L., and Hughes, J.M. 1970. A new technique for sampling duodenal contents. Demonstration of upper small-bowel pathogens. Am. J. Trop. Med. Hyg., 19:349–352.

Beaver, P.C. 1950. The standardization of fecal smears for estimating egg production and worm burden. J. Parasitol., 36:451–456.

——— 1952. The detection and identification of some common nematode parasites of man. Am. J. Clin. Pathol., 22:481–494.

——— 1953. Persistence of hookworm larvae in soil. Am. J. Trop. Med. Hyg., 2:102–108.

———, Malek, E.A., and Little, M.D. 1964. Development of Spirometra and Paragonimus eggs in Harada-Mori cultures. J. Parasitol., 50:664–666.

Chularerk, P., and Desowitz, R.S. 1970. Simplified membrane filtration technique for the diagnosis of microfilaremia. J. Parasitol., 56:623–624.

Dunn, F.L. 1968. The TIF direct smear as an epidemiological tool with special reference to counting helminth eggs. Bull. W. H. O., 39:439–449.

Gelpi, A.P., and Mustafa, A. 1967. Seasonal pneumonitis with eosinophilia. A study of larval ascariasis in Saudi Arabs. Am. J. Trop. Med. Hyg., 16:646–657.

Harada, Y., and Mori, O. 1955. A new method of culturing hookworm. Yonago Acta Medica, 1:177–179.

Hsieh, H.C. 1962. A test-tube filter-paper method for the diagnosis of Ancylostoma duodenale, Necator americanus and Strongyloides stercoralis. W. H. O. Techn. Rept. Ser., 255:27–30.

Katz, N., Chaves, A., and Pellegrino, J. 1972. A simple device for quantitative stool thick-smear technique in schistosomiasis mansoni. Rev. Inst. Med. Trop. S. Paulo, 14:397–400.

Knott, J.I. 1939. A method for making microfilarial surveys on day blood. Trans. R. Soc. Trop. Med. Hyg., 33:191–196.

Martin, L.K. 1965. Randomness of particle distribution in human feces and the resulting influence on helminth egg counting. Am. J. Trop. Med. Hyg., 14:747–759.

———, and Beaver, P.C. 1968. Evaluation of Kato thick-smear technique for quantitative diagnosis of helminth infection. Am. J. Trop. Med. Hyg., 17:382–391.

Melvin, D.M., and Brooke, M.M. 1982. Laboratory Procedures for the Diagnosis of Intestinal Parasites. 3rd ed. Atlanta, Georgia, U.S. Department of Health and Human Services Publication No. (CDC) 82–8282.

Nathan, M.B., Lambourne, A., and Monteil, S. 1982. Evaluation of a membrane (Nuclepore) filtration method using capillary blood for the detection of microfilariae. Ann. Trop. Med. Parasitol., 76:339–345.

Peters, P.A., El Alamy, M., Warren, K.S., and Mahmoud, A.A.F. 1980. Quick Kato smears for field quantification of Schistosoma mansoni eggs. Am. J. Trop. Med. Hyg., 29:217–219.

Proffitt, R.D., and Walton, B.C. 1962. Ascaris pneumonia in a two-year-old girl. Diagnosis by gastric aspirate. N. Engl. J. Med., 266:931–934.

Stoll, N.R., and Hausheer, W.C. 1926. Concerning two options in dilution egg counting: small drop and displacement. Am. J. Hyg., 6 (March Suppl.): 134–135.

Chapter 19

Culture Methods

R. G. Yaeger and M. D. Little

The cultivation of animal agents or vectors of human disease serves a threefold purpose: (1) to supplement other methods of laboratory diagnosis, (2) for use in teaching, and (3) to provide organisms in quantity for investigation. Diagnostically, it is sometimes possible to obtain the parasite or its vector in culture in an identifiable stage when other material for diagnosis may fail to furnish specific evidence. The sections that follow describe media that have been found useful. It is beyond the scope of this book to cover the numerous culture media, both semidefined and defined, that have been developed. Additional information on culture media and methods may be obtained in publications by Jensen (1983) and Taylor and Baker (1978).

CULTIVATION OF PARASITIC PROTOZOA

Intestinal Protozoa

Numerous media have been developed for cultivation of intestinal amebae, flagellates, and the ciliate *Balantidium coli.* To initiate a culture, fresh stools uncontaminated with urine are required. Formed stools containing the cysts may be employed, or liquid specimens with trophozoites. In the latter case, elements of mucus and tissue detritus are more likely to contain the pathogen than the diluted fecal portion. To prevent rapid overgrowth of enteric bacteria, it is frequently helpful to add gentamicin or penicillin plus streptomycin when the stool sample is inoculated into the culture medium, and it is necessary to introduce considerably more inoculum than in bacteriologic cultures. Usually, cultures are not useful in the routine diagnosis of intestinal protozoa. Specimens positive for protozoa by microscopic examination may be negative by culture.

The inoculum should consist of representative portions of the several components of the stool, proctoscopic aspirate, liver aspirate, or other material obtained from the patient. About 0.2 ml of the material is inoculated into the medium and the culture is incubated at 35 to 37°C. Subcultures usually are made at 48-hour intervals. At times no evidence of the suspected organism is found in samplings of the original culture, but subcultures may be positive. The following media are selected from the many good ones that have been developed.

Balamuth's Monophasic Medium

Balamuth's all-liquid medium, easily prepared and long-lasting when stored at about 5°C (Balamuth, 1946), is commonly used for the isolation and maintenance of *Entamoeba histolytica* and some other intestinal amebae. It is also satisfactory for culturing *Balantidium coli,* though the quality and amount of starch in the cultures may need to be more carefully controlled.

The medium is prepared as follows:
1. Weigh 288 g dehydrated egg yolk.
2. Add 288 ml distilled water and 1000 ml 0.85% saline, and with an electric mixer (or similar instrument) emulsify until the suspension is smooth.
3. Heat over an open flame in the top part of a double boiler, stirring constantly until coagulation begins (5 to 10 minutes).
4. Heat the mixture over boiling water, stirring occasionally until coagulation is complete (about 20 minutes). Add 160 ml distilled water to offset loss from evaporation.
5. Filter the mixture through a muslin bag. When the bag cools, it may be squeezed gently to obtain the maximum volume of filtrate.
6. Measure filtrate and add 0.85% saline solution to bring volume to 1000 ml.
7. Dispense the filtrate into 2 1-liter Erlenmeyer flasks. Autoclave for 20 minutes at 15 lb (121°C).
8. Place the flasks in the refrigerator overnight or until the solution is thoroughly chilled.
9. Filter while cold through a Buchner funnel, preferably using negative pressure to facilitate filtration. Use 2 pieces of Whatman qualitative filter paper of suitable size and pour the mixture in small amounts through the funnel, replacing the papers frequently.
10. Measure the filtrate. Add an equal volume of Balamuth's buffer solution (for preparation of the buffer solution, see below).
11. Add 0.5% crude liver extract (Lilly, No. 408), 5 ml per liter of medium.
12. Dispense in 5 to 7 ml amounts in tubes; autoclave for 20 minutes at 15 lb (121°C). Add sterile rice powder and incubate for 24 hours at 37°C before using. The medium may be left in flasks in large amounts, autoclaved, and stored in the refrigerator. It can be kept for a month or more without deterioration, though there may be an accumulation of sediment that should be removed by filtration. Reautoclaving produces no harmful effect and may even be beneficial.

The buffer solution is M/15, prepared as follows. To 174.180 g K_2HPO_4 add distilled water to make 1,000 ml, and to 136.092 g KH_2PO_4 add distilled water to make 1,000 ml. Mix these solutions in a ratio of 4.3 parts of K_2HPO_4 to 0.7 parts KH_2PO_4. To one part of this mixture add 14 parts of distilled water to prepare the M/15 buffer. This final solution is the one used in step 10 above.

Boeck and Drbohlav's Diphasic Medium

The diphasic medium of Boeck and Drbohlav is often used for primary isolation of amebae. It is prepared as follows:

1. Emulsify 4 whole hen's eggs with 50 ml of Ringer's solution (see below).
2. Filter the emulsion through several thicknesses of cheesecloth or surgical gauze.
3. Dispense 2 to 3 ml amounts into 16 × 150 mm Pyrex test tubes.
4. Place several layers of paper in the bottom of the autoclave and slant the tubes at an angle of 30°. (Place the tubes in baskets so that the rows are not more than 2 or 3 deep.)
5. Inspissate for 10 minutes at 15 lb in the autoclave. Cool.
6. Overlay each slant with approximately 5 ml of buffered saline (see below) or normal saline containing 0.5% crude liver extract (Lilly, No. 408).
7. Sterilize slants in the autoclave for 20 minutes at 15 lb (121°C). Wrap the baskets in paper to minimize breaking of the slants during sterilization.
8. Add a loopful of sterile rice powder to each sterile overlaid slant.
9. Incubate medium for 24 hours at 37°C to demonstrate sterility and store at 4°C for later use.

Stock Ringer's solution is prepared by adding NaCl 70.0 g, CaCl 3.0 g, and KCl 2.5 g to 1 liter of distilled water. For use, dilute the stock solution 1:10 with neutral distilled water.

Buffered saline (pH 7.0) is 0.85% saline 450.0 ml and M/15 KH_2PO_4 19.0 ml, combined with M/15 Na_2HPO_4 31.0 ml. The M/15 KH_2PO_4 is KH_2PO_4 9.07 g added to distilled water to make 1 liter. The M/15 Na_2HPO_4 is Na_2HPO_4 9.46 g added to distilled water to make 1 liter.

Diamond (1982) described a liquid medium for the isolation of *Entamoeba histolytica*, *E. coli*, and *Dientamoeba fragilis* from feces. A strain of *E. gingivalis* was also maintained in the medium. The clear medium permits visualization of the protozoa in the test tube, thus eliminating the need for sampling.

Primary Isolation of *Naegleria*

A medium described by Culbertson *et al.* (1968) was recommended as satisfactory for the detection of both *Naegleria* and *Acanthamoeba (Hartmannella)* types of amebae in cerebrospinal fluid or brain tissues.

Medium. Prepare 1.5% Bacto agar in distilled water. Pour 8 ml amounts into plates. Add 0.1 ml saline solution suspension of live *Escherichia coli* at 50°C and mix into the agar, or place that amount of the suspension in the center of the hardened agar plate and spread over the agar surface. Invert the plate to allow evaporation of excess moisture.

Inoculation. Place 0.05 to 0.1 ml of the inoculum in the center of the plate. To avoid irregular spreading and excess moisture that may interfere with examination, place a sterile antibiotic disc in the center of the bacteria-laden agar plate. If the inoculum is expected to be bacteria-free, or nearly so, moisten the disc with 0.05 ml distilled water and place 0.05 ml of suspension of tissue emulsion, tissue particles, or exudate on the disc. If the inoculum is expected or known to be contaminated with bacteria, place 0.05 ml of a solution containing 25 μg neomycin and 2.5 nystatin on the disc, than add the inoculum. Seal the plates and incubate at 37°C, and if the available material is sufficient, make similar preparations and incubate at 23°C.

Examination. The unopened, inverted plate can be examined with the scanning lens (2.5 ×) or low power (10 ×) objective of the microscope, scanning the area around the disc for small, more or less uniform, round or ovoid amebae extending radially from the disc. If the amebae are seen, transfer to fresh plates

to maintain the strain and to a microscope slide in water under a thin coverglass to examine under higher magnification for morphologic features.

Trichomonas vaginalis

Simplified trypticase serum (STS) medium is suitable for isolation of *T. vaginalis* from vaginal exudates and also for the maintenance of bacteria-free cultures for teaching or research. Bacteria can be eliminated by serial transfers in medium containing 500 U of penicillin and 500 mg of dihydrostreptomycin sulfate per ml or 250 μg gentamicin per ml. The medium consists of trypticase (BBL) 20.0 g, cysteine HCl 1.5 g, maltose 1.0 g, and agar (Difco) 1.0 g added to distilled water to make 950.0 ml.

The above ingredients are mixed and heated to boiling to dissolve the agar and filtered while hot through porous Reeves-Angel filter paper No. 845. If desired, add 0.6 ml of 0.5% methylene blue as an indicator for oxygen tension. Cool to 46°C, adjust pH to 6.0 (with HCl or NaOH) if necessary, dilute to 950 ml, and tube in amounts of 9.5 ml. Autoclave the tubed medium for 15 minutes at 15 lb pressure. Store in refrigerator, and prior to inoculation add 0.5 ml of the sterile human or rabbit serum.

Blood and Tissue Flagellates

The inoculum consists of blood, aspirates, or small amounts of biopsy or postmortem samples from glands, spleen, liver, or bone marrow, obtained aseptically from patients suspected of having infection with *Leishmania donovani*, *L. braziliensis*, *L. tropica*, *Trypanosoma gambiense*, *T. rhodesiense*, *T. cruzi*, *T. rangeli*, and other hemoflagellates. To ensure bacterial sterility, it is desirable to introduce 500 U of penicillin plus 500 μg of dihydrostreptomycin sulfate per ml of the liquid phase into each tube at the time of inoculation; 250 μg/ml of gentamicin may be used as an alternative.

Novy, MacNeal, and Nicolle's (NNN) Medium

The NNN medium was developed for cultivation of the leishmanias, but it is equally satisfactory for *Trypanosoma cruzi* and *T. rangeli*. It is prepared from agar 14 g and sodium chloride 6 g added to 900 ml of distilled water. The elements are mixed and brought to the boiling point, then distributed in tubes and sterilized in the autoclave.

In using the tubed medium, it is melted and then cooled to 48°C, and to each tube of medium one third of its volume of sterile defibrinated rabbit blood is added. This is well mixed with the medium by rotating the tube, after which the tubes are slanted and allowed to cool. This is best done on ice, as more water of condensation is obtained, and it is in this supernatant at the bottom of the tubes that the organisms develop most rapidly and in greatest numbers. Before using, the tubes should be tested for sterility by placing them in an incubator at 37°C for 24 hours. If there is insufficient condensate in the tubes, sterile Locke's solution may be added.

Tobie's Diphasic Medium

Tobie's medium is satisfactory for *Trypanosoma cruzi*, *T. rangeli*, *T. gambiense*, *T. rhodesiense*, *Leishmania tropica*, *L. braziliensis*, *L. donovani*, and many nonhuman species of hemoflagellates. It is a diphasic medium.

Solid Phase. Dissolve 1.5 g Bacto-beef (Difco); 2.5 g Bacto-peptone (Difco); 4.0 g sodium chloride; and 7.5 g Bacto-agar (Difco) in 500 ml distilled water. Adjust the pH to 7.2–7.4 with NaOH and autoclave at 15 lb pressure for 20 minutes. Cool this mixture until it can be comfortably held in the hand (about

45°C), then add whole rabbit blood that has been inactivated at 56°C for 30 minutes in the proportion of 25 ml blood to 75 ml base. Coagulation of the whole blood is prevented by using 0.5% sterile sodium citrate. Defibrinated blood may be substituted.

Liquid Phase. Sterile Locke's solution consists of the following composition: NaCl, 8 g; KCl, 0.2 g; $CaCl_2$, 0.2 g; KH_2PO_4, 0.3 g; dextrose, 2.5 g, and distilled water, 1,000 ml.

The base is dispensed in amounts of 5 ml or 25 ml into test tubes or flasks, respectively. The test tubes are kept in a slanted position and the flasks upright until the base has solidified. The the liquid phase is added in amounts of 2 ml and 10 to 15 ml, respectively.

Malarial Parasites

No simple satisfactory culture method has been developed for the diagnosis of malaria by *in vitro* cultivation. Trager (1979) described an *in vitro* system for the continuous cultivation of *Plasmodium falciparum,* but such cultures are primarily for research purposes.

Toxoplasma

T. gondii has been grown in roller tube cultures of mouse and human tissues, but it has not been grown in the absence of living tissue cells.

IN VITRO CULTIVATION OF PARASITIC HELMINTHS

Attempts to culture parasitic helminths through the various stages of their life cycles have become increasingly successful in recent years (Basch, 1981, with *Schistosoma mansoni;* Douvres and Urban, 1983, with *Ascaris suum;* Mak *et al.,* 1983, with *Brugia malayi* and *B. pahangi;* Smyth and Davis, 1974, with *Echinococcus granulosus;* and Thompson *et al.,* 1982, with *Mesocestoides corti). In vitro* cultivation has been used as a means of studying the various aspects of growth and development of the parasitic stages, providing a source of antigens for immunologic studies, and evaluating the efficacy of anthelmintics. In addition, Carvajal *et al.* (1981) and Oshima *et al.* (1982) cultivated anisakid nematode larvae recovered from fish and obtained adult worms that could then be specifically identified.

It is relatively easy to obtain the complete extrinsic, *i.e.,* free-living stages, of strains of *Strongyloides stercoralis* or of other species of this genus exhibting indirect development. Rhabditoid larvae (or eggs) of these strains, recovered from the stools of natural hosts, provide the inoculum. The media consist of host's feces or other suitable nutriment containing the associated enteric bacteria.

REFERENCES

Balamuth, W. 1946. Improved egg yolk infusion for cultivation of *Entamoeba histolytica* and other intestinal protozoa. Am. J. Clin. Pathol., *16*:380–384.

Basch, P.F. 1981. Cultivation of *Schistosoma mansoni in vitro.* I. Establishment of cultures from cercariae and development until pairing. J. Parasitol., *67*:179–185.

Carvajal, J., Barros, C., Santander, G., and Alcalde, C. 1981. *In vitro* culture of larval anisakid parasites of the Chilean hake *Merluccius gayi.* J. Parasitol., *67*:958–959.

Culbertson, C.G., Ensminger, P.W., and Overton, W.M. 1968. Pathogenic *Naegleria* sp.—Study of a strain isolated from human cerebrospinal fluid. J. Protozool., *15*:353–363.

Diamond, L.S. 1982. A new liquid medium for axenic cultivation of *Entamoeba histolytica* and other lumen-dwelling protozoa. J. Parasitol., *68*:958–959.

Douvres, F.W., and Urban, J.F., Jr. 1983. Factors contributing to the *in vitro* development of *Ascaris suum* from second-stage larvae to mature adults. J. Parasitol., *69*:549–558.

Jensen, J.B. (ed.). 1983. *In Vitro Cultivation of Protozoan Parasites.* Boca Raton, Florida, CRC Press.

Mak, J.W., Lim, P.K., Sim, B.K.L., and Liew, L.M. 1983. *Brugia malayi* and *B. pahangi:* Cultivation *in vitro* of infective larvae to the fourth and fifth stages. Exp. Parasitol., *55*:243–248.

Oshima, T., Oya, S., and Wakai, R. 1982. *In vitro* cultivation of *Anisakis* Type I and Type II larvae collected from fishes caught in Japanese coastal waters and their identification. Jpn. J. Parasitol., *31*:131–134.

Smyth, J.D., and Davies, Z. 1974. *In vitro* culture of the strobilar stage of *Echinococcus granulosus* (sheep strain): A review of basic problems and results. Int. J. Parasitol., *4*:631–644.

Taylor, A.E.R., and Baker, J.R. (eds.). 1978. *Methods of Cultivating Parasites in Vitro.* London, Academic Press.

Thompson, R.C.A., Jue Sue, L.P., and Buckley, S.J. 1982. *In vitro* development of the strobilar stage of *Mesocestoides corti.* Int. J. Parasitol., *12*:303–314.

Trager, W. 1979. *Plasmodium falciparum* in culture: Improved continuous flow method. J. Protozool., *26*:125–129.

Chapter 20

Immunologic Diagnosis

S. P. Katz and R. G. Yaeger

Parasites belonging to any of the major animal groups may stimulate an immune response in a given host. The response is more likely to occur when the offending parasite is in intimate contact with host tissue than when it is a lumen dweller or an ectoparasite. Although diagnosis of parasites is most reliably made by direct observation, indirect tests are widely used when demonstration of the parasite is difficult, as in prepatent or other occult infections.

Both humoral and cell-mediated immunity can be induced by parasitic infections, and serologic tests provide a rapid means of detecting them. With serologic tests, detection of either antibodies produced by the host or antigens produced by the parasite is possible. For those procedures in which parasite antigens are required for specific antibody detection, whole organisms, extracts of whole organisms, or extracts fractionated to reduce the number of cross-reacting components may be used. Regardless of the test employed, the interpretation placed on a given test will depend on the stage of the disease. The immunodiagnostic tests used for the detection of parasitic infection follow standard procedures involving routine techniques.

IMMUNOLOGIC TESTS FOR PROTOZOA

Entamoeba histolytica

The most useful serologic test for amebiasis is the indirect hemagglutination test. Others that may be used are indirect immunofluorescence, countercurrent electrophoresis, immunoelectrophoresis, and enzyme-linked immunosorbent assay (ELISA).

Titers obtained with sera from patients with amebic dysentery or amebic liver abscess tend to be very high and those obtained with sera from asymptomatic carriers or uninfected patients tend to be low or negative. The sensitivity of these tests has been enhanced by the use of highly specific commercially available antigens from axenically grown *E. histolytica*.

Naegleria and Acanthamoeba

Immunocytologic techniques for the demonstration and identification of species of the amphizoic free-living amebae, *Naegleria* and *Acanthamoeba*, have been described (Culbertson and Harper, 1984). The procedures may be used on fixed tissues, exudates, discharges, or body fluids.

Giardia lamblia

Serum antibodies to *Giardia lamblia* have been detected by immunofluorescence (Visvesvara *et al.*, 1980) and ELISA (Smith *et al.*, 1980) tests. Their diagnostic value remains to

be determined because of low titers and variable persistence of serum antibodies after loss of infection. A counterimmunoelectrophoresis (CIE) method for detecting *G. lamblia* cyst antigen in fecal samples appears to be sensitive and specific (Craft and Nelson, 1982). However, the CIE test does not detect infection when trophozoites are scant and no cysts are being produced.

Leishmania Species

Diagnosis of visceral leishmaniasis or kala-azar may be accomplished with nonspecific or specific tests.

Nonspecific Tests. Nonspecific immunoglobulin levels rise sharply in visceral leishmaniasis. Addition of a small amount of distilled water, antimony, or formalin to a patient's serum produces precipitation or cloudiness. This is the basis of the serum-euglobulin test of Brahmachari and Sia, the antimony test, and the formal-gel test or aldehyde test of Napier.

Specific Tests. Tests that are specific for leishmaniasis include both an *intradermal skin test* and *serologic procedures*. The intradermal reaction has been used to detect infection with *Leishmania donovani*, *L. tropica*, and *L. braziliensis*. The antigen is obtained by physiologic saline extraction of cultured promastigotes. A delayed hypersensitivity reaction appears within 24 hours of antigen administration and peaks at 72 hours. Skin testing is of particular diagnostic value for *L. braziliensis* after extension of the primary lesion to the mucocutaneous areas.

Serologic Tests. Indirect hemagglutination, indirect immunofluorescence, complement fixation, direct agglutination, and other serologic techniques may be used to diagnose visceral leishmaniasis. Although sensitivity is low with serum from patients with cutaneous leishmaniasis, an immunofluorescent antibody assay and an enzyme-linked immunosorbent assay (ELISA) with amastigote antigen have been reported as giving good results (Anthony *et al.*, 1980). Other techniques useful in the diagnosis of cutaneous leishmaniasis are the direct agglutination test with trypsinized culture forms, complement fixation, and countercurrent electrophoresis.

Trypanosoma rhodesiense and T. gambiense

Infections with *Trypanosoma rhodesiense* and *T. gambiense* are accompanied by marked elevation of IgM, which may be measured in dried blood and used as a nonspecific screening test. Specific diagnosis can be made with a fluorescent antibody test with whole homologous parasites. This technique may be used to survey large populations as well as to diagnose individual cases. A sensitive and specific ELISA for African trypanosomiasis also has been described (Vervoort *et al.,* 1978) but has not come into general use for individual patients.

Trypanosoma cruzi

A number of techniques are useful for the diagnosis of *Trypanosoma cruzi* infection (Chagas' disease), especially in its chronic stage when parasites are otherwise difficult to demonstrate. These tests include direct agglutination, indirect fluorescent antibody, indirect hemagglutination, the soluble antigen fluorescent antibody test, and countercurrent immunoelectrophoresis. The direct agglutination test has been most widely used, but others are now commonly in use. Also described for *T. cruzi* is a method of demonstrating antibodies with antigen-coated nitrocellulose paper strips dipped in the diluted serum sample (Araujo, 1985).

Toxoplasma

Methods of diagnosing toxoplasmosis include serologic tests for specific toxoplasma antibodies. Detection of IgM antibodies is indicative of a recently acquired or reactivated infection. These antibodies, as detected by indirect fluorescent-antibody technique, appear within the first week of infection, peak within a month, and then revert to negative or low levels.

In active infection, IgG antibodies may be revealed with a highly specific complement fixation test developed by Sabin in 1949. The test employs concentrates of organisms grown on chorioallantoic membranes of chick embryos. The Sabin-Feldman dye test as modified by Jacobs and Cook in 1954 also is useful. The test measures the ability of a solution of alkaline methylene blue (pH 10.8) to stain thin wet films of *Toxoplasma gondii* suspended in either normal human serum or serum of a patient. The organisms are obtained from the peritoneal cavity of a mouse on the third day of infection. The cytoplasm and nuclear material of organisms are stained when alkaline methylene blue is added to thin films prepared with normal serum. Neutralizing antibodies in serum from infected patients will prevent staining. The dye test becomes positive earlier than the complement fixation reaction, with long persisting high titers developing in the second week. The complement fixation test, however, is not positive until one month of infection and lasts only a short time. A serial 2-tube rise in titer is indicative of an acute infection.

The indirect fluorescent antibody (IFA) and indirect hemagglutination (IHA) tests with killed antigen are routinely run because they are inexpensive and easy to perform. The IHA tends not to detect acute infections, whereas a single high IgM IFA is indicative of an acute infection. The ELISA and the fluorimmunoassay have been shown to be equivalent in sensitivity to the IFA test, and positive results with these tests as well as the dye test are diagnostic of a chronic infection. A simple and inexpensive direct agglutination test has been described as comparable in sensitivity and specificity to the older standard tests (Desmonts and Remington, 1980).

Pneumocystis

Complement fixation and indirect immunofluorescence tests have been used for the diagnosis of pneumocystosis. These procedures give about 15% false negative results. Antigens for both tests are prepared from infected human or rat lung. With the ELISA for the assessment of antibody and the CIE for the detection of antigen in sera, positive results occur in individuals without clinical evidence of pneumocystosis; therefore, signs and symptoms of disease must be considered in the interpretation of serologic test results (Maddison *et al.,* 1982).

Plasmodium Species

The indirect hemagglutination, indirect immunofluorescence, and enzyme-linked immunosorbent assay have been used for diagnosis of malaria, primarily in surveys and to detect infected blood donors. The indirect fluorescence test is the most widely used test and is highly specific and sensitive when homologous antigen is used (Kagan, 1980). The ELISA test also has been shown to be sensitive and specific.

IMMUNOLOGIC TESTS FOR HELMINTHS

Trichinella spiralis

Trichinella antigen for immunologic tests is usually prepared from larvae digested from the tissues of laboratory infected animals (rats, rabbits, and guinea pigs). The washed larvae may be used intact or lyophilized and used as whole or fractionated worm extracts.

Precipitin Test. There are two types of antibody reaction in trichinosis: one is antilarval and one is antiadult. The antiadult reaction results in an *in vitro* precipitate around the mouth, vulva, and anus of the adult trichinae (Sarles' reaction) and is detectable 15 days after infection; it reaches its maximum about the 25th to 35th day and is negative after about the 50th day. The antilarval type of antibody produces a precipitate that reaches a maximum between the 45th and 60th day.

Intradermal Test. The intradermal test, introduced by Bachman in 1929, uses a fat-free antigen and gives an immediate reaction (10 minutes). It is useful for epidemiologic studies. Positive results occur after 4 to 6 weeks of infection. It is desirable to confirm the positive findings of the intradermal test with one of the serologic tests.

Serologic Tests. The bentonite flocculation test is adequately sensitive and specific for diagnosis of trichinosis and is the procedure of choice. The indirect immunofluorescence test, an indirect hemagglutiation test, and an ELISA test (Van Knapen *et al.,* 1982) also are sensitive and specific. Also available are complement fixation, latex agglutination, and countercurrent immunoelectrophoresis tests. Antibodies in humans become detectable after about 3 weeks of infection, thus preventing detecton of early infection by serologic tests. Titers peak after several weeks and decline slowly, until after 3 years sera usually are negative. Rising titers in repetitive testing indicate an acute or recent infection.

Filariae

Immunodiagnosis of filariasis has relied on antigens of non-human filariae, in particular dog heartworm, *Dirofilaria immitis,* or human filariae, *Brugia malayi,* grown in experimental animals.

Intradermal Tests. Saline extracts of nonhuman and human filariae have been used for skin testing. The reactions are of the immediate type. Because *D. immitis* antigen cross-reacts with other helminth infections, its use is of limited value in regions where such infections as ascariasis, hookworm infection, and strongyloidiasis are present. Skin testing with homologous antigen prepared from *W. bancrofti* or *B. malayi* is sensitive for filariasis but unable to distinguish between filarial infection and filarial disease. Skin testing with crude antigens is simple and economical and is useful in epidemiologic studies. A skin test for *Onchocerca volvulus* with antigen prepared from the excretory-secretory products obtained from *in vitro* cultivation of microfilariae was reported to have a high sensitivity with low levels of cross-reactivity (Schiller *et al.,* 1980).

Serologic Tests. A standard procedure for diagnosis of filariasis has been indirect hemagglutination with antigen prepared from *D. immitis,* although specificity is poor and sensitivity is variable. Indirect immunofluorescence and ELISA tests are sensitive and specific for bancroftian and malayian filariasis (Ottesen *et al.,* 1982). The indirect immunofluorescence test for onchocerciasis has been shown to be sensitive when sections of the worm are used as antigen. A highly sensitive ELISA with excretory-secretory *O. volvulus* antigens has been developed (Ambroise-Thomas, 1980).

Strongyloides stercoralis

Tests described for the diagnosis of strongyloidiasis include ELISA (Neva *et al.*, 1981) and indirect immunofluorescence (Genta and Weil, 1982). *In vitro* lymphoproliferative responsiveness to *S. stercoralis* antigen lacks reliability as a diagnostic test (Genta *et al.*, 1983).

Ascaris lumbricoides

Although *A. lumbricoides* is known to be highly allergenic, practical application of an immunologic test for ascariasis has not been reported.

Toxocara Species

Indirect hemagglutination tests with larval secretory antigens can be useful for the diagnosis of visceral larval migrans caused by *Toxocara*. Improved immunodiagnosis apparently has been achieved by using excretory-secretory antigens in an ELISA test (Van Knapen *et al.*, 1983). *In vitro* lymphocyte proliferative responsiveness to *Toxocara* antigens is diagnostic of infection but it is not done routinely (Caldwell *et al.*, 1980).

Schistosoma Species

Immunodiagnostic tests for schistosomiasis are not as dependable as the demonstration of eggs in excreta or tissue. Such tests are useful for epidemiologic studies, although a correlation between titers and egg excretion levels has not been observed. Almost all stages of the parasite have been used as sources of antigenic materials.

Intradermal Tests. Tests with purified extracts of adults, cercariae, and eggs have proved sensitive and specific. Regardless of the antigenic preparation, responses are not commonly detected prior to maturation of the infection. Both immediate and delayed types of hypersensitivity have been observed in response to schistosome antigens.

Serologic Tests. The most widely used tests for serodiagnosis of schistosomiasis are the indirect immunofluorescence with cercariae or adult worms, slide flocculation, Ouchterlony double diffusion with adult or cercarial extracts, and circumoval precipitin (COP) and ELISA with soluble egg antigens. The COP and the ELISA have proved to be sensitive, specific, and most useful for screening populations for schistosomiasis (Hillyer *et al.*, 1981). The Cercarien-hüllenreaktion of Vogel and Minning and a miracidial immobilization test detect early responses that are sensitive and relatively specific.

Paragonimus westermani

Immunodiagnostic techniques are often needed for the detection of infection with *P. westermani*, since in a large percentage of infections, eggs are not passed in the feces or sputum. Intradermal and complement fixation tests are satisfactorily sensitive. The indirect fluorescence, countercurrent electrophoresis, and indirect hemagglutination techniques also are useful in the diagnosis of paragonimiasis (Kagan, 1980).

Echinococcus (Hydatid)

Several serodiagnostic techniques for hydatid disease are useful (Schantz *et al.*, 1983). In general, the tests are sensitive but relatively nonspecific. High titers indicate infection, but low titers are frequently attributable to cross-reaction with other conditions. Intradermal and complement fixation tests with hydatid fluid employed as antigen have been widely used for many years. However, with the same antigen, immunoelectrophoresis (ARC 5), latex agglutination, indirect hemagglutination, and ELISA tests are now recommended.

Cysticercosis

The intradermal test for cysticercosis in man employs as antigen the fluid taken from cysticerci of domestic animals. This is a group-specific test. Serologic tests used for cysticercosis are complement fixation, indirect hemagglutination, countercurrent electrophoresis, double gel diffusion, immunoelectrophoresis, and immunofluorescence, for which antigens of *Taenia taeniaeformis*, *T. saginata*, *T. solium*, *Cysticercus bovis*, or *C. cellulosae* are used. These tests are poor in specificity because of cross-reactions with other helminth parasites (Kagan, 1980).

IMMUNOLOGIC TESTS INVOLVING ARTHROPODS

Bee and Wasp Venoms

Notable use has been made of the sensitization reaction to the venom of wasps and honeybees. People who develop hypersensitivity to hymenopteran stings can be desensitized and thus freed of the risk of fatal anaphylactic shock (Schwartz *et al.*, 1984).

Precipitin Tests for Blood Ingested by Arthropods

Malariologists and other workers frequently need to know whether a mosquito or other bloodsucking arthropod is selective in its feeding on man or animals in order to determine whether a particular species is important as a transmitter of infectious agents from person to person or from a zoonotic reservoir to humans. The precipitin and other standard tests provide the means of obtaining this information.

The basic serologic test for blood identificaiton is the precipitin reaction, with the passive hemagglutination inhibition test a promising adjunct for discrimination between closely related vertebrates. The hemoglobin crystallization method for blood meal identification is a useful nonserologic supplement in situations in which closely related hosts might otherwise be difficult to separate (Washino and Tempelis, 1983). With the production of monoclonal antibodies, the identification of specific antigens for malaria in mosquito vectors has been accomplished (Burkot *et al.*, 1984). Application of these techniques to the identification of other parasites in arthropod vectors should become possible.

SUMMARY

The parasitic infections for which serologic tests are most helpful in diagnosis of individual cases are amebiasis (amebic liver abscess), Chagas' disease, cysticercosis, echinococcosis (hydatid disease), filariasis, leishmaniasis, paragonimiasis, schistosomiasis, toxocariasis (visceral larva migrans), toxoplasmosis, and trichinosis. Appropriate tests are available at CDC through the State Public Health Laboratories for all of these and for special cases of some other parasitoses.

REFERENCES

Ambroise-Thomas, P.C., Daveau, C., and Desgeorges, P.T. 1980. Serodiagnostic de l'onchocercose par micro-ELISA. Etude de 450 serums et comparaison avec l'immunofluorescence indirecte. Bull. Soc. Pathol. Exot., 73:430–442.

Anthony, R.L., Christensen, H.A., and Johnson, C.M. 1980. Micro enzyme-linked immunosorbent assay (ELISA) for the serodiagnosis of New World leishmaniasis. Am. J. Trop. Med. Hyg., *29*:190–194.

Araujo, F.G. 1985. A method for demonstration of antibodies to *Trypanosoma cruzi* by using antigen coated nitrocellulose paper strips. Am. J. Trop. Med. Hyg., *34*: (in press).

Burkot, T.R., Williams, J.L., and Schneider, I. 1984. Identification of *Plasmodium falciparum*-infected mosquitoes by a double antibody enzyme-linked immunosorbent assay. Am. J. Trop. Med. Hyg., *35*:783–788.

Caldwell, K., Lobell, M., and Coccia, P.F. 1980. Mitogenic response to *Toxocara* antigen and chemotactic defect in visceral larva migrans. Am. J. Dis. Child., *134*:845–847.

Craft, J.C., and Nelson, J.D. 1982. Diagnosis of giardiasis by fecal counterimmunoelectrophoresis. J. Infect. Dis., *145*:499–504.

Culbertson, C.G., and Harper, K. 1984. Pathogenic free-living amebae. Immunocytologic demonstration and species identification. Am. J. Trop. Med. Hyg., *33*:851–856.

Desmonts, G., and Remington, J.S. 1980. Direct agglutination test for diagnosis of *Toxoplasma* infection. Method for increasing sensitivity and specificity. J. Clin. Microbiol., *11*:562–568.

Genta, R.M., Ottesen, E.A., Neva, F.A., Walzer, P.D., Tanowitz, H.B., and Wittner, M. 1983. Cellular responses in human strongyloidiasis. Am. J. Trop. Med. Hyg., *32*:990–994.

Genta, R.M., and Weil, G.J. 1982. Antibodies to *Strongyloides stercoralis* larval surface antigens in chronic strongyloidiasis. Lab. Invest., *47*:87–90.

Hillyer, G.V., Ramzy, R.M.G., El Alamy, M.A., and Cline, B.L. 1981. The circumoval precipitin test for the serodiagnosis of human schistosomiasis mansoni and haematobia. Am. J. Trop. Med. Hyg., *30*:121–126.

Kagan, I.G. 1980. Serodiagnosis of parasitic disease. In *Manual of Clinical Microbiology,* 3rd ed. Edited by E.J. Lennette, A. Balows, J.P. Hausler, Jr., and J.P. Truant. Washington, D.C., American Society for Microbiology, pp. 724–750.

Maddison, S.E., Hayes, G.V., Slemenda, S.B., Norman, L.G., and Ivey, M.H. 1982. Detection of specific antibody by enzyme linked counterimmunoelectrophoresis in humans infected with *Pneumocystis carinii*. J. Clin. Microbiol., *15*:1036–1043.

Neva, F.A., Gam, A.A., and Burke, J. 1981. Comparison of several nematode larval antigens in ELISA test for human strongyloidiasis. J. Infect. Dis., *144*:427–432.

Ottesen, E.A., Weller, P.F., Lunde, M.N., and Hussain, R. 1982. Endemic filariasis on a Pacific island. II. Immunologic aspects: Immunoglobulin complement, and specific antifilarial IgG, IgM and IgE antibodies. Am. J. Trop. Med. Hyg., *31*:953–961.

Schantz, P.M., Wilson, J.F., Wahlquist, S.P., Boss, L.P., and Rausch, R.L. 1983. Serologic tests for diagnosis and post-treatment evaluation of patients with alveolar hydatid disease *(Echinococcus multilocularis)*. Am. J. Trop. Med. Hyg., *32*:1381–1386.

Schiller, E.L., D'Antonio, R., and Figueroa Marroquin, H. 1980. Intradermal reactivity of excretory and secretory products of onchocercal microfilariae. Am. J. Trop. Med. Hyg., *29*:1215–1219.

Schwartz, H.J., Yunginger, J., Teigland, J., Sutheimer, C., and Hiss, Y. 1984. Sudden death due to stinging insect hypersensitivity: Post-mortem demonstration of IgE antivenom antibodies in a fatal case. Am. J. Clin. Pathol., *81*:794–795.

Smith, P.D., Gillin, F.D., Brown, W.R., and Nash, T.E. 1980. IgG antibody to *Giardia lamblia* detected by enzyme-linked immunosorbent assay. Gastroenterology, *80*:1476–1480.

Van Knapen, F., Franchimont, J.H., Verdonk, A.R., Stumpf, J., and Undeutsch, K. 1982. Detection of specific immunoglobulins (IgG, IgM, IgA, IgE) and total IgE levels in human trichinosis by means of the enzyme-linked immunosorbent assay (ELISA). Am. J. Trop. Med. Hyg., *31*:973–976.

Van Knapen, F., Van Leusden, J., Polderman, A.M., and Franchimont, J.H. 1983. Visceral larva migrans: Examinations by means of enzyme-linked immunosorbent assay of human sera for antibodies to excretory-secretory antigens of the second-stage larvae of *Toxocara canis*. Z. Parasitenkd., *69*:113–118.

Vervoort, T., Magnus, E., and Van Meirvenne, N. 1978. Enzyme-linked immunosorbent assay (ELISA) with variable antigen for serodiagnosis of *T. b. gambiense* trypanosomiasis. Ann. Soc. Belge Med. Trop., *58*:177–183.

Visvesvara, G.S., Smith, P.D., Healy, G.R., and Brown, W.R. 1980. An immunofluorescence test to detect serum antibodies to *Giardia lamblia*. Ann. Intern. Med., *93*:802–805.

Washino, R.K., and Tempelis, C.H. 1983. Mosquito host bloodmeal identification: Methodology and data analysis. Annu. Rev. Entomol., *28*:179–201.

Chapter 21

Treatment for Parasitic Diseases

General Considerations

When a parasitic infection has been diagnosed, the next consideration is treatment. The decision of whether treatment is indicated or not, and if so what therapeutic method is to be used, must be based on analysis of numerous factors. These include the severity of the illness, the usual pathogenicity of the etiologic agent, the probability of reinfection or relapse, the efficacy, availability, cost, toxicity, and acceptability of the drugs available for treatment, and the probable compliance of the patient. Often treatment is not indicated because the toxicity of the only available effective drug is more hazardous than the infection or because the existing infection is asymptomatic and the high probability of reinfection makes treatment relatively futile.

Empiric Treatment and Therapeutic Test

Sometimes treatment is carried out without a diagnosis having been scientifically established by the laboratory. Usually this practice is not acceptable, but in the case of some infections adequately sensitive laboratory tests do not exist or may not be available in some areas. Treatment without the benefit of a laboratory diagnosis is called *empiric*. In some instances the response of a specific infection to a certain drug may be so consistent that the drug may be administered as a *therapeutic test*. With the improvement in diagnosis, such cases are increasingly rare, but emetine or metronidazole may be used in this way in the case of amebic liver abscess or ameboma. In other instances, mass treatment may be carried out in a community with known high rates of parasitosis without a diagnosis being established for each individual.

Changes in Drugs of Choice

As scientific knowledge increases and more effective and safer drugs become available, decisions about drug treatment are constantly changing. For example, when gentian violet was the only useful drug against strongyloidiasis, treatment with that toxic drug was often omitted and the patient was given only symptomatic treatment. Since the current chemotherapeutic agent (thiabendazole) is much less toxic and much more effective, and since disseminated strongyloidiasis in immunodeficient patients is more common, there is a much stronger indication for treatment.

Risks in Treatment

In addition to other considerations, the physician must consider the legal liability of treating or not. In geographic areas where amebiasis is highly prevalent, there is little need to treat asymptomatic infections. In the United States, failure to treat such an infection once it has been diagnosed may lead to a judgment against the physician. On the other hand, since the drugs currently available in the United States carry risks, these risks must be explained to the patient, who must then give his informed consent for the treatment or decline it.

Choice of Drugs

New Drugs. Physicians and parasitologists are advised to accept with caution initial reports concerning the marvelous efficacy and minimal toxicity of new drugs. Many drugs once believed to be highly effective and nontoxic have eventually turned out to have serious defects. Enthusiasm as to efficacy is frequently the consequence of inadequate controls in the design of the drug trial. Serious toxic effects may be discovered only after the drug has been widely used for several years. Toxic effects may be overlooked if there is no special effort made to detect them. Many of the antiparasitic drugs cause myocardial damage that is detectable by electrocardiography. If EKG's are not done, neither patient nor physician may be aware of this toxic effect unless a cardiac emergency occurs. Recently it has been found that oxamniquine, an antischistosome drug, can cause electroencephalographic abnormalities as well as seizures (Krajden *et al.*, 1983). Other drugs such as amphotericin B are nephrotoxic and their administration requires close monitoring of renal function. Familiarity with the chemical class to which a drug belongs usually will help one to anticipate its toxic effects.

Preferences in Drugs and Dosage. Table 21–1 shows the preferred treatment for the principal parasitic infections discussed in the earlier chapters. Those consulting the table should use it as a guide but not expect it to provide all essential knowledge of the parasitic infection involved or of the drug to be used. It is impractical to devise a table containing all the information required for intelligent treatment of the patient. The table includes data on side-effects, drug interactions, contraindications, and precautions. When a drug has been selected based on the table, the physician should read pertinent information about the drug in the package insert, the *Physician's Desk Reference* or, if the drug is obtained from the Parasitic Diseases Division of the Centers for Disease Control, the literature sent by that agency before the drug is administered to the patient (Ford, 1983).

The table relies heavily on the *Handbook of Antimicrobial Therapy* of The Medical Letter, which presents recommendations generated by a group of expert consultants. Nevertheless, modifications have been made in those recommendations on the basis of experience and review of the current literature (Most, 1984).

The table does not provide pediatric dosages. These usually can be calculated on a proportional basis according to weight. In any case, dosage and method of administration of the drug

Table 21–1.   Drug Therapy for Parasitic Diseases of Man Listed in Order of Appearance in Text

Parasite	Drug	Dosage
Giardia lamblia	1. Metronidazole	250 mg tid for 5 days
	2. Quinacrine hydrochloride	100 mg tid after meals
	3. Furazolidone	for 5 days
		100 mg qid for 7 days
Trichomonas vaginalis	Metronidazole	250 tid for 7 days
Dientamoeba fragilis	1. Diiodohydroxyquin	650 mg tid for 20 days
	2. Metronidazole	250 mg tid for 7 days
	3. Tetracycline	500 mg qid for 10 days
Leishmania		
L. tropica, L. major (Oriental sore)	Stibogluconate sodium or meglumine antimonate	Not established; varies from 10 mg Sb^v/kg/day IM for 30 days to 30 mg Sb^v/kg/day IM for 10 days*
L. aethiopica (diffuse cutaneous leishmaniasis)	1. Amphotericin B 0.01% in 5% glucose	0.25–1.0 mg/kg daily or on alternate days for 8 weeks (see text, p. 21)
	2. Pentamidine	200 mg IM daily for 10 days; repeat course for relapses
L. mexicana (chiclero ulcer)	1. Stibogluconate sodium or meglumine antimonate	20 mg Sb^v/kg/day (max. 850 mg) IM for 10 days*
	2. Cycloguanil pamoate	350 mg base, IM once
(Diffuse cutaneous leishmaniasis)	Amphotericin B 0.01% in 5% glucose	0.25–1.0 mg/kg by slow infusion daily or on alternate days for up to 8 weeks (see text, p. 23)
L. braziliensis panamensis, guyanensis, peruviana (pian bois, uta)	1. Stibogluconate sodium or meglumine antimonate	20 mg Sb^v/kg/day (max. 850 mg) IM for at least 20 days*
In case of failure of 1.	2. Amphotericin B 0.01% in 5% glucose	0.25–1.0 mg/kg by slow infusion daily or on alternate days for up to 8 weeks (see text, p. 23)
L. braziliensis braziliensis (espundia)	1. Stibogluconate sodium or meglumine antimonate	20 mg Sb^v/kg/day (max. 850 mg) IM for at least 20 days*
	2. Pyrimethamine	25 mg/day po for 2 weeks
In case of failure of 1. and 2.	3. Amphotericin B 0.01% in 5% glucose	0.25–1.0 mg/kg by slow infusion daily or on alternate days for up to 8 weeks (see text, p. 23)
L. donovani (kala-azar or visceral leishmaniasis)	1. Stibogluconate sodium or meglumine antimonate	20 mg Sb^v/kg/day (max. 850 mg) IM for at least 20 days*
	2. Pentamidine	2–4 mg/kg/day IM for up to 15 doses
In case of failure of 1. and 2.	3. Amphotericin B 0.01% in 5% glucose	0.25–1.0/mg/kg daily or on alternate days for 8 weeks (see text, p. 25)
Trypanosoma		
T. rhodesiense and *T. gambiense* (African trypanosomiasis) Early stage (hemolymphatic)	1. Suramin	100–200 mg (test dose) IV, then 1 g IV on days 1, 3, 7, 14, and 21
	2. Pentamidine	4 mg/kg/day IM for 10 days
Late stage with CNS involvement (sleeping sickness)	1. Melarsoprol	2.0–3.6 mg/kg/day IV for 3 doses; then after 1 week 3.6 mg/kg/day IV for 3 doses; repeat after 10–21 days
	2. Tryparsamide	30 mg/kg IV every 5 days to total 12 injections; may be repeated after 1 month (see text, p. 30)
	plus Suramin	10 mg/kg IV every 5 days to total 12 injections; may be repeated after 1 month
T. cruzi (Chagas' disease)	1. Nifurtimox	5 mg/kg/day po in 4 divided doses increasing by 2 mg/kg/day every 2 weeks until dose reaches 15–17 mg/kg/day
	2. Primaquine phosphate	26.3 mg (15 mg base)/day for 7–10 days

Table 21–1. *Continued*

Parasite	Drug	Dosage
Entamoeba histolytica		
Asymptomatic or mild disease	1. Diiodohydroxyquin	650 tid for 20 days
	2. Diloxanide furoate	500 mg tid for 10 days
Dysentery	1. Metronidazole plus diiodohydroxyquin	750 mg tid for 5–10 days 650 mg tid for 20 days
	2. Dehydroemetine	1.0–1.5 mg/kg/day IM (max. 90 mg/day) for up to 5 days
	or	
	Emetine	1 mg/kg/day IM (65 mg/day maximum) for up to 5 days
	plus	
	Diiodohydroxyquin	650 mg tid for 20 days
Hepatic abscess	1. Metronidazole	750 mg tid for 5–10 days
	plus	
	Diiodohydroxyquin	650 mg tid for 20 days
	2. Dehydroemetine	1.0–1.5 mg/kg/day (maximum 90 mg/day) IM for up to 5 days
	or	
	Emetine	1 mg/kg/day (maximum 60 mg/day) IM for up to 5 days
	followed by	
	Chloroquine phosphate	1 g (600 mg base)/day for 2 days, then 500 mg (300 mg base)/day for 2–3 weeks
	plus	
	Diiodohydroxyquin	650 mg tid for 20 days
Naegleria sp. (primary amebic meningoencephalitis)	Amphotericin B 0.01% in 5% glucose	1 mg/kg/day IV for undetermined period
Acanthamoeba sp. (primary amebic meningoencephalitis, uveitis, corneal ulcer)	Not established Amphotericin B *plus* Sulfa drugs may be helpful	 1 mg/kg/day IV for undetermined period Not established
Balantidium coli	1. Tetracycline	500 mg qid for 10 days
	2. Diiodohydroxyquin	650 mg tid for 20 days
Cryptosporidium	No established effective treatment	
Isospora belli (coccidiosis)	Trimethoprim	160 mg qid for 10 days, then bid for 3 weeks
	plus	
	Sulfamethoxazole	800 qid for 10 days, then bid for 3 weeks
Sarcocystis spp.	No effective treatment known	
Toxoplasma gondii	Pyrimethamine	25 mg/day for 3–4 weeks
	plus	
	Trisulfapyrimidines	2–6 g/day for 3–4 weeks
Plasmodium (malaria) (except resistant *P. falciparum*) Treatment of attack:	Chloroquine diphosphate	600 mg base, then in 6 hours 300 mg base (500 mg), then 300 mg base/day for 2 days
If oral dose cannot be given	1. Quinine dihydrochloride	600 mg in 300 ml normal saline IV over at least 1 hour; repeat in 6–8 hours if oral therapy not possible
	2. Chloroquine hydrochloride	200 mg base (250 mg) IM every 6 hours
Ordinary attack, chloroquine-resistant *P. falciparum*	1. Quinine sulfate	600 mg tid for 3 days
	plus	
	Pyrimethamine	25 mg bid for 3 days
	plus	
	Sulfadiazine	500 qid for 5 days
	2. Quinine sulfate	650 mg tid for 3 days
	plus	
	Tetracycline	250 mg qid for 7 days
Severe attack, chloroquine-resistant *P. falciparum*	Quinine dihydrochloride	600 mg in 300 ml normal saline IV over at least 1 hour; repeat in 6–8 hours until oral therapy is possible

Table 21–1. *Continued*

Parasite	Drug	Dosage
Suppression of disease while in endemic area, except for resistant *P. falciparum*	Chloroquine phosphate	500 mg (300 mg base) once weekly from 1 week before exposure and continued for 6 weeks after last exposure
Suppression of disease while in endemic area, resistant *P. falciparum*	Pyrimethamine-sulfadoxine	1 tablet (25 mg pyrimethamine, 500 mg sulfadoxine) once weekly from 1 day before exposure until 6 weeks after last exposure
Prevention of relapse and of delayed primary attack after cessation of suppression of *P. vivax* and *P. ovale*	Primaquine phosphate	15 mg base (26.3 mg) daily for 14 days or 45 mg base (79 mg) weekly for 8 weeks.
Pneumocystis carinii	1. Trimethoprim-sulfamethoxazole	20 mg/kg/day 100 mg/kg/day in 4 divided doses for 14 days
	2. Pentamide isethionate	4 mg/kg IM daily for 12 to 14 days
Fasciola hepatica (sheep liver fluke)	1. Bithionol	30 to 50 mg/kg on alternate days for 10–15 doses
	2. Praziquantel	25 mg/kg tid for 1 day
Fasciolopsis buski (intestinal fluke)	1. Praziquantel	25 mg/kg tid for 1 day
	2. Tetrachloroethylene	0.1–0.12 ml/kg (max. 5 ml)
Clonorchis sinensis (liver fluke)	Praziquantel	25 mg/kg tid for 1 day
Paragonimus westermani (lung fluke)	1. Praziquantel	25 mg/kg tid for 3 days
	2. Bithionol	30 to 50 mg/kg on alternate days for 10–15 doses
Schistosoma		
S. haematobium	1. Praziquantel	40 mg/kg once
	2. Metrifonate	5–15 mg/kg every other week for 3 doses
S. mansoni	1. Praziquantel	40 mg/kg once
	2. Oxamniquine	15 mg/kg once
S. japonicum	Praziquantel	30 mg/kg twice in 1 day
S. mekongi	Praziquantel	20 mg/kg 3 times in 1 day
Taenia saginata, Taenia solium, Hymenolepis diminuta, Dipylidium caninum, Diphyllobothrium latum	1. Niclosamide	4 tablets (2 g) chewed thoroughly in a single dose after a light meal
	2. Praziquantel	15–20 mg/kg once
Hymenolepis nana	1. Niclosamide	2 g chewed thoroughly daily for 5 days
	2. Praziquantel	15–20 mg/kg once
Cysticercus of *Taenia solium* (if surgical removal impossible)	Praziquantel	Dosage not established
Echinococcus granulosus Hydatid (larval) stage (if surgical removal impossible)	Mebendazole	Use is investigational. Dosage not established.
Trichinella spiralis (trichinosis)	Corticosteroids	20 to 40 mg (prednisone) daily, reduced as signs and symptoms decrease
	plus	
	1. Mebendazole	200–400 mg tid × 4 days, then 400–500 mg tid × 10 days
	2. Pyrantel pamoate	10 mg/kg daily for 4 days

Table 21–1. *Continued*

Parasite	Drug	Dosage
Trichuris trichiura (whipworm)	Mebendazole	100 mg bid for 3 days
Enterobius vermicularis (pinworm)	1. Mebendazole 2. Pyrantel pamoate 3. Piperazine citrate 4. Pyrvinium pamoate	100 mg single dose; repeat after 2 weeks 11 mg/kg single dose (max. 1 g), repeat after 2 weeks 65 mg/kg (max. 2.5 g) daily for 7 days; repeat after 2 weeks 5 mg/kg single dose (max. 350 mg); repeat after 2 weeks
Ascaris lumbricoides (roundworm)	1. Mebendazole 2. Pyrantel pamoate 3. Piperazine citrate	100 mg bid for 3 days 11 mg/kg (max. 1 g) single dose 75 mg/kg (max. 3.5 g) daily for 2 days
Necator americanus, Ancylostoma duodenale (hookworm)	1. Mebendazole 2. Pyrantel pamoate	100 mg bid for 3 days 11 mg/kg (max. 1 g) once
Angiostrongylus cantonensis (eosinophilic meningoencephalitis)	Withdrawal of cerebrospinal fluid. Chemotherapy rarely indicated	
Angiostrongylus costaricensis (intestinal angiostrongyliasis)	Thiabendazole	75 mg/kg/day for 3 days
S. stercoralis	1. Thiabendazole 2. Albendazole	25 mg/kg bid (max. 3 g/day) for 2 days 800 mg daily for 3 days (5 days or longer when disseminated)
Ancyclostoma braziliense and other hookworms (cutaneous larva migrans or creeping eruption; dog and cat hookworm larvae in man)	Thiabendazole	Apply topically, or 25 mg/kg bid orally; repeat in 2 days if necessary
Toxocara canis (visceral larva migrans; dog and cat roundworm larvae in man)	Corticosteroids for severe symptoms *or* Diethylcarbamazine *or* Thiabendazole	20 to 40 mg (prednisone) daily, reduced after 3–5 days 2 mg/kg tid for 7–10 days 25 mg/kg bid for 5 days
Wuchereria bancrofti, Brugia malayi, Loa loa, Dipetalonema perstans, Tropical eosinophilia	Diethylcarbamazine	2 mg/kg tid for about 14 days (generally preceded by 3 days of stepwise increments beginning at 50 mg)
Onchocerca volvulus (river blindness)	Diethylcarbamazine *followed by* Suramin	25 mg daily for 3 days, then 50 mg daily for 5 days, then 100 mg daily for 3 days, then 150 mg daily for 12 days 100 to 200 mg (test dose) IV, then 1 g IV at weekly intervals for 5 weeks
Dracunculus medinensis (guinea worm)	1. Thiabendazole 2. Niridazole 3. Metronidazole	25 mg/kg bid for 3 days 25 mg/kg daily (max. 1.5 g) for 10 days 250 mg bid for 10–20 days
Sarcoptes scabei	1. Crotamiton (10%) 2. Lindane (1%) 3. Benzyl benzoate (25%)	Topically Topically (once) Topically
Pediculus capitus, P. humanus	Malathion, lindane, or permethrin in dust	Applied to body and clothing
Phthirus pubis	Lindane, 1% in ointment	Topically (once)

*Sb^v = pentavalent antimony.

to a child should be governed by information gleaned from the above sources.

Drugs of choice are listed in the table in numerical order of preference. Preference is dependent not only on efficacy and safety but also on availability and cost. In at least one instance two drugs, stibogluconate sodium and meglumine antimonate, are about equal in all other respects but differ in their availability in different geographic areas. No preference between these two drugs is indicated. Only stibogluconate sodium is available in the United States.

Availability of Drugs. Many useful antiparasitic drugs are not commercially available in the United States because they have not been approved by the U. S. Food and Drug Administration. A small number of such drugs can be obtained by contacting the Parasitic Diseases Division, Center for Infectious Diseases, Centers for Disease Control, Atlanta, GA 30333 (telephone 404-329-3670). Failure to obtain an indicated drug from commercial sources should be followed by inquiry at this agency (Ford, 1983).

Toxicity. Amphotericin B, tryparsamide, pentamidine, suramin, and emetine are probably the most toxic drugs listed in the table. Special care and monitoring for toxic effects should be used with these drugs. For example, amphotericin B is administered by slow intravenous infusion in 5% dextrose solution in a concentration not exceeding 0.01% (1 mg/10 ml); each dose is given over a period of approximately 6 hours. The dosage must be adjusted to the specific requirements of individual patients, since tolerance to amphotericin B is variable. Beginning with a test dose of 1 mg, if this is tolerated the dose is increased by stepwise increments such as 2 mg, 5 mg, 10 mg, then by 5 mg increments until a dosage of 1.0 mg/kg body weight per day, or the alternate daily dosage of 1.5 mg/kg, is attained. Treatment may be continued at this level for up to 8 weeks. Because the drug is nephrotoxic, monitoring of blood urea nitrogen and creatinine levels and of the urine is required. Intravenous administration of small doses of adrenal corticosteroids immediately before or during the infusion of amphotericin B may decrease the febrile reactions. Similarly, cautious initiation of treatment with suramin is advisable, as well as continuous monitoring for evidences of renal damage during treatment. Lowering the dosage has been reported to be effective in reducing toxicity of suramin without significantly reducing its efficacy.

REFERENCES

Anonymous. 1984. Drugs for parasitic infections. In *Handbook of Antimicrobial Therapy.* New Rochelle, New York, The Medical Letter, pp. 93–110.

Ford, S.L. 1983. Drugs for parasitic diseases. In *Orphan Drugs: Drugs and the Pharmaceutical Sciences,* vol. 13. Edited by F.E. Karch. New York, Marcel Dekker, 1982, pp. 167–180.

Krajden, S., Keystone, J.S., and Glenn, C. 1983. Safety and toxicity of oxamniquine in the treatment of *Schistosoma mansoni* infections, with particular reference to electroencephalographic abnormalities. Am. J. Trop. Med. Hyg., 32:1344–1346.

Most, H. 1984. Treatment of parasitic infections of travelers and immigrants. N. Engl. J. Med., *310*:298–304.

Index

Page numbers in *italics* indicate figures; page numbers followed by "t" indicate tables.

FE